COST-EFFECTIVE DIAGNOSTIC IMAGING
The Clinician's Guide

COST-EFFECTIVE
DIAGNOSTIC
IMAGING
The Clinician's Guide
Third Edition

Zachary D. Grossman, M.D.
Douglas S. Katz, M.D.
Edward D. Santelli, M.D.
Kevin R. Math, M.D.
John J. Wasenko, M.D.

with contributions by
Julie L. Barudin, M.D.
Susan G. Orel, M.D.
Rosalind H. Troupin, M.D.
Nicholas C. Trasolini, M.D.

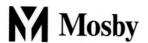 Mosby

St. Louis   Baltimore   Boston   Carlsbad   Chicago   Naples   New York   Philadelphia   Portland
London   Madrid   Mexico City   Singapore   Sydney   Tokyo   Toronto   Wiesbaden

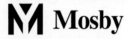

Dedicated to Publishing Excellence

Executive Editor: Susan M. Gay
Developmental Editor: Sandra Clark Brown
Project Manager: Peggy Fagen
Electronic Production Coordinator: Terri Bovay
Manufacturing Supervisor: Kathy Grone

THIRD EDITION

Copyright © 1995 by Mosby–Year Book, Inc.

Printed in the United States of America
Composition by Mosby Electronic Production
Printing/binding by R.R. Donnelley

Mosby–Year Book, Inc.
11830 Westline Industrial Drive
St. Louis, MO 63146

International Standard Book Number ISBN 0-8151-3440-1

95 96 97 98 99 / 9 8 7 6 5 4 3 2 1

The Authors

Zachary D. Grossman, M.D., is Chairman of the
Department of Diagnostic Imaging of the Roswell Park
Cancer Institute, Buffalo, NY, and Professor of Radiology,
School of Medicine, State University of New York at Buffalo,
Buffalo, NY.

Douglas S. Katz, M.D., is Chief Resident in Radiology,
State University of New York Health Science Center,
Syracuse, NY.

Edward D. Santelli, M.D., is Chief Resident in Radiology,
State University of New York Health Science Center,
Syracuse, NY.

Kevin R. Math, M.D., was a Fellow in Musculoskeletal
Radiology at the Hospital for Special Surgery/Cornell
University Medical College, and is now Attending
Radiologist at the Long Island College Hospital,
Brooklyn, NY.

John J. Wasenko, M.D., is Associate Professor of Radiology
(Neuroradiology), State University of New York Health
Science Center, Syracuse, NY.

Julie L. Barudin, M.D., is Assistant Professor of Radiology,
University of Pennsylvania, Philadelphia, PA.

Susan G. Orel, M.D., is Assistant Professor of Radiology,
University of Pennsylvania, Philadelphia, PA.

Rosalind H. Troupin, M.D., is Professor of Radiology and
Section Chief, Mammography/Outpatient Radiology,
University of Pennsylvania, Philadelphia, PA.

Nicholas C. Trasolini, M.D., is Attending Radiologist, St.
Joseph's Hospital and Medical Center, Syracuse, NY.

Preface

WHAT COST-EFFECTIVE DIAGNOSTIC IMAGING REALLY MEANS

Cost-effective diagnostic imaging does not mean doing the cheapest test first.

For two generations skull films were taken after head trauma; **millions** of dollars were wasted on this inexpensive imaging study, which does not address the central clinical issue of head trauma: is the brain injured?

Cost-effective diagnostic imaging does not necessarily mean doing the most accurate test first.

Magnetic resonance imaging (MR) of the long bones is virtually 100% sensitive and 100% specific for fractures, whereas standard x-rays are occasionally falsely negative (and rarely falsely positive), yet the huge cost differential between MR ($850) per exam and bone radiographs ($50 to $120) makes MR cost-ineffective as a screen for fractures. **Cost-effective imaging is a well-thought-out balance between the most accurate and often most expensive tests and less accurate, less expensive tests.** It is easy to see that no purpose is served by inexpensive initial procedures that are inaccurate or irrelevant (like skull films after head trauma) or by expensive tests that are only slightly more accurate than much cheaper exams (like initial magnetic resonance imaging for long

bone fractures). Only upon considerable reflection, however, does one conclude that in certain instances moderately priced tests with intermediate accuracy are more
expensive, in the long run, than expensive tests that are
invariably conclusive. However, moderately expensive tests
that are highly accurate should always precede expensive
tests whose accuracy is only slightly greater.

How is the clinician to choose among imaging exams?

**Clearly, the choice of diagnostic studies, problem
by problem, requires a knowledge of imaging that
is beyond the scope of the already overburdened
primary care physician, not to mention the medical
student, house officer, physician's assistant, and
nurse practitioner. Yet, in the current health care
environment, access to specialists is on the decline,
and even specialists are apt to be best informed
only about their particular area of interest.** Because
disease affects multiple organ systems and because the pace
of imaging development has recently been breathtaking,
specialists also are often out of touch with the best imaging protocols. Compounding this problem is the current
subspecialization of radiology itself, to the extent that even
radiologists are often uninformed about the effectiveness
(and costs!) of imaging procedures outside of their own
subspecialty.

Cost-Effective Diagnostic Imaging: The Clinician's Guide is a
compilation of clear, cogent imaging protocols covering
67 major clinical problems, tailored to the needs of the
practicing clinician. The book is designed for easy reference; therefore, **each chapter stands alone.** Appropriate
chapters are frequently cross-referenced, but **no chapter
assumes knowledge of a previous chapter**. This
approach is well suited to the busy care-giver. We have

eschewed "flow charts" and "decision trees"; life—and medical problems—are seldom so simplistic.

Although *Cost-Effective Diagnostic Imaging: The Clinician's Guide* can also be used as a general text for medical students in clinical diagnosis or radiology rotations and for junior radiology residents, the book is designed primarily for problem-oriented consultation. A cover-to-cover reading will provide an excellent overview, but reconsultation "in the heat of battle" will usually be necessary.

Zachary D. Grossman
Douglas S. Katz
Edward D. Santelli
Kevin R. Math
John J. Wasenko

Acknowledgments

The authors gratefully acknowledge the assistance of many friends and colleagues at the SUNY Health Science Center, Syracuse, in the development of the diagnostic algorithms of this book: Stuart A. Groskin, M.D., Associate Professor of Radiology, Director of Chest Radiology, and Co-Program Director of the Diagnostic Radiology Residency; Ernest M. Scalzetti, M.D., Assistant Professor of Radiology; Beverly A. Spirt, M.D., Professor of Radiology, Director of Diagnostic Ultrasound; Robert B. Poster, M.D., Assistant Professor of Radiology; Larry S. Charlamb, M.D., Fellow in Cardiology; Juan Carlos Lazaro, M.D., Fellow in Nuclear Medicine.

Assistance in developing cost estimates was provided by Andrij R. Wojtowycz, M.D., Assistant Professor of Radiology, Director of Abdominal Imaging, and Director of Diagnostic Radiology, SUNY Health Science Center, and by Susan A. Baran, R.T., Special Procedures Supervisor, SUNY Health Science Center.

Robert Schneider, M.D., Bernard Ghelman, M.D., and Hollis Potter, M.D., of the Hospital for Special Surgery, New York, N.Y., and Carlo Buonomo, M.D., of the Boston Childrens' Hospital, provided valuable input for the Musculoskeletal Sections.

Mrs. Jewel Ann Kramer provided outstanding secretarial assistance.

Contents

Introduction

One of the remarkable paradoxes in contemporary American medicine is the presence of a vague but definite malaise surrounding radiologic diagnosis at a time of unparalleled excitement and accomplishment in the development of imaging hardware and techniques... Too many available choices—especially if imperfectly understood—create confusion and anxiety in the chooser...

The clinical service... enters the radiologic "supermarket," whose shelves are increasingly filled with exotic and expensive studies, and orders tests... It is no indictment of clinical services to say that confusion surrounds the imaging workup.

R. S. Heilman[1]

HOW TO USE THIS BOOK

Cost-Effective Diagnostic Imaging: The Clinician's Guide has been designed as a practical, working manual—a brief text containing state-of-the-art information in the form of clear, cogent imaging protocols covering important medical and surgical problems. Addressed in 67 chapters ranging from "Renovascular Hypertension" to "Blunt Abdominal Trauma," clinical problems are analyzed in terms of the most cost-effective, direct, and efficient route to a diagnosis. Each chapter stands alone; although there is extensive cross-referencing, no chapter requires knowledge of a previous chapter.

We have selected problems whose workup is dominated by imaging and avoided detailed discussion of physical diagnosis and nonimaging diagnostic exams like laboratory tests. Clinicians do not need to be taught clinical medicine by radiologists, and such material is exhaustively covered and readily available in major medical, surgical, and pediatric texts, which devote far too little space to practical modern imaging!

This book is not intended to replace or supersede consultation with the radiologist or nuclear imager; in fact, we encourage such consultation. We stress throughout that communication is the surest means of defining the best imaging solution to a clinical problem. Although our protocols cover many variations and contingencies that affect the workup, unique circumstances inevitably will arise that are best approached through discussion between the imager and the clinician(s). Such communication is most effective when both parties are well informed about the options under consideration.

PROCEDURE COSTS

The procedure costs listed in the beginning of each chapter reflect **total charges to the patient, including all technical, procedural, material, and professional fees.** With the exception of nuclear medicine and angiography, most of the data come from the largest available national database, "Physician's Fees 1994."[2] These fees are derived from a database of over **600 million recently submitted charges** in the United States. Because costs vary from region to region and from imaging department to imaging department, we have used the median (50th percentile) charge for each procedure. The variation in charges for some procedures can be enormous, up to 200%!

A further complication is the substantial markup in many charges from nonteaching hospitals to teaching hospitals, as much as 30% in many parts of the United States.

Of necessity, **we have used charges for outpatient examinations; there is no available national American database for inpatient procedures**. Note that **there is commonly a substantial markup in the total charges (up to 40%) for the same procedures performed on an inpatient. Our cost estimates for angiography and nuclear medicine are particularly tenuous**; procedural charges vary so widely from region to region and hospital to hospital that we opted to use our own data, modified to reflect the lower costs in a nonteaching hospital.

Where nonionic (low-osmolar) contrast material is used, $60/50 ml is added; the total increase can exceed $180.

Thus our figures are intended solely as a basis for *RELATIVE* cost comparisons among various types of imaging studies. Almost invariably, plain films, barium studies, and basic contrast material studies—like an IVP—are less expensive than ultrasound; ultrasound is less expensive than computed tomography; computed tomography, in turn, is less expensive than magnetic resonance imaging. Angiography is usually the most expensive, and nuclear scans can be more or less expensive than computed tomography. **We believe that a knowlege of these generalities only is insufficient and that a list of specific procedure charges at the beginning of each chapter forcefully brings home the high cost of medical imaging.** Although we certainly do not wish to ever discourage the appropriate use of any imaging procedure for diagnostic purposes, we believe that an awareness of the considerable expense involved may stimulate a thoughtful, tempered approach to the imaging workup.

GENERAL CONSIDERATIONS

We assume throughout that modern equipment and radiologic expertise are available. Where special technology that will significantly affect the choice of an exam is mandatory—for example, digitized echocardiography or an endorectal MR coil—that requirement is explained and emphasized in the text.

Although familiarity with imaging techniques is not a prerequisite for understanding individual chapters, the following basic, practical information is included for those who wish to acquaint themselves with the general terminology and methods of modern imaging.

Computed Tomography

Computed tomography (CT) is a radiographic method; however, the X-ray beam is aimed through the patient from many angles to generate each image. The X-rays of standard radiography are detected by film, but for CT they strike radiation detectors, which produce a minute electrical impulse proportional to the intensity of the X-ray beam. The electrical current is quantitated numerically ("digitized") and computer-stored. (Standard X-ray films, of course, record the effect of X-rays as film "blackening.") Unlike standard radiography, CT images can be manipulated and analyzed with the aid of a computer. Sets of photographically optimized images can be subsequently recorded on film for display on standard X-ray film view-boxes. Radiology departments usually retain the original electronic data on magnetic tape.

The standard imaging plane of CT is "axial," and its view of the body is analogous to looking at a slice of bread. Slice thickness can be varied according to the part of the body examined and the purpose of the exam. Most radiologists prefer 10 mm slices for routine studies of the chest, head, and abdomen and much thinner slices (on the order of 1 to 3 mm) for specialized exams, such as the temporal bone. In some cases, axial images can be "reformatted" by the computer into sagittal or coronal images. **The ability of CT to display slices of anatomy without superimposition is the principal basis for its superiority over standard radiography**. Moreover, the data quantitation and the sensitivity of the radiation detectors, as opposed to film, result in greater sensitivity to small density changes. In other words, **CT can detect slight variations in tissue density when standard X-rays do not.** For example, renal stones that are "radiolucent" on an abdominal film are often obviously radiodense on CT.

Traditionally, CT has exquisitely defined the structure of organs, diagnosing disease by the anatomic changes that result from tumor, edema, pus formation, etc. Recently, ultrafast and "spiral" or "helical" CT have been introduced; these systems produce images in less than 1 second, so they can visualize the transit of **intravenously injected contrast material** through the blood vessels of an organ. Because these CT "angiograms" visualize organ blood flow after a **peripheral** contrast material injection, they do not require arterial catheterization. The addition of such data to structural information is an entirely new dimension for CT, much of which has not yet been fully realized. Moreover, spiral CT permits imaging of body parts in a single breath hold, eliminating the motion blur of breathing. An infinite number of slices of various thicknesses can be generated. Finally, three-dimensional reconstructions are feasible, because a "3-D data set" is acquired.

Because CT was originally termed "computed axial tomography" or "computer assisted tomography," the acronyms "CAT" or "CAT scan" appear in portions of the medical literature. "CT" is universally preferred by radiologists. CT is never a portable bedside study.

Sonography or Ultrasound

To generate an ultrasound (US) or sonographic image, a hand-held transducer passes over the skin, gliding along a thin film of acoustical gel applied at the start of the exam. Any skin lesions, surgical dressings, drains, or wounds may interfere with sonography; the sonographer must circumvent these impediments, and sometimes the study is technically limited or completely unfeasible.

The high-frequency sound waves of sonography emanate from the hand-held transducer and bounce off of internal structures. The returning sound beam ("echo") is perceived by the transducer and converted into an image by computer. The contours of many internal structures are well defined by US, and a lesion's ability to reflect echoes (its "echogenicity") is often characteristic.

Sonography delivers no ionizing radiation. Although its complete effects are not fully known, most authorities agree that any risk is minimal compared with that of standard radiography, CT, or nuclear imaging. Thus **sonography is particularly valuable for the study of pregnant women, children, and women of childbearing age.**

Unlike ionizing radiation, the sound-wave frequencies of diagnostic ultrasound cannot penetrate bone and gas. Thus US of the brain after the fontanels have closed is feasible only after craniotomy, and ultrasound of aerated lungs is not possible. Moreover, intestinal gas is an impediment to viewing portions of the abdomen, and portions of the liver and spleen under the ribs may be inaccessible.

Conventional US, like CT, defines the structure of organs. However, newer color Doppler US technology assesses organ perfusion. Perfusion data are particularly useful for differentiating ischemic lesions, like testicular torsion, from inflammatory lesions, like epididymitis. Those situations where color Doppler may be helpful are noted in the text.

Synonyms for sonography include ultrasound, ultra-sonography, medical sonography, "sono," and "echo." In many institutions, US can be a bedside examination.

Nuclear Imaging

Unlike radiography and CT, which **transmit X-rays though** the patient's body, nuclear imaging depends on gamma rays **emitted from** the patient's body; these gamma rays originate from radiopharmaceuticals previous-ly delivered orally or parenterally. Thus nuclear imaging is sometimes called "emission imaging" as opposed to radi-ographic "transmission imaging."

Nuclear images (scans) are almost completely noninva-sive, and they usually—but not always—deliver less radia-tion than standard X-rays or CT. The occasional morbidi-ty and rare mortality associated with radiographic contrast materials are virtually absent with nuclear pharmaceuticals, which are subpharmacologic in dose. With the exception of gamma cisternography, which requires a lumbar punc-ture, radiopharmaceuticals are administered by peripheral intravenous injection or are ingested orally.

Because nuclear imaging utilizes organ- or system-spe-cific radiopharmaceuticals, **the technique excels in functional assessment**; bone-seeking agents accumulate in the skeleton according to osseous blood flow and metabolism, rather than architectural change; renal scans assess glomerular filtration rate and effective renal plasma flow, as well as renal size and contour. However, in most instances, the structural or anatomic information provided by nuclear studies is inferior to that of standard radiogra-phy, CT, magnetic resonance imaging, and US.

Radionuclide imaging uses many isotopes with different half-lives and gamma-ray energies, but by far the most common isotope is technetium-99m (Tc-99m).

Radioisotopes can be bound to many chemicals whose structures determine the in vivo distribution of the resulting radiopharmaceutical compounds. Tc-99m is a component of many radiopharmaceuticals with different biodistributions. **Therefore, from the standpoint of nuclear imagers, "a technetium scan" has little meaning:** Is a Tc-99m-HIDA (hepatobiliary iminodiacetic acid) study for the gallbladder intended, or perhaps a Tc-99m-methylene diphosphonate (MDP) scan for the skeleton? Because it is unreasonable to expect the busy clinician to keep track of the many radiopharmaceuticals available, most nuclear medicine departments urge that the scan be ordered according to the **system** under study for a **given tentative diagnosis; thus an ideal requisition would read, "bone scan, rule out bone metastases" or "gallbladder scan, rule out acute cholecystitis."**

The standard instrument for acquiring nuclear images is the gamma scintillation camera (gamma camera). This device detects the gamma rays emitted by a radiopharmaceutical inside the patient and displays its distribution and intensity as a photograph. Computers assist in the generation of these images and quantification of data.

Synonyms for radionuclide imaging include nuclear medicine, nuclear imaging, isotope imaging, nuclear medicine imaging, scintigraphy, gamma scintigraphy, nuclear scanning, nuclear medicine scanning, isotope scanning, and radionuclide scanning. Nuclear imaging is almost never a portable, bedside examination.

Recently, a variation of nuclear imaging, called single photon emission computed tomography (SPECT), has become widely available. Standard radionuclides are used with SPECT to generate images in "slices," much like those of CT. SPECT markedly increases the sensitivity of nuclear scanning but almost doubles its cost.

Positron emission tomography (PET) is an additional outgrowth of nuclear imaging. Using a PET camera and special cyclotron-produced radionuclides that are produced in a few dozen sites in the United States, the technique generates "slice" images that reflect the biodistribution of compounds containing biologically critical atoms—nitrogen, oxygen, and carbon—as well as other elements like fluorine. Standard nuclear medicine departments cannot use these compounds, because most cyclotron-produced isotopes are too short-lived to survive shipping and storage. In a few important clinical problems, like chronic intractable epilepsy, PET can provide clinically useful information when all other imaging modalities have failed. PET, like SPECT, is never a portable bedside study.

Angiography

Conventional angiography involves injection of radiographic contrast material directly into a blood vessel during rapid-sequence filming. To deliver contrast material to a desired site—for example, the superior mesenteric artery or carotid artery—a catheter is introduced percutaneously, typically via the femoral artery or vein, and is advanced to the appropriate blood vessel. Angiography is thus more invasive than CT, US, magnetic resonance imaging, or nuclear imaging, but the information gained is unique.

Angiography, particularly arteriography, carries a small but significant risk of potentially serious complications including hemorrhage, vascular perforation, embolism, thrombosis, organ infarction, reaction to contrast material, and even death. The exam is usually contraindicated in patients with bleeding diatheses, and most angiographers require a relatively normal platelet count and coagulation profile before proceeding. **Most angiographic studies, including arteriograms, are safely performed on outpatients.** In today's cost-conscious climate, maximal use of outpatient angiography is critical.

A wide variety of specialized catheters and other angiographic devices that allow **intervention and therapy,** as well as diagnosis, are widely available. **In many instances, these procedures are safer, more effective, and less costly than corresponding surgical alternatives,** but great skill is required for consistent success. Interventional procedures that have gained widespread acceptance include dilatation of stenotic vessels (percutaneous angioplasty), dilatation of biliary strictures, percutaneous biliary drainage and calculus removal, percutaneous nephrostomy, percutaneous abscess drainage, and biopsy of almost any organ or mass. Delivery of drugs and embolic material to specific sites through a catheter is appropriate to certain cases. Throughout this book we indicate those situations in which interventional radiologic procedures may be useful and cost-effective.

Magnetic Resonance Imaging

Magnetic resonance imaging (MR) uses signals emitted by the patient's body when placed in a strong magnetic field and perturbed by tiny pulses of radiofrequency energy; a computer processes the signals into images. The MR "scanner" operates by varying magnetic fields and delivering pulses of energy at particular radiofrequencies and particular time intervals. Because these fields and energy pulses are independent of patient orientation, **MR images can be obtained in any plane**; typically, they are axial, sagittal, or coronal. Like CT, MR visualizes a slice of anatomy whose thickness can be varied according to the body part examined and the purpose of the study.

MR reflects the distribution of hydrogen atoms in the body and their molecular surroundings. Although a more detailed discussion is beyond the scope of this book, two different types of images are produced routinely: T1-weighted and T2-weighted. Tl-weighted images tend to show greater anatomic detail, whereas T2-weighted images often highlight specific pathologic processes to a greater degree.

MR devices look like elongated CT scanners. They include a tubular magnet into which the patient is placed. Although the "tube" is open on both ends, some patients experience anxiety in such confined circumstances, and occasionally claustrophobic patients refuse the study. Newer "open bore architecture" units are much less confining, and even in units of standard design thoughtful adaptations (sedation, headphones with music, exam prone rather than supine, anxiolytic drugs, etc.) can make the study compatible for all but the most anxious patients. The magnetic field is of such strength that any local ferromagnetic material is affected; thus patients with conventional life-support equipment or monitoring devices must not enter the field, lest the equipment be rendered nonfunctional or be pulled into the magnet. However, newer MR-compatible life-support systems are now available. **A PACEMAKER IS AN ABSOLUTE CONTRAINDICATION TO MAGNETIC RESONANCE IMAGING**. Patients with any cerebral aneurysm clips should not undergo MR, because of the possibility that clip motion will disrupt the cerebral vasculature. Furthermore, ferromagnetic materials can disturb the field and interfere with the imaging process.

Traditionally, MR images have been degraded by patient motion, because minutes of continuous immobility have been required for each image. Recently, however, newer hardware and software, particularly of the "echo planar" type, have reduced imaging time to **less than 1 second per image**. This development has increased patient "through-put" and reduced patient inconvenience; it has also permitted successful imaging of the beating heart, lungs, and abdomen. Although echo planar technology is not widely available at this time, proliferation of the technology is inevitable. Hopefully, the reduced time requirement for each scan will lower costs, and MR will probably replace US, CT, and nuclear imaging in some situations.

Sophisticated mathematical techniques have recently resulted in the development of MR angiography (MRA), a study in which blood vessels are defined **without the need for vascular puncture or contrast material of any kind.** Currently, the information provided by MRA is less complete than that of angiography, but many investigators believe that in the next decade MRA will replace most cerebral angiography and some peripheral angiography.

Synonyms for MR include nuclear magnetic resonance (NMR) and nuclear magnetic resonance imaging. MR is never a portable examination.

Contrast Material

Traditional radiographic contrast materials for intravenous use are ionic organic molecules containing iodine in hyperosmolar solution. The iodine in contrast material produces radiographic "contrast" by blocking X-rays. As it is excreted by the kidneys, contrast material allows visualization of the urinary tract; in patients with normal renal function, negligible amounts are excreted through the biliary system and gut. **In addition to the urinary tract, intravenous contrast material is crucial for many radiographic exams,** including CT of the liver, some CT of the head, some CT of the chest, and all angiography. Because intravenous contrast material enhances the visualization of many lesions, "CT with intravenous contrast material" is usually termed "enhanced CT." In this text we also refer to "MR with intravenous contrast material" as "enhanced MR." Synonyms for contrast material include contrast medium, contrast agents, and, colloquially, "dye."

Severe, adverse, idiosyncratic reactions to traditional intravenous contrast materials occur with predictable frequency: in 1 to 500 to 1000 doses.[3] Fatal reactions are rare and occur at a rate of 0.9 in 100,000 doses.[3] The precise pathogenesis of contrast material reactions is unknown. A popular theory is that the sudden intravascular load of hyperosmolar solution triggers a rapid influx of intravascular fluid; an overreaction to this fluid load causes abrupt vasodilatation, resulting in cardiovascular collapse. Alternatively, some investigators postulate that contrast materials are directly cardiotoxic or that major reactions are truly anaphylactic. **There is no reliable way to identify all patients at high risk.** The widely held belief that iodine allergy or seafood allergy (seafood contains iodine) predisposes to a major reaction has recently been challenged. In addition to the severe adverse reactions, most patients report a feeling of heat, and many develop transient nausea, flushing, or even hives.

Reactions to the traditional contrast materials has led to the development of newer, safer, low osmolarity, so-called nonionic contrast agents. These agents reduce the incidence of mild to moderate reactions but probably do not reduce the incidence of rare, fatal reactions. Although routine use of these agents on **every patient who requires intravenous contrast material** has been advocated by some, others have taken a more cautious approach. The cost of traditional agents has added little to each examination, but **the cost of low osmolarity and/or nonionic agents is significant, sometimes virtually dou-**

bling the cost of the procedure. Therefore, **we advo-cate the use of traditional contrast materials except for:**

1. Patients who have had a significant previous contrast material reaction—e.g., cardiovascular collapse, laryn-gospasm, or bronchospasm.
2. Asthmatics or those with atopic or allergic disease requiring medication or hospitalization.
3. Patients with severe respiratory compromise, includ-ing pulmonary hypertension or adult respiratory dis-tress syndrome.
4. Patients with significant cardiovascular disease, including congestive heart failure, recent myocardial infarct, unstable angina, or severe cardiac arrhythmias.
5. All children up to 2 years of age.
6. Patients with sickle cell disease.
7. Patients with renal failure, with serum creatinine equal to or greater than 2.5 mg/dl.
8. Major trauma with one or more or the following: hypotension or shock or unstable vital signs, neuro-trauma, unavailable past medical history, spinal pre-cautions, disorientation.
9. Angiography, including pulmonary angiography, peripheral arteriography, bronchial/spinal angiogra-phy, peripheral venograms, and neurovascular arteri-ography.

Admittedly, this list is long, but even if nonionic or low-osmolar agents were used in all of these circumstances, many patients would be studied with traditional contrast materials at a substantial saving.[3]

Prophylactic treatment with the following simple, inexpensive drug regimen can offer the same level of protection against ionic contrast material ana-phylactoid reaction as the use of low-osmolarity,

nonionic contrast agents themselves: 50 mg prednisone orally 13, 7, and 1 hour before the study **and** 50 mg diphenhydramine 1 hour before the study.[3] This prophylactic regimen is a viable alternative to the more expensive contrast agents in asthmatics and those patients with a history of multiple allergies; however, the prednisone/diphenhydramine regimen will not protect against the toxicity of contrast materials in other circumstances (like renal failure or cardiovascular disease).

MR contrast materials, unlike radiographic contrast materials, are gadolinium-based rather than iodine-based. Several forms of MR contrast agents are available; all are administered intravenously, and although generally safe even in the presence of renal failure, they can rarely be associated with adverse reactions and even death.

Any organization or institution that administers either iodine-based or gadolinium-based contrast materials intravenously should be fully prepared for resuscitative efforts and emergency life support.

Risks of Ionizing Radiation

Half of the ionizing radiation dose received by the United States population is due to medical diagnostic or therapeutic irradiation. The risks from this radiation exposure are very low but real. They include genetic defects, carcinogenesis, and developmental defects (in exposed fetuses). For all but moderately high rates of exposure to fetuses, the risks are exceedingly small when compared with spontaneous rates of mutation, cancer, and birth defects. There is general agreement that the benefits from appropriately ordered diagnostic exams far outweigh the risks. If a diagnostic exam is really needed, the fact that radiation exposure will occur should not override clinical judgment.

A WORD ABOUT CITED LITERATURE

In keeping with the brief, concise nature of this book, we have limited references to those necessary to document newer findings and controversial statements. Therefore some chapters include a list of references, others include "suggested additional reading," and a few include both.

REFERENCES

1. Heilman RS: What's wrong with radiology. N Engl J Med 1982; 306:447–449.
2. Context Physicians Fees 1994, Practice Management Information Corp, Los Angeles, CA, 1994.
3. Manual on Iodinated Contrast Media, Committee on Drugs and Contrast Media of the American College of Radiology, published by the American College of Radiology, 1991.

Part I
GASTROINTESTINAL

1

Acute Cholecystitis

INTRODUCTION

The initial study of choice in suspected acute cholecystitis depends to a very great extent on the clinician's level of diagnostic confidence. When the diagnosis is tentative, a right upper quadrant imaging survey is appropriate, and ultrasound (US or sonography) is ideal. However, when acute cholecystitis is the sole serious consideration, a nuclear Tc-99m-hepatobiliary iminodiacetic acid study (HIDA), which addresses the issue of cystic duct patency, is best, because acute cholecystitis is **almost always** associated with cystic duct occlusion (usually by a gallbladder stone). In reality, the clinical status is often poorly defined; therefore, **the majority of patients with right upper quadrant pain should initially undergo sonography.**

A vexing diagnostic dilemma is the problem of acute **acalculous cholecystitis**, a condition in which **the gallbladder is inflamed but the cystic duct is not necessarily obstructed.** This state has been attributed to reflux of pancreatic juice into the gallbladder, vasculitis of the gallbladder wall (especially following surgery involving cardiopulmonary bypass), seeding of the gallbladder in generalized bacteremia, or intermittent obstruction from a moving stone in the gallbladder neck. In such cases, **the sonogram can strongly suggest acute cholecystitis, yet**

HIDA may prove that the cystic duct is patent. (The cystic duct can be patent or obstructed, depending on the degree of duct wall edema.) The ultimate decision as to the presence or absence of acute cholecystitis is then a clinical one.

Costs: abdominal US, $201; HIDA, $225.

PLAN AND RATIONALE

When the diagnosis is tentative and a right upper quadrant survey is indicated:

Step 1: Sonogram

US virtually always localizes the gallbladder; therefore, the sonographer can usually tell whether the abdominal tenderness is really over that organ. This "sonographic Murphy's sign" is extremely valuable, especially if the patient can cooperate. The sonographer asks the patient to localize the site of maximum tenderness and places the sonographic probe there, to confirm that it overlies the gallbladder.

Calculi and gallbladder wall thickening are also defined, and the latter, in the proper clinical context (especially right upper quadrant tenderness), strongly suggests acute cholecystitis. Moreover, fluid around the gallbladder—"pericholecystic edema"—is highly supportive (although it may also result from other conditions like ascites).

When **calculi** and **either wall thickening or a positive Murphy's sign** coexist, **acute cholecystitis is extremely likely**, and the imaging workup ends. Sometimes, however, only one or two of these findings are present, along with a confusing clinical picture; in these circumstances, HIDA can be an extremely effective follow-up.

Step 2: Nuclear Technetium-99m-Hepatobiliary Iminodiacetic Acid Scan

After intravenous injection, HIDA is cleared from the circulation and rapidly excreted by the liver into the biliary tree, filling the gallbladder by retrograde passage through the cystic duct and entering the duodenum via the common duct. Injection of morphine IV is usually part of the procedure, to encourage gallbladder filling (see **Additional Comments**). **HIDA can establish whether the cystic duct is patent, because gallbladder filling proves cystic duct patency. Cystic duct patency is very strong evidence against acute obstructive cholecystitis, because cystic duct obstruction by a stone is the hallmark of that condition.**

If US suggests acute cholecystitis **and HIDA fails to fill the gallbladder**, **acute obstructive cholecystitis is highly likely**, and the workup ends.

If US suggests acute cholecystitis **and HIDA fills the gallbladder,** cystic duct patency is proven, and **acute obstructive cholecystitis is excluded**. The imaging workup ends, but the unlikely possibility of **acalculous** cholecystitis remains; the diagnostic decision is then a clinical one.

When acute cholecystitis is strongly suspected and cystic duct patency is the primary issue:

Step 1: Nuclear Technetium-99m-Hepatobiliary Iminodiacetic Acid Scan

If HIDA fills the gallbladder, cystic duct patency is proven with absolute certainty, and **acute obstructive cholecystitis is excluded.** Nearly always, the workup for acute cholecystitis ends; however, the unlikely possibility of acute acalculous cholecystitis remains, because in that condition the gallbladder may fill with HIDA (the cystic duct may be patent) despite gallbladder inflammation. When acute acalculous cholecystitis remains suspect despite gallbladder filling by HIDA, US is an excellent follow-up study.

If HIDA fails to fill the gallbladder, acute obstructive cholecystitis is highly likely. Because clinical suspicion of acute cholecystitis would invariably be strong in cases where HIDA was the primary imaging study for right upper quadrant pain, the gallbladder imaging workup almost always ends, but, if for some reason significant doubt remains, US is an excellent follow-up. **This circumstance is most uncommon and usually occurs when the accuracy of the HIDA study is in question, for example, in patients with TPN who cannot tolerate intravenous morphine as part of the procedure** (see Additional Comments).

Step 2: Sonogram

Point tenderness over the gallbladder, pericholecystic edema, gallbladder wall thickening, and stones support the clinical impression of acute cholecystitis.

SUMMARY AND CONCLUSIONS

1. The initial study of choice for suspected acute cholecystitis is usually sonography, because the usual clinical situation calls for an imaging survey of the right upper quadrant.
2. If sonographic and clinical findings strongly support the diagnosis of acute cholecystitis, further imaging is usually unnecessary. However, if the diagnosis is equivocal after US, HIDA is appropriate to establish whether the cystic duct is patent.

3. HIDA is an excellent follow-up, because failure to fill the gallbladder supports a sonographic impression of acute obstructive cholecystitis, whereas gallbladder filling establishes cystic duct patency with certainty and excludes **acute obstructive cholecystitis**. Note, however, that occasional cases of **acute acalculous** cholecystitis do occur, **especially after surgery involving cardiopulmonary bypass. In these cases US will be strongly suggestive of acute cholecystitis, whereas HIDA may establish cystic duct patency, and a decision as to the presence or absence of cholecystitis is a clinical one.**

4. When the initial clinical question is narrowly focused on the presence or absence of acute cholecystitis, HIDA is the appropriate first study, because it determines whether the cystic duct is patent, and sonography does not directly address that issue.

5. US is an excellent follow-up to an initial HIDA when (a) acute acalculous (nonobstructive) cholecystitis is suspected, despite gallbladder filling by HIDA, or (b) when supporting evidence of acute cholecystitis is required after HIDA fails to fill the gallbladder (a rare circumstance).

ADDITIONAL COMMENTS

• When HIDA was initially introduced, the gallbladders of patients who had fasted for 12 hours or who had a history of alcoholism and/or pancreatitis sometimes failed to fill with HIDA, **despite a patent cystic duct,** probably because they were already filled with viscous, static bile, allowing no room for HIDA. Similarly, persistent problems with nonfilled gallbladders occurred in patients on total parenteral nutrition (TPN). In an attempt to fill such gallbladders—i.e., to reduce the number of "false positive" cases in which nonfilling was due to causes other than cystic duct obstruction—a highly effective and safe pharmacologic strategy was devised: **when the common duct is visualized, 3 mg of morphine is administered intravenously.** Morphine constricts the sphincter of Oddi, raising pressure in the common duct, forcing the gallbladder to fill if the cystic duct is patent, **even in the presence of viscous, static gallbladder bile.** Therefore many departments of nuclear medicine request that inpatients and emergency room patients be sent for their HIDA study **along with 3 mg of morphine ready for IV injection.** (Because a narrow temporal "window" exists for the IV morphine injection—i.e., the interval between common duct visualization and biliary tree emptying—a wait for later delivery of morphine from a nursing unit or an emergency room would usually be too long.)

• The oral cholecystogram has no place in the evaluation of acute cholecystitis.

SUGGESTED ADDITIONAL READING

Krishnamurthy GT, Turner FE. Pharmacokinetics and clinical application of technetium-99m-labeled hepatobiliary agents. Semin Nucl Med 1990; 20:130-149

Mettler FA, Guiberteau MJ. Essentials of Nuclear Medicine Imaging, 3rd ed. Philadelphia, 1991, Saunders, pp 196-200.

Palmer EL, Scott JA, Strauss WH. Practical Nuclear Medicine. Philadelphia, 1992, Saunders, pp 275-280.

Rumack CM, Wilson SR, Charboneau WJ. Diagnostic Ultrasound, vol 1. St Louis, 1991, Mosby, pp 115-118.

2

Gallbladder Stones

INTRODUCTION

For a generation, the oral cholecystogram (OCG) was the screen for gallbladder stones and chronic cholecystitis, because it is noninvasive and highly effective; however, sonography (ultrasound or US) has long since replaced the OCG as a first-line test for detecting calculi. Moreover, sonography may define a thickened gallbladder wall, sometimes a sign of chronic cholecystitis.

Costs: abdominal sonogram, $201; OCG, $151.

PLAN AND RATIONALE

Step 1: Sonogram

The sensitivity of meticulous sonography for detecting gallbladder stones is extremely high, in good hands approaching 100%. False positives are quite uncommon.

If the screening sonogram is of good quality and is normal or demonstrates calculi, the search for calculi or chronic cholecystitis ends. **Very rarely**, however, a gallbladder sonogram cannot be performed adequately, usually because of massive patient obesity or the patient's unwillingness to cooperate; in these cases an OCG is appropriate.

Step 2: Oral Cholecystogram

After oral ingestion of contrast material in capsule form, X-ray films of the abdomen 24 hours later reveal an opacified gallbladder; calculi appear within the galbladder as radiolucencies.

If the follow-up OCG is normal or demonstrates calculi, the imaging workup ends.

Approximately 20% of all OCGs fail to demonstrate an opacified gallbladder. These cases are associated with a high incidence of underlying calculi and/or chronic cholecystitis. In such cases, when the sonogram was suboptimal, sonography may be attempted again.

SUMMARY AND CONCLUSIONS

1. US is the appropriate initial exam. A normal study virtually excludes calculi or chronic cholecystitis. The need for an OCG is rare.
2. Oral cholecystography is an appropriate follow-up in those **most uncommon** cases when the sonogram was suboptimal or unfeasible.
3. If the follow-up OCG fails to visualize the gallbladder, a repeat sonogram should be attempted, because these cases are associated with a high incidence of stones or chronic cholecystitis.

ADDITIONAL COMMENTS

- Sonography is particularly worthwhile as an initial study, because, unlike the oral cholecystogram, the sonogram is a multi-organ exam. The sonographer examining the gallbladder also studies the common duct, head of the pancreas, intrahepatic ducts, liver parenchyma, and porta hepatis. Findings in these areas may reveal the cause of chronic right upper quadrant pain.

- CT is poorly suited to the demonstration of gallbladder calculi, and HIDA studies are essentially worthless in this regard.
- Some studies have indicated that **delayed gallbladder filling** with HIDA is a reliable sign of *chronic* cholecystitis, and such a finding may be reported during a HIDA study for *acute* cholecystitis, but HIDA is never an appropriate screening study for gallbladder stones.
- The fact that sonography delivers no ionizing radiation is particularly important in the context of gallbladder stones/chronic cholecystitis, because many patients studied for this problem are young women.

SUGGESTED ADDITIONAL READING

Rummack CM, Wilson SR, Charboneau, WJ. Diagnostic Ultrasound, vol 1. St Louis, 1991, Mosby, pp 109-111.

3

Appendicitis

INTRODUCTION

Appendicitis is the most common indication for emergency abdominal surgery in the Western world. Although it can occur at any age, appendicitis is most frequent during the second decade.[1] The lifetime risk of appendicitis is about 7%.[2]

The diagnosis is confidently established preoperatively about 80% of the time by the history, physical exam, and laboratory values, without imaging. In the other 20%, particularly in the elderly, women of childbearing age, infants, and young children[2], the diagnosis of appendicitis is often difficult.[3] Elderly patients with appendicitis often manifest few clinical signs and symptoms; gynecologic disease in women of childbearing age (particularly pelvic inflammatory disease, ovarian torsion, and rupture of an ovarian cyst) commonly mimics appendicitis; infants and young children give no history and are prone to appendiceal perforation. **In these circumstances imaging is valuable** and can decrease the rate of negative exploratory surgery, which is 20% to 25% percent in many surgical practices.[4] Also, accurate early diagnosis decreases the incidence of appendiceal perforation and abscess.

Both computed tomography (CT) and ultrasound (US) can confirm the diagnosis or reveal other processes that mimic appendicitis, like gynecologic or bowel disease or even renal calculi. The barium enema is reserved for those few cases in which CT or US is equivocal.

Costs: plain abdominal films, $57; US, abdomen and pelvis, $385; CT, abdomen and pelvis, $840; BE, $147; labeled leukocyte scan, $505.

PLAN AND RATIONALE

If the diagnosis of appendicitis is equivocal:

Step 1: Plain Abdominal Films, Supine and Erect

Plain abdominal films are often normal or relatively non-specific. **An appendicolith, a calcification in the appendix, is the only specific plain film finding of appendicitis;**[1] these are discovered about 10% of the time. Appendicoliths may be multiple, are virtually diagnostic of appendicitis in the correct clinical setting, and are associated with a high likelihood of appendiceal perforation.[1] Occasionally, an additional oblique film is necessary to clarify the position of a calcification and to prove that it truly represents an appendicolith.[5]

If the appendix has perforated, the clinical diagnosis is more difficult, **but the radiographs are usually more suggestive;** small bowel obstruction, a soft tissue mass (inflammatory edema and pus around the perforation), or air outside the bowel lumen (either loculated air from perforation or air within an abscess) may appear.[1]

In the presence of an appendicolith, further imaging is usually unnecessary. Without an appendicolith, further imaging is appropriate. (However, the presence or absence of perforation may alter management; CT should be considered the next diagnostic step if perforation is a possibility [see below, Step 2b: Computed Tomography].)

If the patient is an infant or young child, a pregnant woman, or a woman of childbearing age, US is next when plain films are negative or equivocal (see below, Step 2a). For other patients and/or if perforation is likely, CT is appropriate (see below, Step 2b).

Step 2a: Ultrasound

US now plays an important role in the workup of appendicitis. Although less accurate than CT,[6] it is more appropriate when CT is especially difficult (infants and young children) and when ionizing radiation to the abdomen and pelvis is best avoided (pregnant women and women of childbearing age). Moreover, US is less expensive than CT.

To perform US of the right lower quadrant in suspected appendicitis, a "graded compression" technique is used. A linear (rectangularly shaped) transducer is placed over the point of maximal tenderness. The underlying bowel is slowly and gently compressed and displaced. The normal appendix is seen as a tubular, compressible structure, with a transverse diameter of 6 mm or less. A noncompressible appendix with a transverse diameter of more than 6 mm (in adults or children) is very suggestive of appendicitis. An appendicolith is also very strong evidence of appendicitis; **because appendicoliths may be non-calcified, they are seen more frequently on US than on plain films.**[7]

An appendiceal abscess may also be defined; if an abscess is suspected, CT is indicated for further evaluation (see below, Step 2b).

If the appendix is not seen, the remainder of the abdomen and the pelvis are examined, to seek other possible explanations for the symptoms.[8]

Successful right lower quadrant US is operator-dependent and often fails when the appendix is retrocecal, when multiple dilated bowel loops are present, and when the patient is either obese or is extremely tender in the right lower quadrant and cannot tolerate the exam.[4] Also, a perforated appendix is harder to detect by US than by CT.[3,4]

If US is equivocal or demonstrates a right lower quadrant mass, CT is warranted.

Step 2b: Computed Tomography

CT is the test of choice to evaluate patients (other than infants, young children, pregnant women, and women of childbearing age) when the diagnosis of appendicitis is equivocal. A recent prospective study showed that CT is more accurate than US in this context.[6] A proper CT requires thin (5 mm) sections through the right lower quadrant. Two findings strongly suggest appendicitis: an abnormal appendix or an appendicolith with surrounding inflammatory change/abscess.[6] If **only** inflammatory change or an abscess in the right lower quadrant is seen—without an abnormal appendix or an appendicolith—appendicitis is likely but not confirmed.[6]

CT clearly reveals the complications of appendiceal perforation—phlegmon or abscess—better than US.[6] **Preoperative differentiation between phlegmon and abscess is desirable,** because a phlegmon increases the risk of postoperative complications when surgery is immediate; many surgeons treat a phlegmon with antibiotics for several days before operating. If an abscess is discovered, initial imaging-guided percutaneous drainage is often feasible (see Chapter 61, Percutaneous Invasive Guided Biopsy).[9,10]

If ultrasound and computed tomography are equivocal:

Step 3: Barium Enema

To exclude appendicitis by barium enema, the entire appendix, including its bulbous tip, must be filled with barium. Frequently, the **normal** appendix cannot be filled; therefore, nonfilling or incomplete filling, by itself, does not constitute a positive sign of appendicitis. Suggestive but nondiagnostic indicators of appendicitis include a right lower quadrant mass compressing the cecum and/or terminal ileum.

SUMMARY AND CONCLUSIONS

1. The diagnosis of appendicitis is confidently established on clinical grounds in about 80% of individuals, without imaging.
2. In the remaining 20%, plain abdominal films are appropriate. If these are negative or equivocal, US is best for infants, young children, pregnant women, and women of childbearing age; CT is appropriate for all others.
3. Ultrasound has a high positive predictive value for appendicitis; however, if US is equivocal or demonstrates a mass or if perforation is suspected, CT is warranted.
4. If the diagnosis remains in doubt, **a few** patients will benefit from a barium enema.

ADDITIONAL COMMENTS

- An appendicolith incidentally discovered on a radiograph of a child or young adult is frequently associated with the later development of appendicitis. Prophylactic appendectomy should be considered.[5]

- When CT is equivocal, a technetium-99m-HMPAO-labeled white blood cell scan may be helpful. Scanning can be performed within 1 to 2 hours after WBC injection and is sensitive and specific for bowel inflammation.[11]
- Color Doppler augments US examination of the appendix.[9,12] The inflamed appendix often has increased blood flow in its wall, easily demonstrated by color Doppler.
- CT is better than US for demonstrating conditions in the abdomen and pelvis that mimic appendicitis.[6]

REFERENCES

1. Skucas J, Spataro RF. Appendix. In Radiology of the Acute Abdomen. New York, 1986, Churchill Livingstone, pp 249-259.
2. Balthazar EJ. Disorders of the appendix. In Gore RM, Levine MS, Laufer I, eds. Textbook of Gastrointestinal Radiology, vol. 1. Gore RM, Levine MS, Laufer I, eds. Philadelphia, 1994, Saunders, pp 1310-1341.
3. Sherman NH, Rosenberg HK. The pediatric pelvis. In Rumack CM, Wilson SR, Charboneau JW, eds. Diagnostic Ultrasound, vol. 2. St Louis, 1991, Mosby, pp 1235-1236.
4. Skaane P, Amland PF, Nordshus T, Solheim K. Ultrasonography in patients with suspected acute appendicitis: a prospective study. Br J Radiol 1990; 63:787-793.
5. Kirks DR, Caron KH. Gastrointestinal tract. In Kirks DR, ed. Practical Pediatric Imaging: Diagnostic Radiology of Infants and Children. Boston, 1991, Little, Brown, pp 798-808.
6. Balthazar EJ, Birnbaum BA, Yee J, et al. Acute appendicitis: CT and US correlation in 100 patients. Radiology 1994; 190:31-35.
7. Silverman FN, Kuhn JP, eds. Caffey's Pediatric X-ray Diagnosis, 9th ed. St Louis, 1993, Mosby, pp 1109-1113.
8. Gaensler EHL, Jeffrey RB Jr, Laing FC, Townsend RR. Sonography in patients with suspected acute appendicitis: value in establishing alternative diagnoses. AJR 1989; 152:49-51.
9. Federle MP. Tender right lower quadrant mass: rule out appendiceal abscess. In Thompson WM, ed. Common Problems in Gastrointestinal Radiology. St Louis, 1989, Mosby, pp 344-351.
10. Borushok KF, Jeffrey RB Jr, Laing FC, Townsend RR. Sonographic diagnosis of perforation in patients with acute appendicitis. AJR 1990; 154:275-278.

11. Allan RA, Sladen GE, Bassingham A, et al. Comparison of simul-
    taneous Tc-99m-HMPAO and In-111-oxine labelled white cell
    scans in the assessment of inflammatory bowel disease. Eur J Nucl
    Med 1993; 20:195-200.
12. Quillin SP, Siegel MJ. Appendicitis in children: color doppler
    sonography. Radiology 1992; 184:745-747.

SUGGESTED ADDITIONAL READING

Brown JJ. Acute appendicitis: the radiologist's role. Radiology 1991;
    180:13-14.
Vignault F, Filiatrault D, Brandt ML, et al. Acute appendicitis in chil-
    dren: evaluation with US. Radiology 1990; 176:501-504.

4

Biliary Tract Obstruction

INTRODUCTION

Jaundice or right upper quadrant pain often results from biliary tract obstruction. The goal of diagnostic imaging is to establish whether obstruction is present and, if so, to determine its cause.

Stones in the biliary tree usually pass distally, to the sphincter of Oddi, where they lodge. Tumors of the pancreatic head or ampulla of Vater also can cause distal obstruction.

The extrahepatic ducts are more compliant than the intrahepatic ducts and dilate early in obstruction. Later, intraductal pressure rises as bile is produced, and the intrahepatic ducts dilate. If the obstruction is relieved—e.g., an obstructing stone passes—the intrahepatic ducts decompress first.

In the initial workup of the aseptic patient without previous biliary tract surgery, three noninvasive imaging methods are applicable: ultrasound (US or sonography), computed tomography (CT), and nuclear imaging with Tc-99m-hepatobiliary iminodiacetic acid (HIDA). Some cases call for more invasive techniques, including percutaneous transhepatic cholangiography (PTC) and endoscopic retrograde cholangiopancreatography (ERCP).

Costs: abdominal US, $201; abdominal CT, unenhanced, $362; HIDA, $225; PTC, $518; ERCP, $820; endoscopic US, $484.

PLAN AND RATIONALE

Step 1: Ultrasound

US is the best initial exam because it visualizes the intrahepatic ducts, gallbladder, and common bile duct and is less costly than CT.

If sonography reveals normal ducts, the workup usually ends. However, **rarely clinical evidence suggests ongoing obstruction** in the presence of sonographically normal ducts. This pattern usually results from very recent obstruction; obstructed bile ducts may not have had sufficient time to dilate. A nuclear scan can reveal an obstruction before ductal dilatation has occurred.

If US reveals dilated extrahepatic or intrahepatic ducts, obstruction is likely. The most common cause is a gallstone in the common duct.

If stones in the gallbladder are found and the pancreatic head is sonographically normal, some clinicians end the workup, presuming that a calculus is responsible for the obstruction. This school of thought contends that additional imaging is necessary only if additional clinical signs need explanation or if sonographic findings are equivocal. However, the rationale for further imaging is that treatment of a common duct stone differs radically from treatment of a tumor, and therefore an effort to differentiate between these conditions is worthwhile. Stones are often endoscopically or percutaneously extractable, whereas tumors require resection or, if unresectable, palliative biliary drainage. Thus, regardless of the presence or absence of gallbladder stones, many clinicians pursue the cause of common duct blockage.

If clinical evidence suggests obstruction despite a normal sonogram:

Step 2: Nuclear Tc-99m Hepatobiliary Iminodiacetic Acid

After intravenous injection, HIDA is cleared from the circulation by the liver and excreted into the biliary tree. The intrahepatic ducts are not visualized. Very early in the course of biliary tract obstruction there is usually enough hepatic function for adequate HIDA excretion by the liver into the bile ducts. Visualization of the duodenum indicates that the common duct is patent. If HIDA enters the duodenum and the biliary tree is not sonographically dilated, the workup ends.

Failure of HIDA to enter the duodenum confirms obstruction. As an alternative to HIDA, a repeat sonogram may document progressive ductal dilatation.

If HIDA fails to enter the duodenum or if repeat sonography reveals ductal dilatation without a cause, CT is an appropriate follow-up (see Step 2: Computed Tomography, below).

If ultrasound reveals dilated ducts without a cause:

Step 2: Computed Tomography

CT can sometimes define a distal common bile duct calculus even when the pancreatic head is sonographically normal and, if the sonogram was technically limited, can define pancreatic head tumors missed by sonography.

If CT reveals an obstructing tumor or calculus, the workup usually ends. If CT fails to define the cause of obstruction, somewhat more invasive techniques, PTC or ERCP, are available.

Step 3: Endoscopic Retrograde Cholangiopancreatography or Percutaneous Transhepatic Cholangiography

During percutaneous transhepatic cholangiography (PTC) or endoscopic retrograde cholangiopancreatography (ERCP), the bile ducts are filled with contrast material, so that the site of obstruction and often its cause are visible. Subsequently, calculus extraction may be feasible.

ERCP involves passage of an endoscope through the mouth and into the duodenum, cannulation of the common duct under direct visualization, and retrograde contrast material injection. The duct is defined distal to an obstruction and often proximal to an incomplete obstruction. Moreover, the pancreatic duct is usually visualized. Various interventions are feasible, including stone extraction, biopsy, and papillotomy. In skilled hands, the procedure is safer than surgical exploration.

PTC involves a percutaneous needle puncture through the abdominal wall into the liver, followed by injection of contrast material into an intrahepatic duct, defining ducts proximal to an obstruction but not usually the pancreatic duct. PTC with a thin (22 gauge) needle has a low morbidity. The interventional radiologist can place a percutaneous drainage tube, dilate strictures, and place ductal stents to bypass various types of obstruction.

SUMMARY AND CONCLUSIONS

1. US is the most appropriate initial imaging study for suspected biliary tract obstruction.
2. If US is normal, the imaging workup usually ends.
3. If US reveals dilated ducts and a normal pancreatic head, a common bile duct calculus can be differentiated from tumor by CT.

4. PTC and ERCP are excellent but more invasive methods for visualizing intermittently obstructing intraductal calculi, ductal strictures, and tumors involving the bile ducts. They should follow less invasive procedures.
5. Occasionally, the initial US is normal, but early obstruction is suspected. Liver function is usually preserved in early obstruction, so HIDA can be useful. Alternatively, a repeat sonogram may show progressively dilating ducts.

ADDITIONAL COMMENTS

- Uncommonly, US reveals dilated ducts yet clinical and laboratory evidence does not suggest obstruction. This pattern can result from recently relieved obstruction or cholecystectomy. In recently relieved obstruction, a follow-up sonogram in several days will clarify the issue as the ducts decompress. Alternatively, HIDA will reveal a patent system, because hepatic function is usually sufficient to excrete HIDA as bilirubin falls.
- A new imaging modality called endoscopic ultrasound can evaluate the region of the pancreatic head, pancreatic duct, and distal common bile duct. This procedure involves placing an endoscope into the duodenum, where a built-in transducer generates images. The exact role of endoscopic ultrasound in the evaluation of biliary obstruction has not yet been defined.
- HIDA excretion depends on liver function, but bilirubin levels of 10 to 15 mg/dl usually are *not* a contraindication to the study, and HIDA may even work with bilirubin levels of 20 to 25 mg/dl. While some nuclear physicians advocate HIDA as the initial screen to confirm biliary obstruction, the great majority of imagers continue to favor ultrasound, because independent of hepatic function it provides anatomic detail and examines the pancreatic head.

- In addition to very early obstruction and intermittent obstruction, a rare cause of normal-sized but obstructed ducts is obstruction superimposed on sclerosing cholangitis. In this condition, chronic inflammation renders the bile ducts nondistensible, so a distal obstruction might not be followed by typical ductal dilatation. HIDA may clarify the issue, assuming sufficient liver function; otherwise, the diagnosis may require ERCP or PTC.

SUGGESTED ADDITIONAL READING

Akiyama H et al. Percutaneus treatments for biliary diseases. Radiology 1990; 176:25-30.

Ferucci JT, Mueller PR, van Sonnenberg E. Transhepatic cholangiography. In Berk RN, Ferucci JT, Leopold GR, eds. Radiology of the Gallbladder and Bile Ducts, Philadelphia, 1983, Saunders, pp 314-364.

Leopold GR. Biliary ultrasonography. In Berk RN, Ferucci JT, Leopold GR, eds. Radiology of the Gallbladder and Bile Ducts. Philadelphia, 1983, Saunders, pp 201-238.

Pasanen P, Partanen K, Pikkarainen P, Alhava E, Pirinen A, Janatuinen E. Ultrasonography, CT, and ERCP in the diagnosis of choledochal stones. Acta Radiol 1992; 33:53-56

5

Hepatic Metastases

INTRODUCTION

Computed tomography (CT), magnetic resonance imaging (MR), sonography (ultrasound or US), and nuclear imaging can detect hepatic metastases.

MR can be equivalent to or better than CT for detection of hepatic lesions, but MR's cost is greater.[1] **US is an ineffective screen**, because parts of the liver may be inaccessible. Nuclear scanning, even with single photon emission tomography (SPECT), is inferior to CT in spatial resolution and images only the liver and spleen, whereas CT evaluates the entire abdomen. Therefore, in the routine evaluation of possible hepatic metastatic disease, **CT is the modality of choice. However, CT for hepatic screening requires an intravenous injection of contrast material (contrast enhancement). Without contrast material, CT is less effective than the other modalities.**

Although evaluation of the liver for metastatic disease is the focus of this chapter, the problem of incidentally discovered hepatic masses is relevant, because the liver is very often examined by CT or US for nonmalignant disease, during which solitary or even multiple lesions are identified. Unless these are clearly cysts, they must be further characterized by imaging or biopsy.

Costs: abdominal CT, enhanced, $433; liver scan, SPECT,

$387; abdominal MR, unenhanced, $823; abdominal MR, enhanced, $943; liver scan with labeled RBCs, SPECT, $410; liver biopsy, CT-guided, $802; liver biopsy, US-guided, $511.

PLAN AND RATIONALE

When the patient has NO documented contraindication to intravenous contrast material:

Step 1: Computed Tomography with Intravenous Contrast Material

When a primary tumor is abdominal—or is extraabdominal but may well involve abdominal organs or spaces—abdominal CT is appropriate to search for metastases, adenopathy, and ascites. With intravenous contrast material the study can exclude hepatic metastases with a high level of confidence, and when hepatic lesions (especially cysts) are discovered they sometimes can be fully characterized, obviating biopsy.

Multiple hepatic masses (especially new masses) are presumed to represent metastatic disease in the proper clinical context. **A solitary mass** may require biopsy (see Chapter 61, Percutaneous Invasive Guided Biopsy) or another imaging study for clarification.

A normal enhanced CT usually ends the workup, unless strong clinical suspicion of hepatic tumor persists.

When intravenous contrast material is contraindicated, or when computed tomography is normal but clinical suspicion of hepatic tumor persists:

Step 1a: Magnetic Resonance Imaging (if available, otherwise see Step 1b, below)

MR technology has largely overcome problems related to motion artifacts from breathing, bowel peristalsis, and vascular pulsations, and the study does not require the iodinated intravenous contrast material used for CT. Thus MR is an excellent initial screen for patients who cannot tolerate iodinated contrast material, particularly those with proven allergy to contrast material or with renal failure.[3] Furthermore, MR can sometimes detect small metastatic lesions missed by CT; **therefore, it is an appropriate follow-up to a normal CT when suspicion of hepatic metastases persists**. Finally, MR characterizes many liver masses as hemangiomas, eliminating the need for biopsy.[2,4]

If MR is normal, the imaging workup for hepatic metastases ends.

If modern MR software and hardware are not available, nuclear liver-spleen scanning with SPECT is a reasonable alternative.

Step 1b: Radionuclide Liver-Spleen Scanning with SPECT

Despite its sensitivity, CT can miss occasional **diffusely infiltrative lesions**, particularly infiltrating hepatoma and lymphoma, which may approximate hepatic density. However, **in diffuse liver involvement, when enhanced CT is normal, nuclear imaging is usually grossly abnormal.** Nuclear scanning, however, is very unlikely to reveal **discrete lesions** too small for detection by contrast enhanced CT.

The scan involves intravenous injection of technetium-99m (Tc-99m) labeled sulfur colloid or microaggregated albumin. This particulate radiopharmaceutical is rapidly cleared from the circulation by the reticuloendothelial system (RES) of the liver and spleen, revealing lesions as "cold" areas. SPECT technology markedly increases spatial resolution. **The technique is nonspecific, because virtually**

any hepatic space-occupying lesion—cyst, abscess, hematoma, etc.—that displaces or replaces reticuloendothelial cells will be cold.

If nuclear imaging with SPECT is normal, the imaging workup ends.

When a solitary hepatic lesion of uncertain nature is detected by CT during a metastatic screen or incidentally discovered liver lesions detected by CT or US must be characterized:

Step 1: Nuclear Scan with Labeled RBCs or Dynamic Gadolinium Enhanced Magnetic Resonance Imaging

Hemangiomas are common benign hepatic lesions. In patients with a malignancy, hepatic masses that **may** represent hemangiomas (based on their CT or US appearance) must be further characterized, because the staging and prognosis of the primary cancer differ radically according to whether there is liver involvement. Similarly, **incidentally discovered** liver masses must be further characterized. Both nuclear scanning and MR are extremely effective for characterizing hemangiomas, but **nuclear scanning is generally preferred, because of its lower cost.**

Hepatic hemangiomas are so vascular that their blood pool is easily differentiated from other solid hepatic masses by nuclear scanning with labeled red blood cells (RBCs). The labeled RBCs are injected intravenously; resolution is markedly improved by SPECT.

MR rivals nuclear imaging for characterizing hepatic hemangiomas, because of their unique "signal characteristics" when imaged with certain pulse sequences.

If the lesion is not a hemangioma or if it is very small and difficult to characterize with certainty, percutaneous guided needle biopsy can be definitive.

Step 2: Percutaneous Guided Needle Biopsy

Imaging-guided biopsy can often provide sufficient tissue for histologic diagnosis (see Chapter 61, Percutaneous Invasive Guided Biopsy).

SUMMARY AND CONCLUSIONS

1. **Contrast enhanced CT is the appropriate screen for hepatic metastatic disease**, unless contrast material is contraindicated. Modern MR scanning is as effective, but updated MR scanners are less available and MR is more expensive.
2. A normal contrast enhanced CT is sufficient—when combined with normal liver function tests—to end the workup.
3. Multiple hepatic lesions, in the proper context, are considered metastatic.
4. Contrast enhanced CT may rarely miss metastatic disease. Therefore, if clinical data suggest metastatic disease despite a normal contrast enhanced CT or if the patient cannot tolerate intravenous contrast material, MR or a nuclear liver-spleen scan with SPECT is appropriate. **MR is favored, because of its far superior spatial resolution.**
5. Contrast enhanced CT can often fully characterize hepatic lesions as cysts, but where a confirmation of hemangioma is necessary, a nuclear study with RBCs or an MR is appropriate. The two exams are approximately equal in sensitivity and specificity, yet the nuclear study is less expensive.
6. Percutaneous imaging-guided needle biopsy can provide tissue, if a lesion requires further characterization.

ADDITIONAL COMMENTS

- As fast-scan MR units using "echo planar" technology proliferate, MR may well replace CT as the primary screen for hepatic metastatic disease.

- If hepatic arterial chemotherapy is under consideration, a hepatic arteriogram may be indicated, as a "roadmap" for placement of the intrahepatic arterial infusion catheter. Furthermore CT may be performed in conjunction with injection of contrast material directly into the superior mesenteric artery. The liver is imaged by CT during the portal venous phase of the injection. This is known as CT arterial portography (CTAP) and requires an angiographer to place the catheter. **This technique further increases the sensitivity of CT for the detection of metastatic disease but is somewhat invasive.** CTAP is used when surgical resection of hepatic metastases is a consideration or when resection of a solitary liver tumor is contemplated, to ensure that no other hepatic lesions are present.

- Spiral CT is a new technology that generates rapid high-resolution scans of the liver. Its sensitivity and specificity are greater than those of conventional CT.

REFERENCES

1. Vassiliades VG, Foley WD, Alcaron J, et al. Hepatic metastases: CT versus MR imaging at 1.5T, Gastrontest Radiol 1991; 16:159–1631.
2. Semelka RC, Shoenut JP, Kroeker MA, et al. Comparison of dynamic contrast-enhanced CT and T2-weighted fat suppressed, FLASH, and dynamic gadolinium-enhanced MR Imaging at 1.5T. Radiology 1992; 184:687–694.
3. Stark DD, Wittenberg J, Butch RJ, Ferrucci JR Jr. Hepatic metastases: randomized, controlled comparison of detection with MR imaging and CT. Radiology 1987; 165:399–406.
4. Hamm B, Fischer E, Taupitz M. Differentiation of hepatic hemangioma from metastases by dynamic contrast enhanced MR imaging. J CAT 1990; 14:205–216.

6

Bile Leak

INTRODUCTION

Imaging can detect, define, and follow bile leaks following trauma or surgery or occurring as a complication of laparoscopic cholecystectomy. Computed tomography (CT) and ultrasound (US or sonography) detect abnormal fluid collections in the abdomen but do not differentiate bile collections from blood or pus. Also, they cannot determine whether a leak is ongoing or whether a fluid collection is the result of a previous leak that has sealed.

Nuclear biliary tract imaging with Tc-99m-hepatobiliary iminodiacetic acid (HIDA) can document on active leak at the time of the study. After intravenous injection, HIDA is rapidly cleared from the circulation, accumulated by the liver, and excreted into the biliary tree. The abdomen is imaged, with visualization of the common duct, cystic duct, gallbladder, and duodenum. Imaging can continue until all of the HIDA has been excreted (usually less than 2 hours, but occasionally 12 to 24 hours).

If the problem is postsurgical and a T-tube remains in place, then the most direct approach is T-tube cholangiography; contrast material is injected directly into the T-tube under fluoroscopic control, and the biliary tree is well defined. The procedure is also excellent for detecting stenoses and biliary duct calculi.

Costs: T-tube cholangiogram, $90; abdominal CT, enhanced, $433; abdominal US, $201; HIDA, $225.

PLAN AND RATIONALE

If the suspected leak is postsurgical and a T-tube remains in place:

Step 1: T-Tube Cholangiogram

Direct injection of contrast material under fluoroscopic control, through a T-tube, produces excellent filling and visualization of the extrahepatic biliary tree and much of the intrahepatic tree. Active leaks are almost always defined. If the T-tube cholangiogram is normal, then the workup ends unless there is compelling clinical evidence of an *intermittent* leak.

Step 2: Nuclear Hepatobiliary Iminodiacetic Acid Scan

In occasional cases a T-tube cholangiogram is normal yet signs and symptoms suggest an **intermittent** leak. Because HIDA is excreted over a period of hours, the "window" during which this study can detect an intermittent leak is longer than that of T-tube cholangiogram. Therefore, when an intermittent leak is nonetheless suspected, a normal T-tube cholangiogram is often followed by HIDA imaging.

Although intraductal lesions and calculi are not well defined by HIDA, the presence of HIDA outside of the normal biliary tree or gut is easily detected. When bile leaks are sought, the T-tube is clamped after intravenous HIDA injection, and often the patient is imaged in the position most likely to elicit pain or leak. Sometimes follow-up images at 24 hours are obtained to establish whether a slow leak has occurred overnight.

If an active leak appears, **the diagnostic workup ends**, unless follow-up HIDA studies are required to determine whether the leak has stopped. For purposes of anticipated intervention—either surgical repair/drainage or radiologic "guided" transcutaneous drainage—CT is often required.

Step 3: Computed Tomography

CT can define the three-dimensional anatomy of a bile collection; without this information transcutaneous drainage is nearly impossible. Furthermore, surgical intervention is greatly expedited by foreknowledge of the extent of the fluid collection.

When no T-tube is in place:

Step 1: Nuclear Hepatobiliary Iminodiacetic Acid Scan

Although intraductal lesions and calculi are not well defined by HIDA imaging, the presence of HIDA outside of the normal biliary tree or gut is easily detected. Often the patient is imaged in the position most likely to elicit pain or leak, and sometimes follow-up images at 24 hours are obtained to establish whether a slow leak has occurred overnight.

If the HIDA study is normal, then the diagnostic workup ends unless clinical suspicion of an intermittent leak persists. In this very uncommon situation, the HIDA scan can be repeated.

If an active leak appears, the **diagnostic workup** ends unless follow-up HIDA studies are required to determine whether the leak stops. For purposes of anticipated intervention—either surgical repair/drainage or radiologic "guided" transcutaneous drainage—CT is often required.

Step 2: Computed Tomography

CT defines the three-dimensional anatomy of a bile collection; without this information transcutaneous drainage is nearly impossible. Furthermore, surgical intervention is greatly expedited by foreknowledge of the extent of the fluid collection.

SUMMARY AND CONCLUSIONS

1. When a T-tube is in place, direct injection of contrast material through the tube—a T-tube cholangiogram— is the first-line procedure for bile leak. Intermittent leaks may remain undetected.
2. When no T-tube is in place or when a T-tube cholangiogram fails to define a suspected intermittent leak, HIDA imaging is appropriate.
3. CT reveals abnormal fluid collections, defines their three-dimensional anatomy, and provides essential information before transcutaneous or surgical drainage; therefore, CT sometimes follows a positive T-tube cholangiogram or HIDA study. CT cannot prove that a bile leak is ongoing.

ADDITIONAL COMMENTS

- Patients with suspected bile leak are often postsurgical; dressings, drains, and wounds may inhibit sonography.

SUGGESTED ADDITIONAL READING

Palmer El, Scott JA, Strauss WH. Practical Nuclear Medicine. Philadelphia, 1992, Saunders, pp 280-283.

7

Malignant Pancreatic Tumor

INTRODUCTION

Pancreatic carcinoma is responsible for 5% of all cancer-related deaths in the United States. It is highly lethal, with a mortality of at least 95%; 90% are unresectable at presentation. Extension to peripancreatic soft tissues, adjacent organs, and regional lymph nodes is common. Recent therapeutic progress has been essentially nil, despite earlier and better diagnosis.

Computed tomography (CT) and transabdominal ultrasound (US) can define a pancreatic mass and surrounding abdominal structures. Endoscopic retrograde cholangiopancreatography (ERCP) and endoscopic ultrasound (EUS) can, in selected cases, detect small pancreatic tumors when CT and US are normal or equivocal. Angiography serves as a "road map" before surgical resection.

Costs: abdominal US, $201; abdominal CT, enhanced, $433; ERCP, $820; endoscopic US, $484; pancreatic biopsy, CT-guided, $861; pancreatic biopsy, US-guided, $571.

PLAN AND RATIONALE

For suspected pancreatic carcinoma in the jaundiced patient:

Step 1: Ultrasound

Lesions producing jaundice are most likely to occur in the **pancreatic head**. US detects pancreatic head tumors as well as CT and can define other causes of jaundice, like a gallstone in the common bile duct or a tumor of the ampulla of Vater. It also detects bile duct dilatation, **differentiating obstructive from nonobstructive jaundice** (see Chapter 4, Biliary Tract Obstruction).

If US of the pancreatic head and bile ducts is normal and the study is of good quality, the imaging workup for suspected pancreatic cancer in the jaundiced patient ends.

If US is equivocal or the study is technically limited, CT is appropriate; if US detects a pancreatic mass, the lesion should be studied by CT for staging.

If US reveals ductal dilatation with no apparent cause, yet the pancreatic head is sonographically normal, ERCP or EUS may be appropriate, to seek a very small tumor (of the ampulla of Vater involving the distal common bile duct or the distal pancreatic duct) or ductal stenosis. (See *If no pancreatic mass is found, yet clinical suspicion is compelling, or if computed tomography is equivocal*, below).

Step 2: Computed Tomography

CT is noninvasive and **reliably images the entire pancreas and adjacent structures**.[1-4] The study is most revealing when thin sections through the pancreas are obtained during rapid intravenous infusion of contrast material.

If CT demonstrates a large mass (> 3 cm), invasion of adjacent soft tissues, encasement of blood vessels, local lymphadenopathy, or liver metastases, **the tumor is very likely unresectable.** Unfortunately, CT less accurately predicts **the resectability of pancreatic tumors** if these findings are absent, since small metastases to the liver and peritoneum are often detected at surgery or autopsy but not by CT.[5]

If CT reveals a **small pancreatic mass,** CT- or US-guided biopsy is frequently appropriate, to confirm the diagnosis before surgery.

If CT of the pancreas is normal and the biliary tract is not obstructed, the imaging workup for pancreatic carcinoma in the jaundiced patient ends.

For suspected pancreatic carcinoma in the nonjaundiced patient:

Step 1: Computed Tomography (see above, *For suspected pancreatic carcinoma in the jaundiced patient,* **Step 2).**

If a potentially resectable pancreatic mass is defined by computed tomography:

Step 2: Imaging-Guided Biopsy

CT- or US-guided biopsy of all potentially resectable pancreatic masses should be considered, because **false positive CTs do occur**; in particular, focal pancreatitis can simulate cancer, and guided biopsy may avoid unnecessary exploratory surgery. The procedure is accurate and safe; serious complications are very uncommon.[6] (See Chapter 61, Percutaneous Invasive Guided Biopsy.)

If no pancreatic mass is found, yet clinical suspicion is compelling, or if computed tomography is equivocal:

Step 2: Endoscopic Retrograde Cholangiopancreatography, Endoscopic Ultrasound, or Imaging-Guided Biopsy for Selected Patients

If CT demonstrates a **slight** abnormality in pancreatic contour or a **slight** increase in pancreatic size, a small tumor or anatomic variation may be responsible. ERCP or CT-guided percutaneous needle biopsy may be definitive. CT-guided biopsy is an alternative to ERCP (see Chapter 61, Percutaneous Invasive Guided Biopsy). Similarly, if CT or US demonstrate **biliary obstruction but an otherwise normal pancreas**, a small pancreatic head or ampullary tumor may be responsible. ERCP may be helpful, and EUS may also play a role (see additional comments).

ERCP involves the passage of an endoscope through the mouth into the duodenum, where the ampulla of Vater is visualized and cannulated. Under fluoroscopy, contrast material is injected, filling the pancreatic duct and the biliary tree. This study reveals fine anatomic detail of the duct system and can define very small pancreatic carcinomas, **because these carcinomas originate from the pancreatic ducts**. Ampullary and distal common bile duct tumors, as well as ductal stenoses, are also defined. Small tissue samples or brushings can be obtained through the endoscope.

SUMMARY AND CONCLUSIONS

1. US is the appropriate first study in jaundiced patients. It accurately determines whether the biliary system is dilated, may detect nonneoplastic causes of jaundice,

effectively reveals tumors of the pancreatic head, and is less expensive than CT. If US finds a lesion in the pancreatic head, CT is appropriate for staging; if US is inconclusive or technically limited, CT is also appropriate.

2. CT is the initial test of choice for imaging nonjaundiced patients with suspected pancreatic carcinoma, because the entire pancreas and peripancreatic tissues are defined.

3. A normal CT or US ends the workup for pancreatic carcinoma **in the jaundiced patient** *without* **biliary dilatation.**

4. If CT reveals a suspicious contour abnormality or if pancreatic cancer is suspected despite a normal CT in the nonjaundiced patient, ERCP or percutaneous imaging-guided biopsy may confirm the presence of tumor.

5. Pancreatic tumor may cause pancreatitis by obstructing the pancreatic duct. Unexplained pancreatitis that fails to respond to conservative therapy should be studied by ERCP, because ductal obstruction and encasement by a small tumor may be responsible.

ADDITIONAL COMMENTS

- Fast (spiral or helical) CT scanners reduce respiratory motion artifact, improving image quality. These scanners are more effective than conventional CT for staging pancreatic cancer, especially in terms of vascular invasion. This technology is rapidly proliferating but is not yet universally available.

- When resection of a pancreatic tumor is planned, angiography can provide a presurgical road map, if the surgeon requires one. Angiography no longer plays a routine diagnostic role in the evaluation of pancreatic tumors.

- ERCP is a somewhat invasive procedure that requires a gastroenterologist with special expertise. The examination is sometimes unsuccessful because of variations in anatomy, regardless of the skill and experience of the endoscopist. The procedure can be augmented by endoscopic ultrasound, during which the tip of the endoscope contains a rotating transducer. EUS visualizes the pancreas through the stomach and is best performed jointly by the endoscopist and radiologist. While EUS may detect small pancreatic tumors, the role of EUS has not been fully defined, and EUS is not widely available.

- MR is more expensive than CT and does not offer any major advantages. However, it is an excellent alternative to CT for patients in whom intravenous iodinated contrast material is contraindicated—e.g., those with renal failure. Recent technical advances in MR have significantly improved its ability to detect pancreatic tumors. In selected patients in whom CT findings of resectability are inconclusive, recent work suggests that MR may be helpful.

- CT may be performed after selective catheterization of the arterial supply to the pancreas (CT angiography). While this converts a noninvasive procedure into an invasive one, it can be used in selected instances to detect islet cell neoplasms.

- If a pancreatic pseudocyst is suspected, ultrasound should be performed first. Pseudocysts are easily localized and characterized by ultrasound, which is less expensive than CT.

- Although the detection of pancreatic cancer with modern imaging techniques has not been proven to prolong survival, imaging plays an important role in securing the correct diagnosis and in planning supportive therapy—palliative surgery and radiation therapy.[7,8]

- ERCP may be used to place a stent into the common bile duct, to relieve jaundice in a patient with an unresectable pancreatic tumor.

REFERENCES

1. Fishman EK, Jones B, Siegelman SS. The indeterminate pancreatic mass: carcinoma versus focal pancreatitis. In Siegelman SS, ed. Computed Tomography of the Pancreas. New York, 1983, Churchill Livingstone, pp 157-177.
2. Fishman EK, Siegelman SS. Computed tomography of pancreatic carcinoma. In Siegelman SS, ed. Computed Tomography of the Pancreas. New York, 1983, Churchill Livingstone, pp 123-156.
3. Haaga JR. Magnetic resonance imaging of the pancreas. Radiol Clin North Am 1984; 22:869-877.
4. Clark LR, Jaffe MH, Choyke PL, Grant EG, Zeman RK. Pancreatic imaging. Radiol Clin North Am 1985; 23:489-501.
5. Reznek RH, Stephens DH. The staging of pancreatic adenocarcinoma. Clin Radiol 1993; 47:373-381.
6. Neuerburg J, Gunther RW. Percutaneous biopsy of pancreatic lesions. Cardiovasc Intervent Radiol 1991; 14:43-49.
7. Semelka RC, Kroeker MA, Shoenut JP, et al. Pancreatic disease: prospective comparison of CT, ERCP, and 1.5-T MR imaging with dynamic gadolinium enhancement and fat suppression. Radiology 1991; 181:785-791.
8. Mitchell DG, Shapiro M, Schuricht A, et al. Pancreatic disease: findings on state-of-the-art MR images. AJR 1992; 159:533-538.

SUGGESTED ADDITIONAL READING

Brandt KR, Charboneau JW, Stephens DH, Welch TJ, Goellner JR. CT- and US-guided biopsy of the pancreas. Radiology 1993; 187:99-104.

Federle MP, Goldberg HI. The pancreas. In Moss AA, Gamsu G, Genant HK, eds. Computed Tomography of the Body with Magnetic Resonance Imaging, vol. 3. Philadelphia, 1992, Saunders, pp 869-932.

Freeny PC. Radiologic diagnosis and staging of pancreatic ductal adenocarcinoma. Radiol Clin North Am 1989; 27:121-128.

Kloppel G, Maillet B. Classification and staging of pancreatic nonendocrine tumors. Radiol Clin North Am 1989; 27:105-120.

Megibow AJ. Pancreatic adenocarcinoma: designing the examination to evaluate the clinical questions. Radiology 1992; 183:297-303.

Reimer P, Saini S, Hahn PF, Mueller PR, Brady TJ, Cohen MS. Techniques for high-resolution echo-planar MR imaging of the pancreas. Radiology 1992; 182:175-179.

Thoeni RF, Blankenberg F. Pancreatic imaging: computed tomography and magnetic resonance imaging. Radiol Clin North Am 1993; 31:1085-1113.

Vellet AD. Characterization of pancreatic adenocarcinoma by magnetic resonance imaging. J Can Assoc Radiol 1991; 42:180-184.

Vellet AD, Romano W, Bach DB, et al. Adenocarcinoma of the pancreatic ducts: comparative evaluation with CT and MR imaging at 1.5 T. Radiology 1992; 183:87-95.

8

Increased Hepatic/Splenic Size

INTRODUCTION

Liver size is proportional to height and body surface area; the liver decreases in size with increasing age.[1] Because the liver may extend below the right costal margin in normal individuals, a palpable liver is not necessarily enlarged. A mildly or moderately enlarged spleen may be difficult to detect on physical exam, particularly in obese patients.[2] Complicating matters further, the shape and size of the normal spleen are highly variable; however, in 95% of normal adults the length of the spleen is less than 12 cm and the width of the spleen is less than 7 cm.[2,3]

Nuclear scanning, computed tomography (CT), and ultrasound (US) are useful in determining whether the liver or spleen is actually enlarged.

Costs: abdominal CT, unenhanced, $362; abdominal US, $201; liver-spleen scan, $212.

PLAN AND RATIONALE

For confirmation of hepatomegaly or hepatosplenomegaly:

Step 1: Nuclear Liver–Spleen Scan

The nuclear liver–spleen scan is the simplest study for **suspected hepatomegaly or hepatosplenomegaly.** After intravenous injection, technetium-99m-labeled colloid particles are almost immediately phagocytized by the liver and spleen. Images of the abdomen in various projections clearly reveal the size and shape of the liver and spleen and their relationship to the rib cage.

Step 2: Computed Tomography

CT is appropriate if **the etiology** of suspected hepatomegaly or hepatosplenomegaly is at issue. An experienced observer can estimate the degree of enlargement solely by image inspection, without measurement.[4]

CT demonstrates focal or diffuse hepatic and/or splenic abnormalities and lesions elsewhere in the abdomen, which may help explain the organomegaly, like primary or secondary tumors, fatty infiltration of the liver, lymphadenopathy (e.g., in lymphoma), and varices (in portal hypertension).

For determination of splenic size only:

Step 1: Ultrasound

Ultrasound almost always accurately estimates splenic size, and **because it is less expensive than either the nuclear liver–spleen scan or CT, US is the study of choice when splenomegaly alone is at issue.** As with CT, image inspection is as accurate as measurement.

US can also detect focal splenic abnormalities (e.g., infarct, abscess, tumor).

SUMMARY AND CONCLUSIONS

1. The nuclear liver-spleen scan provides a good estimateof **both hepatic and splenic size** and is a good intial test for confirming hepatomegaly or hepatosplenomegaly.
2. CT is appropriate if **the etiology** of suspected hepatomegaly and/or splenomegaly is at issue.
3. Ultrasound is the initial study of choice **for sizing the spleen alone.** It is less expensive than either liver-spleen scanning or CT.

ADDITIONAL COMMENTS

- US generates superb images that are unsurpassed for evaluating bile duct size and are useful for evaluating diffuse and focal liver abnormalities, but its inability to image the entire liver on a single "slice" prevents a very reliable measurement of liver length.[1]
- CT, US, and the liver-spleen scan can all characterize splenic enlargement as mild, moderate, or massive. This can help narrow the huge differential diagnosis of splenomegaly.[2]

REFERENCES

1. Rumack CM, Wilson SR, Charboneau JW. Diagnostic Ultrasound. Mosby, 1991, St Louis pp 51, 91-93.
2. Wilson JD, Braunwald E, Isselbacher KJ, et al., eds. Harrison's Principles of Internal Medicine, 12th ed. New York, 1991, McGraw Hill, pp 268-269, 357-358.
3. Frank K, Linhart P, Kortsik C, et al. Sonographic determination of spleen size: normal dimensions in adults with a healthy spleen. Ultraschall Med 1986; 7:134-137.
4. Moss AA, Gamsu G, Genant HK. Computed Tomography of the Body with Magnetic Resonance Imaging, 2nd ed. Philadelphia, 1992, Saunders, pp 1062-1064.

SUGGESTED ADDITIONAL READING

Eichner ER, Whifield CL. Splenomegaly: an algorithmic approach to diagnosis. JAMA 1981; 246:2858.

Hendersen JM, Heymsfeld SB, Horowitz J, Kutner MH. Measurement of liver and spleen volume by computed tomography. Radiology 1981; 141:525.

9

Acute Gastrointestinal Bleeding in the Adult

INTRODUCTION

Acute bleeding, indicated by grossly bloody gastric aspirate, hematemesis, hematochezia, or severe melena, must be differentiated from chronic bleeding, usually indicated by iron deficiency anemia or stools positive for occult blood. These clinical problems require different imaging approaches (see Chapter 10).

When endoscopy identifies a bleeding site, emergency diagnostic imaging is unnecessary, but when endoscopy is technically unfeasible or fails because of excessive hemorrhage, emergency imaging plays a key role. Nuclear imaging demonstrates active bleeding and, if possible, localizes its **approximate** site, so that selective angiography for more precise localization can be performed. However, massive or life-threatening hemorrhage in a patient not taken directly to the operating room is frequently studied only by angiography.

Barium in the intestinal lumen hinders subsequent endoscopic, angiographic, and nuclear investigations. Therefore, if any of these studies are contemplated in acute GI bleeding, an upper GI series or barium enema should be delayed (see "Additional Comments" for the **later** role of barium studies; in the acute setting, barium examinations have virtually no role).

Costs: Tc-99m-RBC bleeding study, $247; visceral angiogram, $2979; Meckel's diverticulum nuclear scan, $177.

PLAN AND RATIONALE

Step 1: Technetium-99m-labeled Red Blood Cell Study

The goal of the nuclear exam is to document active bleeding as a precursor to angiography, which, performed during an active bleed, is a high-yield procedure.

A few milliliters of the patient's own red blood cells (RBCs) are removed, labeled with technetium-99m (Tc-99m), and reinjected. The labeled RBCs circulate normally. If bleeding is present, serial images of the abdomen usually reveal focal accumulation of labeled RBCs in the gut lumen. The labeled RBC technique can detect bleeding rates as low as 0.05 to 0.1 ml/min. Accurate **localization** of the bleeding site, as opposed to **detection** of bleeding, requires **recognition of specific bowel segments** as extravasated radiopharmaceutical enters the bowel lumen and moves, driven by peristalsis.

Because labeled red cells in the gut lumen are not resorbed, bleeding that occurs at any time between radiopharmaceutical injection and imaging may be identified. In this respect, the nuclear scan differs markedly from the angiogram, **because active bleeding must exist at the time of contrast material injection for angiographic detection.**

If the nuclear study documents and approximately localizes active bleeding, angiography is appropriate for therapy (vasopressin infusion or embolization) or to better localize the lesion and its vascular anatomy, as a presurgical "road map."

If nuclear imaging documents the presence of active bleeding but does not localize its site, angiography can often identify the site and even the cause.

If nuclear imaging fails to document active bleeding, most angiographers are reluctant to proceed, because angiography without documentation of an ongoing bleed is a low-yield procedure.

Step 2: Angiogram

Angiography is usually performed by a percutaneous transfemoral arterial puncture. Under fluoroscopic guidance a catheter is positioned in the vessel to be studied, usually the superior mesenteric, inferior mesenteric, or celiac artery. Then, over several seconds, contrast material is injected and serial films are obtained. Bleeding points are defined as the contrast material extravasates from the vascular space into the gut lumen; a bleeding rate of at least 0.5 to 1.0 ml/min is required at the time of contrast material injection.

About two-thirds of upper GI bleeds originate in the stomach or first portion of the duodenum, and one-third result from ruptured esophageal varices. Angiography successfully localizes the source of bleeding in the majority of patients with duodenal and gastric lesions but seldom demonstrates bleeding varices, because the contrast material is usually very dilute in the late stages of an arteriogram when varices are best visualized. If the gastric aspirate contains blood and gastroesophageal varices are identified, the varices are usually assumed to represent the bleeding site, even if no contrast material extravasation is seen. Vascular ectasia (angiodysplasia) of the cecum and ascending colon characteristically presents as small, dilated clusters of arteries and veins on angiography; a specific diagnosis can be made even in the absence of acute bleeding.

SUMMARY AND CONCLUSIONS

1. When endoscopy defines a bleeding source, emergency imaging is usually unnecessary, unless a specific angiographic intervention can treat the hemorrhage.
2. Massive or life-threatening GI hemorrhage not immediately treated surgically should be studied by angiography.
3. When endoscopy fails to find a bleeding source, nuclear imaging is often useful to document (and sometimes approximately localize) active bleeding as a precursor to angiography.
4. Angiography may be invaluable for therapy or more precise localization before surgery, once nuclear imaging has confirmed ongoing hemorrhage. If nuclear imaging reveals no active bleeding, neither will angiography, unless the patient coincidentally rebleeds at the time of the angiogram.
5. Barium studies have no role in the initial evaluation of acute GI bleeding.

ADDITIONAL COMMENTS

- Barium studies do not actually demonstrate bleeding itself, and barium in the GI tract interferes with subsequent angiographic, nuclear, and endoscopic procedures. Therefore barium exams are best avoided in the initial evaluation of acute bleeding.
- A Meckel's diverticulum may acutely bleed, especially in children. A nuclear study can localize a Meckel's diverticulum, regardless of whether bleeding is active. Tc-99m pertechnetate is injected intravenously and the abdomen is imaged. The radiopharmaceutical concentrates in the ectopic gastric mucosa commonly present in symptomatic Meckel's diverticula.

- Angiographic treatment of acute GI bleeding is often effective when more conservative therapies have failed. This method is ideal for high-risk surgical candidates; in other patients, it is an important temporizing measure, permitting surgery at the most opportune time, rather than as an emergency.

- The angiographic technique most commonly used is intraarterial infusion of vasopressin. Vasopressin infusion requires an indwelling arterial catheter and careful monitoring for 24 to 48 hours, usually in an intensive care unit. Its effectiveness is probably due to smooth muscle contraction of both the GI tract wall and the vascular tree, reducing blood flow and promoting thrombosis. The complications of vasopressin therapy are usually minor and easily managed. Bowel infarction is very unusual if excessive vasospasm is avoided.

- Another technique to control GI bleeding is transcatheter arterial embolization, although it is technically difficult and the risk for infarction is significant. Several materials have been used to embolize and subsequently clot bleeding vessels, including autologous thrombi, Gelfoam particles, steel coils, and even synthetic glue. The technique requires great skill, because the angiographer must place the catheter tip into the bleeding vessel and avoid embolizing neighboring normal vessels.

- Angiographic treatment of bleeding esophageal varices is different. Vasopressin is often infused through a catheter in the superior mesenteric artery, with the goal of diminishing portal blood flow and hence blood flow through the bleeding esophageal varices. Alternatively, vasopressin may be infused through a peripheral vein. This technique avoids the occasional complications of arterial catheters, but it has the disadvantage of requiring higher infusion rates, thereby increasing the frequency of dose-related side effects. A third technique, performed in a few centers, involves the percutaneous transhepatic puncture of portal vein branches and selective placement of a catheter into the coronary veins. The bleeding esophageal varices may then be embolized. The results of treatment have been disappointing, and most patients can be treated with endoscopic sclerotherapy.

- A relatively new treatment for refractory variceal bleeding is the transjugular intrahepatic portosystemic shunt (TIPS). This involves a puncture of the right internal jugular vein and production of a communication between major branches of the hepatic and portal veins. This communication is maintained via a metallic mesh stent, which is subsequently dilated to an appropriate size using a balloon catheter. Central venous and portal venous pressures are measured before and after stent placement; a drop in the pressure gradient indicates successful shunting.

- A variation in angiographic diagnosis involves the infusion of agents such as heparin, streptokinase, or urokinase **that provoke or prolong bleeding!** This technique, diagnostic pharmacoangiography, is sometimes useful when bleeding has stopped by the time of diagnostic angiography. The short-term resumption of bleeding permits precise localization.

SUGGESTED ADDITIONAL READING

Baum S. Arteriographic diagnosis and treatment of gastrointestinal bleeding. In Abrams HL, ed. Abram Angiography: Vascular and Interventional Radiology, 3rd ed. Boston, 1983, Little, Brown, pp 1669-1700.

Bunker SR, Lull RJ, Tanasescu DE, Redwine MD, Rigby J, Brown JM, Brachman MB, McAuley RJ, Ramanna L, Landry A, Waxman AD. Scintigraphy of gastrointestinal hemorrhage: superiority of 99mTc red blood cells over 99mTc sulfur colloid. AJR 1984; 143:543-548.

Maurer AH, Rodman MS, Vitti RA, Revez G, Krevsky B. Gastrointestinal bleeding: improved localization with cine scintigraphy. Radiology 1992; 185:187.

Rosch J, Keller FS, Wawrukiewicz AS, Krippaehne WW, Dotter CT. Pharmacoangiography in the diagnosis of recurrent massive lower gastrointestinal bleeding. Radiology 1982; 145:615-619.

Winzelberg GG, McKusick KA, Froelich JW, Callahan RJ, Strauss HW. Detection of gastrointestinal bleeding with 99mTc-labeled red blood cells. Semin Nucl Med 1982; 12:139-146.

Zuckerman DA, Bocchini TP, Birnbaum EH. Massive hemorrhage in the lower gastrointestinal tract in adults: diagnostic imaging and intervention. AJR 1993; 161: 703-711.

10

Chronic Gastrointestinal Bleeding in the Adult

INTRODUCTION

Chronic gastrointestinal (GI) bleeding usually presents with iron deficiency anemia or stools positive for occult blood. Sigmoidoscopy often detects a lesion in the distal colon; imaging may be required to assess the extent of the lesion, to find additional lesions, or to locate a lesion if sigmoidoscopy is normal.

Colonoscopy and upper intestinal tract endoscopy are approximately as sensitive as barium exams but involve more patient discomfort, risk, and expense. Therefore they usually follow barium exams in the evaluation of **chronic bleeding. Sigmoidoscopy, however, should precede any barium studies.**

Costs: sigmoidoscopy, $91; BE, $147; UGI with small bowel follow-through, $192; enteroclysis, $295; visceral angiogram, $2979; Meckel's diverticulum nuclear scan, $177.

PLAN AND RATIONALE

Step 1: Barium Studies

When the entire GI tract is surveyed for bleeding sources, the barium enema (BE) is usually performed before the upper gastrointestinal (UGI) series, because residual barium from a BE is easily evacuated and does not interfere with further studies; after a UGI series, barium can remain in the gut for 1 to 3 days, **delaying the next study.**

Although the BE and UGI series are relatively standard, techniques for study of the small intestine vary. Many institutions administer additional oral barium immediately after a UGI series and radiographically follow its progress through the jejunum and ileum. Others perform a separate examination of the small bowel, called "enteroclysis" (see **Step 2, Enteroclysis**, below).

"Air contrast" barium exams excel in detecting small mucosal lesions. After barium, air is introduced into the colon or stomach via enema tube or oral administration of gas-forming tablets respectively. Air distends the gut lumen, exquisitely defining the mucosa.

Step 2: Enteroclysis

The standard small-bowel series is notorious for missing small lesions. Although meticulous technique may improve the sensitivity of standard exams, some institutions use "enteroclysis" as their primary small-bowel study in patients with a high likelihood of disease.

For enteroclysis, a nasoduodenal tube is inserted and positioned with its tip near the ligament of Treitz, and a small balloon is inflated to maintain this position. Barium is introduced at about 100 ml/min. The distal progression of barium is followed fluoroscopically. Air, water, or even methylcellulose may be added through the tube after barium for better mucosal coating.

Enteroclysis is available in only a limited number of centers. Because the exam is lengthy and requires a nasoduodenal tube, it is somewhat uncomfortable, although with-

out major risk. Where available, enteroclysis should precede gastroscopy and colonoscopy according to some
authorities, but others, knowing that the yield of lesions in
the small intestine is low, even with enteroclysis, recommend endoscopy first.

Negative sigmoidoscopy and barium studies are usually
followed by colonoscopy and upper gastrointestinal tract
endoscopy. If these studies are also negative, angiography
may be appropriate in selected patients.

Step 3: Angiography

Angiography can occasionally identify lesions that cause
chronic blood loss.

After percutaneous transfemoral introduction, a catheter
is advanced up the aorta, retrograde. The major feeding
vessels of the GI tract are catheterized and contrast material is injected, defining the vascular pattern of the gut and
any lesions. Extravasation of contrast material into the
bowel lumen is typically **not** seen, because the rate of
bleeding is too slow and usually intermittent (below 1.0
ml/min). Arteriovenous malformations, including
angiodysplasia of the colon, are most frequently identified,
especially in the elderly; **they are assumed to represent
the bleeding source when other abnormalities are
not defined.** Occasionally, small neoplasms undetected
by both barium exams and endoscopy are discovered.

Step 4: Radionuclide Meckel's Diverticulum Scan

A Meckel's diverticulum may **rarely** produce chronic GI
bleeding in adults. The lesion can sometimes be identified,
because its ectopic gastric mucosa concentrates a radiopharmaceutical, technetium-99m-pertechnetate, within 2
hours of intravenous injection. Sensitivity of the pertechnetate scan is approximately 75% when ectopic gastric

mucosa is present.[1] This study is usually performed after more common lesions have been excluded. Although noninvasive, a Meckel's scan usually follows endoscopy and an angiogram, except in children, in whom the lesion is much more common.

SUMMARY AND CONCLUSIONS

1. Endoscopy and barium exams of the upper and lower GI tract identify the majority of lesions responsible for chronic bleeding. **Sigmoidoscopy should precede all barium exams, but the BE and UGI series come before other more demanding forms of endoscopy.**
2. Enteroclysis is a barium study of the small intestine. It involves less risk than colonoscopy and gastroscopy and if available may be considered after negative BE and UGI studies. Some centers substitute enteroclysis as their usual small-intestinal series, whereas others perform a routine small-bowel study first.
3. Colonoscopy and gastroscopy usually precede angiography, if sigmoidoscopy and barium studies are normal.
4. **In chronic bleeding, angiography does not define an active bleeding site but locates abnormal vascular patterns, such as angiodysplasia, arteriovenous malformation, and neoplasm,** which may produce chronic blood loss.
5. Meckel's pertechnetate scans are sometimes useful, especially in children.

ADDITIONAL COMMENT

- Nuclear medicine techniques for evaluation of **acute** gastrointestinal bleeding are not useful in chronic bleeding, because the rate of blood loss in chronic bleeding is too low.

REFERENCE

1. Herlinger H. Small bowel. In Laufer I, ed. Double Contrast Gastrointestinal Radiology with Endoscopic Correlation. Philadelphia: 1979; Saunders, pp 423-494.

SUGGESTED ADDITIONAL READING

Baum S, Athanasoulis CA, Waltman AC. Angiodysplasia of the right colon as a cause of chronic gastrointestinal bleeding (abstract). Gastroenterology 1975; 68:A-5/862.

Conway J. The sensitivity, specificity and accuracy of radionuclide imaging of Meckel's diverticulum. J Nucl Med 1976; 17:553.

Jaramillo E, Slezak, P. Comparison between double-contrast barium enema and colonoscopy to investigate lower gastrointestinal bleeding. Gastrointest Radiol 1991; 17:81.

Miller RE, Sellink JL. Enteroclysis: the small bowel enema, how to succeed and how to fail. Gastrointest Radiol 1979; 4:269-283.

Rollens ES, Pincus D, Hicks ME, et. al. Angiography is useful in detecting the source of chronic gastrointestinal bleeding of obscure origin. AJR 1991; 156:385.

11

Blunt Abdominal Trauma

INTRODUCTION

Several techniques apply to the study of blunt abdominal trauma: plain films, computed tomography (CT), angiography, retrograde urethrography/cystography, and fluoroscopic studies of the intestine. Moreover, nuclear liver-spleen scans and intravenous pyelography (IVP) are sometimes helpful as follow-up exams.

Costs: plain abdominal films, $69; retrograde urethrogram/cystogram, $197; abdominal and pelvic CT, enhanced, $840; visceral angiography, $2979; HIDA, $225; IVP, $168; liver/spleen scan, $212; chest CT, $498; thoracic angiogram, $1278; UGI without small bowel follow-through, $160; gastrograffin enema, $147.

PLAN AND RATIONALE

In the clinically unstable patient:

Emergency life-saving surgery takes precedence; delay for diagnostic imaging may be inappropriate, but if there is time for limited, portable exams, plain films of the chest, abdomen, and pelvis are most important.

In the clinically stable patient:

Step 1: Plain Films of the Abdomen and Pelvis

Plain films exclude most fractures and may detect gross intraperitoneal air or fluid. However, **normal plain films do not eliminate the need for further imaging.**

Step 2: Computed Tomography

CT of the abdomen with intravenous contrast material is the central study in blunt abdominal trauma. The exam often takes less than 30 minutes and is available virtually everywhere on an emergency basis. Newer "spiral" or "helical" CT dramatically reduces imaging time; a complete abdominal and pelvic exam requires only 5 to 10 minutes from start to finish, with actual scanning times much shorter.

CT accurately defines a wide variety of injuries, including intra- and retroperitoneal hemorrhage; hepatic, splenic, and pancreatic laceration/hematoma; bowel laceration; renal contusion/hematoma; skeletal fractures; and fluid and/or air near the lung bases. Most often CT ends the workup. However, further imaging is appropriate in specific circumstances:

Liver. If a bile leak is suspected after abdominal CT, a nuclear HIDA scan is appropriate (see Chapter 6, Bile Leak).

Spleen. Although nuclear spleen scanning is probably as sensitive as CT for detecting splenic laceration/hematoma, **it is inappropriate in the acute setting**, because abdominal CT provides key information about many other organs. However, **to follow the course of a splenic laceration, once other abdominal injuries are no longer of concern, the nuclear liver–spleen scan is preferred, because of its lower cost.** (Of course, if injuries to multiple organs must be followed, follow-up CT is appropriate.)

Pancreas. Pancreatic injuries are usually defined in the acute setting; however, if the initial exam is equivocal yet suspicion of pancreatic injury persists, a follow-up study may be useful, because peripancreatic inflammation/hemorrhage may have increased to diagnostic levels by the time of the later study.

Kidneys. Absent renal excretion of intravenously administered contrast material strongly raises the possibility of renovascular compromise, and a detailed study of the renal arteries may be required, so that surgical salvage can be attempted. Multiple factors determine whether angiography is appropriate; the decision is best left to the angiographer and vascular surgeon.

When extravasation of contrast material from the renal collecting systems and/or ureters indicates ureteropelvicalyceal laceration, follow-up IVPs are appropriate to monitor the process.

Lower Thorax. Abdominal CT always includes the lower thorax, where pleural fluid, unsuspected pneumothorax, or parenchymal lung injury may be defined. Unless there is also suspected aortic injury, these findings can usually be followed by chest films, but if the mediastinum is suspicious for hematoma, separate thoracic CT or angiography is mandatory (see Chapter 28, Aortic Injury in Blunt Chest Trauma).

Bladder. Hematuria in the presence of normal kidneys and ureters raises the question of urethral or even bladder trauma. A retrograde urethrogram and cystogram is then appropriate. The urethra is catheterized and filled with contrast material; if the urethra is intact, the bladder is catheterized, filled, and studied.

Intestine. Suspected duodenal hematoma and colonic laceration can be confirmed by a tailored upper gastrointestinal series (UGI) and gastrograffin enema, respectively.

SUMMARY AND CONCLUSIONS

1. **CT is the definitive study for blunt abdominal trauma.**
2. Plain films of the abdomen, pelvis, and chest are helpful and should not be skipped.
3. Other specific exams can be directed to sites of suspected injury, based on the initial CT findings: HIDA scan for bile leak, angiography for injury of the renal vasculature, retrograde urethrography and cystography for urethral or bladder trauma, UGI series for duodenal hematoma, and gastrograffin enema for colonic laceration.

ADDITIONAL COMMENTS

- In the patient with trivial abdominal trauma and hematuria, an IVP is preferred to a renal scan, because it provides much better anatomic detail of the renal contours, pelvicalyceal systems, and ureters.
- In blunt abdominal trauma, sonography is inferior to CT and may be technically difficult because of rib fractures, skin injuries, or ileus.
- Magnetic resonance imaging currently has no role in abdominal trauma.

SUGGESTED ADDITIONAL READING

Federle MP. CT of abdominal trauma. In Federle MP, Brant-Zawadzki M, eds. Computed Tomography in the Evaluation of Trauma, 2nd ed. Baltimore, 1986, Williams & Wilkins, pp 191-273.

Federle MP. CT in the evaluation of pelvic trauma. In Federle MP, Brant-Zawadzki M, eds. Computed Tomography in the Evaluation of Trauma, 2nd ed. Baltimore, 1986, Williams & Wilkins, pp 274-302.

Kuligowska E, Mueller PR, Simeone JF, et al. Ultrasound in upper abdominal trauma. Semin Roentgenol 1984; 19:281-295.

Lang EK, Sullivan J, Frentz G. Renal trauma: radiological studies. Radiology 1985; 154:1-6.

Sandler CM, Phillips JM, Harris JD, et al. Radiology of the bladder and urethra in blunt pelvic trauma. Radiol Clin North Am 1981; 19:195-211.

12

Small Bowel Obstruction

INTRODUCTION

Small bowel obstruction (SBO) is common. Eighty percent of all intestinal obstructions occur at the level of the small bowel,[1] and 80% of these result from adhesions or hernias. Another common cause of SBO is malignancy, usually metastatic, while abdominal or pelvic abscess and small bowel tumor are much less frequent.

The clinical and radiographic diagnosis of SBO can be difficult.[2] **SBO must be differentiated from ileus**, which may follow any abdominal insult or result from a wide variety of extraabdominal or systemic diseases. Ileus usually responds to conservative therapy and nasogastric tube drainage, whereas mechanical obstruction often requires surgical intervention.

Costs: plain abdominal films and upright chest film, $69; BE, $147; UGI with small bowel follow-through, $192; enteroclysis, $295.

PLAN AND RATIONALE

Step 1: Plain Radiographs

Supine, upright, and decubitus films of the abdomen are essential. If the patient is too ill for an upright radiograph, decubitus films (the patient lies on his/her side) or a cross-table lateral film (the patient is supine) is acceptable. Upright films can exclude free intraperitoneal air, which, if present, almost always indicates bowel perforation. If feasible, an **upright chest film** is also strongly recommended; **the upright chest film is the best view to detect free intraperitoneal air.**

The plain film diagnosis of bowel obstruction rests on the fact that proximal to an obstruction the bowel distends, usually with fluid and air, whereas distal to the obstruction it empties of both. Initially, peristalsis continues proximal to the obstruction. Thus typical findings in complete or "high-grade" SBO include multiple dilated, air-filled small bowel loops, with decreased or absent colonic gas. Early on, air-fluid levels of unequal heights in each dilated small bowel loop appear on upright or decubitus films.

Despite the value of plain films, **the diagnosis of SBO is often tenuous**: ileus may be resemble a partial SBO, dilated small bowel loops filled with fluid (but not air) may be radiographically invisible, and air-fluid levels of unequal heights can result from other conditions.[3] Moreover, a very proximal SBO may present with few dilated bowel loops, and the bowel proximal to the obstruction may be empty of air, as a result of repeated vomiting. Therefore **plain films for SBO have a high false positive and false negative rate.**[4]

A particularly difficult diagnostic problem is "closed loop" obstruction. When obstruction occurs at two separate points, the process can lead to bowel strangulation, decreased blood supply, and bowel infarction. Closed loop obstruction and strangulation often remain undiscovered until surgery,[5] because there is insufficient gas trapped in the closed loop to produce the characteristic air-fluid levels of obstruction. The fluid-filled bowel loops may produce a radiographic sign known as "pseudotumor," but this appearance is not specific. **In fact, the abdominal films of patients with life-threatening closed loop obstruction can even be normal.**[2,6,7]

If plain films are equivocal for obstruction or **if the site of an obstruction must be better defined before therapy**, barium studies of the bowel are required. (In practical terms, most patients are placed on nasogastic suction and plain films are repeated to follow the course of the process; surgery often follows without further imaging.)

All barium studies are contraindicated if free intraperitoneal air is visible on plain films.

When the obstruction may be in the distal small bowel or the colon:

Step 2: Barium Enema

If colonic obstruction is a serious consideration, a barium enema should precede any oral barium study, because orally administered barium may harden proximal to an obstructing colonic lesion.

Barium without air (a "single-contrast study") is introduced per rectum. If no obstruction is encountered in the colon, barium can often be refluxed into the distal small bowel until the obstruction is reached. If reflux of barium into the distal small bowel is unrevealing, then a barium study of the lesion from above is justified.

When the colon has been exonerated by a barium enema or the initial plain films indicate obstruction in the small bowel:

Step 3: Oral Barium Studies

The conventional upper gastrointestinal (UGI) series and small bowel follow-through involve oral administration of barium and sequential fluoroscopic and radiographic study of the barium column as it progresses distally. The study may define the level of an obstruction but rarely its specific cause, because the barium column is progressively diluted by intraluminal fluid as it progresses, reducing its visibility. For better definition and for patients with partial acute or intermittent small–bowel obstruction, particularly if the physical exam and plain radiographs are inconclusive, a technique called "enteroclysis" can be more precise.

Enteroclysis can detect even subtle lesions like minimal adhesions and can contribute significantly to major decisions in terms of surgery or conservative therapy. Intraluminal masses and abnormalities of the intestinal wall are also sometimes discovered.[5,6] Nonetheless, enteroclysis is underutilized, because the study is somewhat demanding for the patient and because it requires special radiologic expertise.

Enteroclysis is contraindicated if complete obstruction or bowel strangulation is suspected.

Under fluoroscopic control, a long tube is placed from above into the proximal jejunum. Barium, followed by a solution of methylcellulose, is infused (either by hand injection or by mechanical pump) directly into the jejunum. The barium-methylcellulose column is followed as it progresses to the site of obstruction. The study requires less than 30 minutes and is preferable to a small bowel follow-through, because it is briefer, avoids the need for serial films, **and delivers a bolus directly into the small bowel without significant dilution of barium.**

After barium studies the workup usually ends. However, recent reports suggest that computed tomography (CT) or ultrasound may be effective **in certain specific circumstances**. Please see **ADDITIONAL COMMENTS**, below.

SUMMARY AND CONCLUSIONS

1. Small bowel obstruction is common. Plain films of the abdomen are the best initial study. Although plain films may be definitive, they are often falsely positive or negative. Therefore, follow-up barium studies are frequently required. **All barium studies are contraindicated if plain films demonstrate free intraabdominal air.**

2. To differentiate between a proximal colonic obstruction and a distal SBO, a "single-contrast" barium enema is appropriate. Usually barium can be refluxed into the distal small bowel if no colonic obstruction is present. The exact site and cause of the obstruction can be demonstrated.

3. If the colon is exonerated and **intermittent or partial small bowel obstruction** is present or strongly suspected, enteroclysis may be helpful in determining the exact site and nature of an obstructing lesion. Enteroclysis is almost always superior to a standard small bowel follow-through. **Enteroclysis should not be performed in complete SBO or if strangulation is likely.**

4. CT and possibly ultrasound can be helpful in selected patients (see **ADDITIONAL COMMENTS**) but are not routinely indicated in the SBO workup.

ADDITIONAL COMMENTS

- **Water–soluble contrast materials like gastrograffin are inappropriate** in patients with SBO. **They are not**

effective in this setting and are potentially danger-ous; **their hypertonicity draws additional fluid and electrolytes into the small bowel. Furthermore, these contrast materials can be fatal if aspirated.**

- Recent reports have suggested a possible role for CT in certain patients with SBO.[4,8,9] CT may confirm the presence or absence of SBO in equivocal cases and can sometimes determine its etiology (e.g., tumor, occult internal or external hernia, or abscess). The study can be especially useful when there is a history of abdom-inal cancer. Moreover, the absence of a defined lesion may imply that adhesions are responsible.

- In chronic obstruction the bowel wall becomes hypo-tonic; decreased peristalsis causes enteroclysis to fail. In this setting CT can be particularly useful. CT has also been effective in patients with closed loop obstruction and/or strangulation.

- Despite its success **in selected cases**, CT's exact role in SBO is currently unclear, and CT cannot routinely be recommended until further prospective outcome analyses are available: does the additional information provided by CT affect patient management sufficiently to justify its cost **on a routine basis?** Nonetheless, in specific patients—if the standard plain film and barium workup is not decisive—the option of CT should be discussed with the radiologist before surgery is consid-ered the sole diagnostic option.

- Ultrasound may also have a limited role in the evalua-tion of SBO. Hyperperistaltic, dilated, and fluid-filled small bowel loops are directly visualized. Ultrasound can sometimes identify a closed loop obstruction, identify a proximal SBO, and determine the presence, site, and etiology of SBO, despite the presence of con-siderable bowel gas.[10] However, the sensitivity and specificity of ultrasound for SBO are unknown, and like CT, its the cost–effectiveness is unproven. The option of ultrasound should be considered along with CT when plain film and barium workups have failed.

REFERENCES

1. Chen MYM, Ott DJ, Kelley TF, Gelfand DW. Impact of the small bowel study on patient management. Gastrointest Radiol 1991; 16:189-192.
2. Eisenberg RL. Gastrointestinal Radiology: A Pattern Approach, 2nd ed. Philadelphia, 1990, Lippincott, pp 411-440.
3. Harlow CL, Stears RLG, Zeligman BE, Archer PG. Diagnosis of bowel obstruction on plain abdominal radiographs: significance of air–fluid levels at different heights in the same loop of bowel. AJR 1993; 161:291-295.
4. Fukuya T, Hawes DR, Lu CC, Chang PJ, Barloon TJ. CT diagnosis of small bowel obstruction: efficacy in 60 patients. AJR 1992; 158:765-769.
5. Maglinte DDT, Lappas JC, Kelvin FM, Rex D, Chernish SM. Small bowel radiography: how, when, and why? Radiology 1987; 163:297-305.
6. Herlinger H, Maglinte DDT. Clinical Radiology of the Small Intestine. Philadelphia, 1989, Saunders, pp 49-65, 479-506.
7. Balthazar EJ, Birnbaum BA, Megibow AJ, Gordon RB, Whelan CA, Hulnick DH. Closed-loop and strangulating intestinal obstruction: CT signs. Radiology 1992; 185:769-775.
8. Megibow AJ, Balthazar EJ, Cho KC, Medwid SW, Birnbaum BA, Noz ME. Bowel obstruction: evaluation with CT. Radiology 1991; 180:313-318.
9. Maglinte DDT, Gage SN, Harmon BH, et al. Obstruction of the small intestine: accuracy and role of CT in diagnosis. Radiology 1993; 188:61-64.
10. Ko YT, Lim JH, Lee DH, Lee HW, Lim JW. Small bowel obstruction:sonographic evaluation. Radiology 1993; 188:649-653.

13

Dysphagia

INTRODUCTION

Dysphagia is the subjective awareness of difficulty swallowing. Classically, dysphagia for liquids is associated with motor disorders, while dysphagia for solids is associated with either motor or structural disorders.[1] Swallowing problems may also present as coughing, choking, nasal regurgitation, or hoarseness.

The swallowing mechanism is extremely complex. Thus dysphagia has numerous causes, including neurologic disease (stroke, Alzheimer's, Parkinson's, head trauma), muscle disorders (myasthenia gravis), anatomic lesions (esophageal web, Zenker diverticulum), tumors (oral cavity, pharynx, esophagus, or gastric cardia), prior surgery and/or radiation therapy, and medications. In addition, swallowing difficulty may be the presenting symptom of systemic diseases like scleroderma.

The patient's impression of the level of a swallowing blockage is often unreliable, because the sensation of dysphagia is often referred from the lesion to another level. Clinical exam is also unreliable; for example, an intact gag reflex does not necessarily mean that the pharyngeal phase of swallowing is intact.[2]

A barium swallow is the initial exam of choice for most patients with dysphagia. Endoscopy is more expensive and more invasive and does not evaluate the motility of the upper gastrointestinal tract.

Costs: barium swallow with videofluoroscopy, $107; endoscopic US, $484.

PLAN AND RATIONALE

For the evaluation of patients presenting with dysphagia:

Step 1: Barium Swallow with Videofluoroscopy

The patient drinks liquid barium under fluoroscopy, in both the upright and the supine positions, and the study is videotaped. The oral cavity, pharynx, and esophagus are examined. For detailed mucosal evaluation "spot" images are also obtained.

The exam can be individually tailored to the patient's symptoms or ability to cooperate. When there is a history of dysphagia for solids and the routine study with liquid barium is normal, thicker barium followed by a barium tablet or barium-coated marshmallow is then administered. Abnormalities like subtle esophageal strictures can be detected by this technique.

If the barium swallow is normal, the workup ends, but if lesions that require biopsy, cytology, or clarification are detected, endoscopy is appropriate.

Step 2: Endoscopy

Endoscopy is usually required to further evaluate esophageal strictures, webs, ulcerations, and tumors. Biopsy or therapeutic intervention is often feasible through the endoscope.

In selected patients, endoscopic ultrasound, a new technique available in some centers, can help to determine if there is extension of esophageal mucosal tumor through the esophageal wall; this information is helpful for staging. A tiny ultrasound transducer is introduced through the endoscope and images are displayed on a television screen. The technique can define details of the esophageal wall better than any other imaging method.

For the evaluation of patients with dysphagia or suspected aspiration resulting from known neurologic, neuromuscular, or other disorders, to help design their "swallowing reeducation" therapy:

Step 1: Tailored Barium Swallow with Videofluoroscopy

Dysphagia is common in patients with neurologic disorders, particularly stroke. Aspiration often results, and up to 40% of such patients who aspirate are not recognized as such clinically.[3] Management may be significantly improved by a **tailored** barium swallow with videofluoroscopy.[2,4]

Optimally, these studies are performed by a radiologist together with a speech pathologist. A special chair supports patients who are unable to sit upright. Oral, pharyngeal, and esophageal phases of swallowing are examined under fluoroscopy, and the study is videotaped.

Thin barium, then thicker barium, and finally a variety of barium-impregnated solids of different consistencies are swallowed. The exam is stopped if there is any substantial aspiration. The study can help to determine if the patient is really aspirating, the consistency of food that he or she aspirates, and the phase of swallowing during which aspiration occurs. Various patient positions (e.g., head flexed during swallowing) and specialized maneuvers (e.g., coughing after swallowing, to clear the larynx) are tried under fluoroscopy, in an attempt to eliminate aspiration;

these positions and maneuvers may then be applied routinely by the patient during eating and drinking.

SUMMARY AND CONCLUSIONS

1. Dysphagia has numerous causes and may be the presenting symptom of a systemic disease or local malignancy. Therefore, it should be considered a potentially serious condition until proven otherwise.[1] **Dysphagia that worsens over several months is particularly worrisome for an obstructing esophageal stricture or tumor.**[1]
2. The exam of choice for patients who present with dysphagia is a barium swallow with videofluoroscopy.
3. Any definite or suspected local lesion may then be studied by endoscopy, which is more invasive and expensive than a barium swallow. In many cases brushings, biopsies, or intervention is feasible through the endoscope. Endoscopic ultrasound can define tumor extension through the esophageal wall, for staging.
4. A tailored barium swallow for patients with dysphagia and/or suspected aspiration from neurologic, neuromuscular, or other conditions who are undergoing "swallowing reeducation" can be very helpful in planning patient management.

ADDITIONAL COMMENTS

- Patients should fast overnight before a barium swallow.
- While lower esophageal and gastric cardia abnormalities may refer dysphagia to the pharynx, pharyngeal abnormalities almost never refer dysphagia to the thorax. A detailed pharyngeal study is usually not needed in patients with low substernal symptoms, but a thorough esophageal study is appropriate.[5]

- Substernal pain may be due to esophageal motility abnormalities. Painful swallowing in general may be due to esophageal or pharyngeal infection, ulceration, or tumor. The barium study can be very helpful in evaluating such patients.
- The barium swallow effectively evaluates children with swallowing problems like gagging, vomiting during feeding, or suspected aspiration. The etiology of dysphasia is very different in children than in adults; children should be studied in their usual feeding position.

REFERENCES

1. Pope CE II. Diseases of the esophagus. In Wyngaarden JB, Smith LH Jr, eds. Cecil Textbook of Medicine, 18th ed. Philadelphia, 1988, Saunders, p 679.
2. Dodds WJ, Logemann JA, Stewart ET. Radiologic assessment of abnormal oral and pharyngeal phases of swallowing. AJR 1990; 154:965-974.
3. Jones B, Kramer SS, Donner MW. Dynamic imaging of the pharynx. Gastrointest Radiol 1985; 10:213-224.
4. Chen MYM, Ott DJ, Peele VN, Gelfand DW. Oropharynx in patients with cerebrovascular disease: evaluation with videofluoroscopy. Radiology 1990: 176:641-643.
5. Levine MS, Rubesin SE. Radiologic investigation of dysphagia. AJR 1990; 154: 1157-1163.

SUGGESTED ADDITIONAL READING

Feinberg MJ, Ekberg O. Videofluoroscopy in elderly patients with aspiration: importance of evaluating both oral and pharyngeal stages of deglutition. AJR 1991; 156: 293-296.

Jones B, Donner MW. Examination of the patient with dysphagia. Radiology 1988; 167:319-326.

Kramer SS. Special swallowing problems in children. Gastrointest Radiol 1985; 10: 241-250.

Siebens AA, Linden P. Dynamic imaging for swallowing reeducation. Gastrointest Radiol 1985; 10:251-253.

14

Screening for Colorectal Cancer and Polyps

INTRODUCTION

Colorectal cancer (CRC) is the second most common cancer in American adults; the disease kills 60,000 people in the United States annually. Almost all CRCs begin as adenomatous polyps. Thus **polyp detection is cancer prevention.**[1,2] There is bitter controversy, however, as to which tests are best to screen for colorectal cancer and polyps.

Costs: sigmoidoscopy, $91; barium enema, $147; colonoscopy, $618; colonoscopy with polypectomy, $856.

PLAN AND RATIONALE

The American Cancer Society recommends annual fecal occult blood testing (FOBT) and sigmoidoscopy every 3 to 5 years for each person over 50 years of age.[3,4] Both FOBT and sigmoidoscopy have limits as screening tests. FOBT is cheap, simple, and safe; yet, even correctly performed, it fails to detect up to 50% of all colorectal carcinomas and polyps.[1] Flexible sigmoidoscopy (even with some of the newer, long endoscopes) may find less than half of all colonic adenomas and carcinomas.[1,3]
Combined FOBT and sigmoidoscopy may miss up to one-third of all colorectal carcinomas.[3] An

effective screening test for polyps and colorectal cancer should **examine the entire colon**. Moreover, a logical approach would customize the screening process to each population subgroup on the basis of risk.

Screening patients at average risk for developing colorectal cancer, starting at age 50:

Step 1: Fecal Occult Blood Testing and Digital Rectal Exam Annually

Step 2: Sigmoidoscopy AND Barium Enema every 3 to 5 years

Some authorities recommend colonoscopy (endoscopic exam of the entire colon) to screen individuals at average risk for colorectal carcinoma.[4] However, colonoscopy costs much more than a barium enema, often requires patient sedation, and has a much greater incidence of complications (especially bowel perforation) than either sigmoidoscopy or a barium enema. Also, in more than 25% of patients, the colonoscope is unable to reach the right side of the colon.[3] (On the other hand, lesions that are detected can also be biopsied and removed.) A barium enema, performed with careful bowel preparation and meticulous technique, is as accurate as colonoscopy in detecting lesions 1 cm or more in diameter throughout the colon, with a sensitivity of greater than 90%.[1,5] However, barium studies of the colon can miss rectal lesions, and the highest incidence of undetected polyps by both barium enema and endoscopy is in the rectosigmoid region (presumably a result of commonly coexistent diverticular disease, which causes interpretation errors on barium enemas and perception errors on endoscopy).[6]

We believe that colonoscopy is too expensive and

invasive for mass screening of patients at average risk for colorectal cancer, whereas the less expensive and invasive barium enema and sigmoidoscopy are complementary. Therefore, we recommend that all such individuals over age 50 have yearly FOBT and digital rectal exam, along with sigmoidoscopy AND a barium enema every 3 to 5 years. Our protocol slightly modifies the most recent guidelines of the American College of Radiology (also accepted by the American College of Physicians), which recommends yearly FOBT and every 3 to 5 years, sigmoidoscopy WITH OR WITHOUT a barium enema.[4] Our rationale for modifying the American College of Radiology guidelines rests on the fact that FOBT and sigmoidoscopy OR a barium enema will miss some colonic lesions, whereas the combination of a barium enema AND sigmoidoscopy screens the entire colon.

Screening patients at high risk (positive family history), starting at age 40:

Step 1: Fecal Occult Blood Testing and Digital Rectal Exam Annually

Step 2: Colonoscopy, OR Barium Enema AND Sigmoidoscopy Every 3 to 5 Years

The risk of developing CRC in individuals whose first-degree relatives have had the disease increases three- to four-fold.[7] The American College of Radiology has developed guidelines for screening these individuals (also accepted by the American College of Physicians). Starting at age 40, FOBT and a digital rectal exam are recommended annually, with colonoscopy OR a barium enema every 3 to 5 years. **Colonoscopy is justified in these individuals, because the procedure's risk is outweighed by the potential benefit of screening the entire colon and concurrently removing any lesions, which are much more prevalent in this group than in the general population. As an alternative to colonoscopy, we suggest BOTH a barium enema AND flexible sigmoidoscopy every 3 to 5 years. The combination of these two tests screens the entire colon.**

SUMMARY AND CONCLUSIONS

1. Colorectal cancer is the second most common cause of cancer in American adults; 60,000 individuals will die annually in the United States of this disease. Colorectal cancer is known to develop almost exclusively within benign adenomatous polyps. Effective screening may save many lives.

2. We support the recent screening guidelines of the American College of Radiology for CRC, with some important modifications. Individuals at no increased risk of developing CRC should have fecal occult blood testing and digital rectal exams annually, starting at age 50, as well as sigmoidoscopy AND a barium enema every 3 to 5 years.

3. Individuals at increased risk of developing CRC—namely, people with a first-degree relative who have developed the disease—should have fecal occult blood testing and digital rectal exam annually starting at age 40, along with colonoscopy or a barium enema AND flexible sigmoidoscopy every 3 to 5 years.

4. The barium enema has been underutilized as a screening test for colorectal cancer. Unlike flexible sigmoidoscopy, it examines the entire colon. It is safer,

cheaper, and as effective as colonoscopy in detecting colonic polyps or carcinomas greater than or equal to 1 cm in diameter.

ADDITIONAL COMMENTS

- Both double-contrast (barium and air introduced into the colon) and single-contrast (barium only) enemas can be very effective in detecting colonic lesions 1 cm or more in diameter.[2] Most radiologists now perform double-contrast enemas routinely. Single-contrast examinations may be indicated if the patient is very elderly or is infirm and has limited mobility (the double-contrast study is more demanding for the patient). Double-contrast examinations are more sensitive than single-contrast examinations for the detection of lesions less than 1 cm in diameter, and colonoscopy may be more sensitive than either barium enema technique for such small lesions. However, carcinoma rarely occurs in polyps less than 1 cm in diameter, and screening efforts should be directed toward detecting lesions 1 cm or greater in diameter.[1]
- Endoscopy should follow the detection of any colonic lesion on a barium enema.
- The importance of proper colonic preparation for a barium enema cannot be overemphasized. Patients (or their referring physicians) should contact the office of the radiologist who will be performing the exam regarding the proper bowel preparation.

REFERENCES

1. Ott DJ. Role of the barum enema in colorectal carcinoma. Radiol Clin North Am 1993; 31:1293-1313.
2. Rice RP. Lowering death rates from colorectal cancer: challenge for the 1990s. Radiology 1990; 176:297-301.
3. Gelfand DW, Ott DJ. The economic implications of radiologic screening for colonic cancer. AJR 1991; 156:939-943.

4. Ferrucci JT. Screening for colon cancer: controversies and recommendations. Radiol Clin North Am 1993; 31:1189-1195.
5. Jaramillo E, Slezak P. Comparison between double-contrast barium enema and colonoscopy to investigate lower gastrointestinal bleeding. Gastrointest Radiol 1992; 17:81-83.
6. Margulis AR, Burhenne HJ, eds. Alimentary Tract Radiology, 4th ed. St Louis, 1989, Mosby, pp 2017-2022.
7. Ransohoff DF, Lang CA. Screening for colorectal cancer. N Engl J Med 1991; 325: 37-41.

SUGGESTED ADDITIONAL READING

Eddy DM. Screening for colorectal cancer. Ann Intern Med 1990; 113:373-384.
Levin B, Murphy GP. Revision in American Cancer Society recommendations for the early detection of colorectal cancer. CA 1992; 42:296.
Thoeni RF, Margulis AR. The state of radiographic technique in the examination of the colon: a survey in 1987. Radiology 1988; 167:7-12.

Part II
GENITOURINARY

15

Renal Mass in the Adult

INTRODUCTION

In adults, renal masses are often discovered on an intravenous pyelogram (IVP) during the workup of urinary tract problems like hematuria or calculi.

The goal of renal imaging is to differentiate between simple cysts on the one hand and solid or complex (partly cystic and partly solid) masses on the other hand. Simple renal cysts are benign lesions that require no treatment and are found in up to 50% of the population over age 50. While there are many potential causes of solid or complex masses, both benign and malignant, **they must be considered malignant until proven otherwise.**

Imaging options include intravenous pyelography (IVP), sonography (ultrasound or US), computed tomography (CT), nuclear scanning, magnetic resonance imaging (MR), and angiography. **The IVP cannot reliably differentiate simple cysts from other lesions; ultrasound and CT, however, differentiate them.** Nuclear imaging and angiography have no primary role in the study of renal masses yet in select cases may be helpful. The role of MR in evaluating adult renal masses remains somewhat limited.

Because simple cysts are so common and sonography is less expensive than CT, sonography is the

preferred initial exam when a mass is detected on an IVP, unless certain worrisome characteristics are present.

Costs: abdominal US, $201; abdominal CT, enhanced, $433; renal biopsy, CT-guided, $901; renal biopsy, US-guided, $609.

PLAN AND RATIONALE

If the initial IVP detects a mass without worrisome characteristics:

Step 1: The Sonogram

The sonographic appearance of a simple cyst is virtually pathognomonic. **If sonography proves that a lesion is a simple cyst, the workup stops.**

If sonography reveals a lesion that is solid or is a cyst(s) that is "indeterminate" (i.e., does not meet all criteria for benignity), then CT is the next step. (See **"If the initial IVP detects a mass with worrisome characteristics," Step 1: Computed Tomography,** below)

If the initial IVP detects a mass with worrisome characteristics:

Step 1: Computed Tomography

CT is the diagnostic "gold standard" for renal masses. A study without contrast material (unenhanced) is performed first, to demonstrate calcification or hemorrhage, immediately followed by a study with intravenous contrast material (enhanced).

If a renal mass has typical benign cystic features or can be characterized as a specific benign solid lesion, like an angiomyolipoma, the workup stops. If CT reveals a solid mass or a complex cystic mass with irregular calcifications and thick septations, it is considered malignant until proven otherwise.

CT has an accuracy rate of over 90% for staging renal tumors. Although it cannot provide a histologic diagnosis, it reveals the relationship of a renal mass to adjacent structures, the degree of renal tumor extension, and the status of the contralateral kidney. CT almost always ends the presurgical workup, but in selected cases, especially when the patient is a poor surgical risk, needle aspiration can be helpful.

Step 2: Percutaneous Guided Needle Aspiration/Biopsy

Under CT or sonographic guidance, the renal mass is punctured percutaneously and aspirated or biopsied for cytology/histology.

When infection is suspected, guided aspiration can confirm the diagnosis and obtain material for culture. Catheters may be placed in a renal or perirenal abscess for drainage.

SUMMARY AND CONCLUSIONS

1. **Although the IVP often initially demonstrates a mass, it cannot unequivocally diagnose a simple cyst and has no utility in the workup beyond initial mass detection.**
2. When the IVP detects a mass without worrisome characteristics, sonography is appropriate.
3. **When the renal mass is clearly a simple cyst on sonography, the workup ends.** If the mass is not a simple cyst on sonography, CT is mandatory.

4. **When the IVP detects a mass with worrisome characteristics, CT is mandatory.**
5. Complex cystic or solid masses on CT are considered malignant until proven otherwise, unless they have specific benign characteristics like an angiomyolipoma.
6. Many radiologists believe that percutaneous aspiration is rarely indicated and should be reserved for the evaluation of renal masses in patients who are poor surgical risks or have suspected renal abscesses or infected cysts.

ADDITIONAL COMMENTS

- **A normal IVP does not exclude a renal mass.** An IVP detects only half of all renal tumors between 2 and 3 cm in diameter that are detected by CT. **If there is a strong clinical suspicion of a renal tumor—for example, because of hematuria—and the IVP is negative, CT is mandatory.**
- Although recent advances have improved MR's ability to detect renal lesions, its role in the workup of renal masses remains somewhat limited, and it is more expensive than CT. Where available, MR angiography can assist in the staging of renal cell carcinoma, because it accurately demonstrates tumor invasion of the renal veins and/or inferior vena cava. Also, MR can substitute for CT in patients who cannot tolerate contrast material because of renal failure or allergy.
- Angiography is usually reserved for suspected vascular masses like arteriovenous malformations or to demonstrate tumor invasion of the renal veins and/or inferior vena cava, if enhanced CT or MR is inconclusive. Moreover, some surgeons request angiography as a presurgical "road map" or to have a hypervascular lesion embolized before surgery.

- The nuclear renal scan is useful in clarifying the rare borderline IVP or sonogram where a variation in renal contour could represent a small solid parenchymal mass, a normal parenchymal bulge, or a "column of Bertin." (A column of Bertin is normal renal cortical tissue that extends between renal pyramids, appearing as a mass.) Normal parenchymal function on a nuclear renal scan in the area of interest excludes a neoplasm. For this uncommon study, a special renal cortical radiopharmaceutical, Tc-99m-dimercaptosuccinic acid (DMSA) is best.
- The standard Tc-99m-DTPA nuclear scan is also useful for **assessing renal function in a contralateral kidney before surgery.**

SUGGESTED ADDITIONAL READING

Bosniak MA. The current radiological approach to renal cysts. Radiology 1986; 138:1-10.

Choyke PL. MR imaging in renal cell carcinoma. Radiology 1988; 169:572-573.

Davidson AJ. Radiology of the kidney. Philadelphia, 1985, Saunders.

Dunnick NR. Renal lesions: great strides in imaging. Radiology 1992; 182:305-306.

Dunnick NR, McCallum RW, Sandler CM. Textbook of Uroradiology. Baltimore, 1991, Williams & Wilkins, pp 96-134.

Fein AB, Lee JKT, Balfe DM, et al. Diagnosis and staging of renal cell carcinoma: a comparison of MR imaging and CT. AJR 1987; 148:749-753.

Hartman DS. Cysts and cystic neoplasms. Urol Radiol 1990; 12:7-10.

Johnson CD, Dunnick NR, Cohan RH, et al. Renal adenocarcinoma: CT staging of 100 tumors. AJR 1987; 148:59-63.

Lee JKT. Recent advances in magnetic resonance imaging of renal masses. J Can Assoc Radiol 1991; 42:185-189.

Smith SJ, Bosniak MA, Meigbow AJ, et al. Renal cell carcinoma: earlier discovery and increased detection. Radiology 1989; 170:699-703.

Zeman RK, Cronan JJ, Rosenfield AT, et al. Imaging approach to the suspected renal mass. Radiol Clin North Am 1985; 23:503-529.

16

Renal Failure

INTRODUCTION

The initial radiologic evaluation of renal failure, acute or chronic, requires a determination of renal size, exclusion of urinary tract obstruction, and an evaluation of each individual kidney's function. Plain films of the abdomen and pelvis, a renal sonogram (ultrasound or US), and computed tomography (CT) accomplish these ends. A nuclear renal scan is sometimes also useful.

Costs: abdominal plain films, $45; renal US, $201; pelvic CT, unenhanced, $372; nuclear renal scan, $257.

PLAN AND RATIONALE

Step 1: Plain Film of the Abdomen and Pelvis ("KUB")

A plain film of the abdomen and pelvis (a "**KUB**," for kidneys, ureters, and bladder) reveals renal and ureteral stones and other soft tissue calcifications, as well as bony abnormalities associated with chronic renal failure.[1,2] A rough estimate of renal size is also possible.

Step 2: Renal Sonogram

Sonography is the main imaging exam in the evaluation of renal failure. The study is quick, uncomplicated, noninvasive, and relatively inexpensive. Ultrasound measures renal size and parenchymal thickness accurately, evaluates the pelvicalyceal systems for dilatation, and can detect other morphologic lesions like cysts and tumors. Moreover, a skilled sonographer can sometimes discern an abnormal parenchymal "echo texture" (echogenicity). **Unlike the IVP and nuclear renal scan, the sonogram is independent of renal function.**

History primarily determines the chronicity of renal failure, but renal size helps in the determination; normal–sized or enlarged kidneys usually indicate an acute process; small kidneys, a more chronic process. Increased echogenicity suggests chronic disease.

Less than 5% to 10% of renal failure (acute or chronic) is due to urinary tract obstruction and is almost always bilateral. However, obstruction is generally the most easily correctable cause of renal failure, so excluding obstruction is a priority.[1,3] Risk factors for bilateral obstruction include recent pelvic surgery, pelvic malignancy, prostatic hypertrophy, and bilateral renal and/or ureteral stones. **Pelvicalyceal dilatation is the hallmark of obstruction, and therefore a normal sonogram effectively excludes this condition, except in rare cases (see ADDITIONAL COMMENTS).**

When sonography reveals no pelvicalyceal dilatation, "medical renal disease" (i.e., parenchymal disease unrelated to urinary tract drainage) exists in the overwhelming majority of cases. An enormous variety of conditions, like diabetic nephropathy, collagen vascular disease, drug toxicity, and infectious nephritis, can be responsible.

The role of imaging in these conditions is limited to determining the glomerular filtration rate, if necessary (see **ADDITIONAL COMMENTS**) and guiding renal biopsy. If a histologic diagnosis is necessary for therapeutic or prognostic puposes, sonography is the best guidance method (see Chapter 61, Percutaneous Invasive Guided Biopsy).

When sonography demonstrates bilateral hydronephrosis, the bladder should be sonographically evaluated immediately after the patient voids. If the bladder remains full after voiding, the kidneys should be reevaluated after the bladder is emptied by a Foley catheter, because an overdistended or obstructed bladder may cause collecting system dilatation by exerting back-pressure on the distal ureters.[3] In the presence of an empty bladder and persistent bilateral pelvicalyceal dilation, the pelvis is sonographically examined for masses, which often cause ureteral obstruction, especially in females.

If exam of the pelvis is unrevealing, equivocal, or suboptimal, the pelvis and retroperitoneum require further study.

Step 3: Computed Tomography

CT effectively examines the pelvis and retroperitoneum between the kidneys and bladder. (Frequently, portions of this anatomic region are inaccessible to ultrasound because of bowel gas.)

If necessary, retrograde ureteral stenting or percutaneous nephrostomy can relieve bilateral renal obstruction (see Chapter 18, Obstructive Uropathy).

SUMMARY AND CONCLUSIONS

1. A plain radiograph of the abdomen and pelvis (KUB) is a valuable, inexpensive exam for the initial evaluation

of patients with renal failure. Urinary tract calcifications and valuable adjunctive information about the soft tissues and bones may be visible.

2. **Sonography is the imaging study of choice for the evaluation of renal failure, because it is rapid, noninvasive, uncomplicated, and relatively inexpensive.** Renal size and pelvicalyceal status are accurately determined. **Urinary tract obstruction, a relatively uncommon cause of renal failure, is excluded with a very high degree of accuracy. If no obstruction exists, imaging is limited to guiding a biopsy or determining the GFR.**

3. If sonography reveals bilateral obstruction but cannot define its cause, CT is usually successful.

ADDITIONAL COMMENTS

- **Rarely, sonographically normal pelvicalyceal systems may be present with complete acute obstruction, because the sonogram has been performed before the pelvicalyceal systems have had time to dilate. In such cases, where obstruction is suspected, a repeat sonogram is appropriate in 1 or 2 days, or a nuclear renal scan can be performed immediately.**

- Renal arterial occlusion is an uncommon cause of renal failure. If renal artery occlusion by emboli is suspected, especially if there are predisposing medical conditions, like atrial fibrillation, a nuclear renal scan can document perfusion to one or both kidneys.

- The nuclear scan can also measure **the total GFR and the individual GFR of each kidney.** This measurement is sometimes considered more useful than the BUN or serum creatinine, because it is more accurate and **can be partitioned between the kidneys individually.**

Unlike a creatinine clearance, which requires meticulous 24-hour urine collection, the nuclear GFR measurement is rapidly generated.

- The intravenous pyelogram (IVP) is not recommended in the workup of renal failure. The IVP in this condition is usually nonspecific, and **the contrast material is potentially toxic to poorly functioning kidneys. Sonography has replaced the IVP as the imaging test of choice in renal failure.**
- Sonography may occasionally be falsely positive for obstruction (see Chapter 18, Obstructive Uropathy).
- While all imaging findings in renal failure are usually nonspecific, in selected instances the findings may be diagnostic or greatly narrow the differential diagnosis. For example, renal cortical calcification may be due to prior acute cortical necrosis or oxalosis; a diffusely calcified kidney suggests tuberculous autonephrectomy; and enlargement of both kidneys by numerous cysts is characteristic of polycystic renal disease.
- Occasionally, because of factors such as obesity, sonography is technically limited. The kidneys may be difficult to find, particularly if they are small. CT is helpful in such circumstances.
- Angiography is rarely needed to evaluate patients with renal failure,[1] unless acute renal arterial obstruction and major arterial stenosis are considerations.
- MR is not indicated in the evaluation of renal failure.

REFERENCES

1. Dunnick NR, McCallum RW, Sandler CM. Textbook of Uroradiology. Baltimore, 1991, Williams & Wilkins, pp 437–438.
2. Curry NS. Genitourinary tract. In Griffiths HJ. Radiology of Renal Failure, 2nd ed. Philadelphia, 1990, Saunders, pp 1–58.
3. Rumack CM, Wilson SR, Charboneau JW, eds. Diagnostic Ultrasound. St Louis, 1991, Mosby, pp 236–243.

SUGGESTED ADDITIONAL READING

Davidson AJ. Radiology of the Kidney, 2nd ed. Philadelphia, 1994, Saunders.

Freeman LM, Lutzker LG. The kidneys. In Freeman LM, ed. Freeman and Johnson's Clinical Radionuclide Imaging, 3rd ed. Orlando, Florida, 1984, Grune & Stratton, pp 725-834.

17

Renovascular Hypertension

INTRODUCTION

Hypertension is a major health problem affecting nearly 60 million Americans. The vast majority of patients have primary or essential hypertension; renovascular disease accounts for only 1% to 4%.

Clinical signs that suggest a renovascular cause include (1) uncontrolled blood pressure despite maximal doses of antihypertensives, (2) malignant hypertension with evidence of encephalopathy or retinopathy, (3) onset of hypertension in persons under 30 years or greater than 50 years of age, (4) abrupt onset of hypertension, (5) rapid worsening of pre-existing hypertension, (6) decreased renal function after treatment with angiotension converting enzyme (ACE) inhibitors, and (7) a flank or abdominal bruit.

Most renovascular lesions are atherosclerotic. However, in young women fibromuscular dysplasia is more common. Rare causes of high-renin hypertension without a renovascular lesion include renal cysts, renal neoplasms, polycystic renal disease, and even calyceal dilatation secondary to obstruction.

No purpose is served by expensive workups to establish the presence or absence of renovascular lesions unless vascular repair is contemplated. The following plan presupposes that the clinician is enthusiastic about surgery or percutaneous transluminal angioplasty

(PTA), both of which can be very successful in treating this disease. Nuclear renal scans, renal vein renin sampling, and arteriography have a diagnostic role.

Costs: renal scan, with and without captopril, $357; renal vein renins, $3028; renal arteriogram, $1006; renal arteriogram with angioplasty, $3719.

PLAN AND RATIONALE

If renal function is not significantly compromised:

Step 1: Captopril Radionuclide Renal Scan

In patients with good or mildly compromised renal function, the initial examination is the captopril renal nuclear scan. The study can employ radiopharmaceuticals that are excreted by glomerular filtration, like technetium-99m-diethylenetriaminepenta-acetic acid (Tc-99m-DTPA), or by tubular secretion, like technetium-99m-mercapto-acetyltriglycine (Tc-99m-MAG-3).

An initial intravenous injection of Tc-99m-DTPA or Tc-99m-MAG-3 is followed by rapid-sequence "flow" images and later "static" images. The uptake of radiopharmaceutical by each kidney is quantitated, providing an indicator of renal function (glomerular filtration [GFR] if Tc-99m-DTPA is used or effective renal plasma flow [ERPF] if Tc-99m-MAG-3 is used). The GFR or ERPF for each kidney is calculated **individually**. Subsequently, an angiotensin converting enzyme (ACE) inhibitor, like captopril, is administered, and a second dose of radiopharmaceutical is injected; the patient is reimaged, and the renal function for each kidney is recalculated.

A stenotic renal artery decreases blood flow to the **afferent** arterioles of the glomeruli of the affected kidney.

In response to this ischemia, to maintain its GFR, the kidney attempts to preserve glomerular filtration pressure by constricting its **efferent** arterioles and by increasing renal arterial blood flow. The mechanism through which these adaptations occur is the angiotensin-renin axis; the ischemic kidney releases renin, a powerful hypertensive agent that also constricts the efferent arterioles. **ACE inhibitors block the effect of renin**, so that blood pressure falls and the compensatory vasoconstriction of the efferent arterioles abates. Because the arterioles of the ischemic kidney are in a state of maximal constriction to maintain filtration pressure, relaxation causes a precipitous fall in filtration pressure, **dropping that kidney's GFR**. Thus a positive Tc-99m-DTPA captopril study is indicated by a change in the **comparative GFRs of each kidney** by about 20% after the drug is administered.

Because the sensitivity of the exam depends on reliable GFR or ERPF measurements, it is most valuable when renal function is relatively well preserved. The function of severely failing kidneys cannot be as reliably quantitated.

If the captopril renal scan is normal, the workup usually ends. If the scan is equivocal or if clinical suspicion of a renovascular etiology remains high despite a normal exam, renal vein renins should be assessed. (Uncommonly, **bilateral** renal stenoses produce severe high-renin hypertension that will not respond to captopril with a unilateral sharp drop in GFR, because both kidneys are affected equally.)

If the renal scan is strongly positive, renal arteriography is appropriate directly, without the necessity of renal vein renins.

If the captopril study is equivocal, if the captopril study is normal yet renovascular hypertension remains suspect, or if renal function is significantly compromised:

Step 2: Renal Vein Renin Sampling

Renal vein renin levels are determined by withdrawing blood directly from the renal veins, under fluoroscopic control, after percutaneous puncture of the common femoral vein and renal vein catheterization. The renin levels of each kidney are compared; a ratio of 1.5:1.0 (stenotic side : normal side) supports a diagnosis of high-renin hypertension, usually secondary to unilateral renal artery stenosis.

If renal vein renin levels are similar in each kidney, renal arterial stenosis is unlikely. Most of the time the workup ends unless there is overwhelming clinical evidence, in which case arteriography is appropriate. Uncommonly, bilateral renal arterial stenoses can produce high-renin hypertension without asymmetry in renal vein renin levels.

A positive renal vein renin study should be followed by a renal arteriogram, with the possibility of therapeutic intervention by PTA.

Step 3: Renal Arteriogram

The common femoral artery is punctured percutaneously, and a catheter is advanced up the aorta and into the renal arteries; contrast material is injected as films are exposed.

While the renal nuclear scan can quantitate the GFR and suggest high-renin hypertension, **the arteriogram directly visualizes the renal arteries and parenchyma.** Arterial stenoses and other lesions, including tumors, cysts, and parenchymal scarring, are clearly defined. The arteriogram is essential for planning PTA, which sometimes can directly follow the diagnostic arteriogram, without the need for an additional procedure.

Step 4: Percutaneous Transluminal Angioplasty or Surgical Repair

The choice of interventional method is best jointly determined by the clinician and angiographer, because certain arterial lesions are amenable to PTA, **which is usually less expensive than surgical repair**. PTA requires catheterization of the renal arteries, in the manner of diagnostic arteriography (see Step 3 above). A balloon at the end of the catheter is inflated at the site of the stenosis, widening the artery. A repeat aortogram is then performed to evaluate the degree of dilatation and serve as a post-PTA baseline.

Long- and short-term outcomes of angioplastied lesions are quite favorable; fibromuscular dysplasia responds especially well. The procedure is safe and well tolerated in most cases. However, rare complications, like renal arterial rupture or uncontrolled renal arterial dissection, require that emergency surgical backup be available.

In some institutions PTA is performed at the same "sitting" as the renal arteriogram; a dual procedure is convenient and cost effective but is not always feasible, because some initial patient preparation before PTA (like ingestion of aspirin, to reduce thrombosis) is usually required. Therefore, if a patient with high-renin hypertension is to undergo diagnostic renal angiography, the angiographer and clinician should confer on the possibility of a dual procedure in the event that a stenosis is demonstrated.

SUMMARY AND CONCLUSIONS

1. The captopril radionuclide study is the initial imaging procedure for renovascular hypertension, if renal function is not significantly compromised.

2. If renal function is significantly compromised, renal vein renin sampling should be performed directly.
3. Angiography is the definitive study **to characterize renal arterial stenoses**.
4. Most renovascular lesions are amenable to PTA, which is usually less expensive than surgical repair.

ADDITIONAL COMMENTS

- The availability of carefully performed diagnostic **non-imaging** pharmacologic tests for high-renin hypertension, using ACE inhibitors, is limited; if readily available, they should precede imaging. They are quite specific for high-renin hypertension, yet, like the nuclear renal scan or even renal vein sampling, they can be falsely positive because of calyceal obstruction, renal tumor, or renal cysts. (Such space-occupying lesions may induce renal ischemia by direct pressure, resulting in high unilateral renin output, without a renovascular lesion.) Rarely, severe essential hypertension may also produce false positives in pharmacologic testing.
- Some authors favor intravenous digital angiography at the time of renal vein renin sampling, providing images of the renal arteries without the need for a separate aortic catheterization. Contrast material is injected into the inferior vena cava as a bolus, and the renal arteries are visualized as the bolus arrives via the aorta. The contrast material is dilute, but images produced can be quite good and demonstrate arteriosclerotic lesions most accurately. This exam does not replace a conventional renal arteriogram, but it can suggest a lesion that should be studied further.
- The hypertensive IVP has no place in the modern workup for renovascular hypertension.

SUGGESTED ADDITIONAL READING

Dunnick NR, Svetkey LP, Cohan RH, et al. Intravenous subtraction renal angiography: use in screening for renovascular hypertension. Radiology 1989; 171:219-222.

Hillman BJ. Imaging advances in the diagnosis of renovascular hypertension. AJR 1989; 153:5-14.

Klinge J, Mali WP, Puijlaert CB, et al. Percutaneous transluminal renal angioplasty: initial and long-term results. Radiology 1989; 171:501-506.

Sfakianakis GN, Bourgoignie JJ, Georgiou M, et al. Diagnosis of renovascular hypertension with ACE inhibition scintigraphy. Radiol Clin North Am 1993; 31:4.

Streeten DHP, Anderson GH, Freiberg JM, et al. Use of an angiotensin II antagonist in the recognition of "angiotensinogenic hypertension." N Engl J Med 1975; 292:657-662.

Tegtmeyer CJ, Selby JB. Renal angioplasty. In Syllabus: A Categorical Course in Diagnostic Radiology-Interventional Radiology. Radiological Society of North America, December 1-6, 1991.

Wilms GE, Baert AL, Amery AK, et al. Short-term morphologic results of percutaneous transluminal renal angioplasty as determined with angiography. Radiology 1989; 170:1019-1021.

18

Obstructive Uropathy

INTRODUCTION

Many imaging techniques apply to suspected obstructive uropathy. A high-quality abdominal film is always first; it may detect calcifications within the urinary tract or obvious masses.

The goal of imaging is to establish the presence or absence of obstruction, define its anatomic level, and suggest a cause. After an initial plain film, an intravenous pyelogram (IVP), sonogram (ultrasound or US), computed tomography (CT), and voiding cystourethrogram (VCUG) can all play a role.

Costs: abdominal plain film, $45; IVP, $168; abdominal US, $201; abdominal and pelvic CT, enhanced, $840; VCUG, $121; antegrade pyelogram, $339; retrograde pyelogram, $489; nuclear renal scan, without and with Lasix, $353.

PLAN AND RATIONALE

In the absence of anuria or advanced renal disease, when acute obstructive uropathy with no known probable cause extrinsic to the urinary tract is suspected:

Step 1: Intravenous Pyelogram

If renal function is sufficient, an intravenous pyelogram (IVP) is usually best for confirming or excluding obstruction and defining its level and cause. The IVP provides a rough index of renal function and defines renal size, parenchymal thickness, and anatomic detail of the pelvicalyceal systems and ureters. Poorly functioning kidneys, however, may not excrete enough contrast material for diagnostic renal and ureteral visualization. A normal IVP excludes obstruction.

If the IVP reveals pelvicalyceal widening and defines its cause—most commonly, a ureteral calculus—the imaging workup ends.

Further imaging is necessary when the IVP reveals pelvicalyceal widening but does not reveal its cause or when a lesion that requires further clarification is defined.

In anuria or advanced renal disease, or when acute obstructive uropathy with a known probable extrinsic cause (e.g., a pelvic mass) is suspected, or when chronic obstruction is suspected:

Step 1: Renal Sonogram

In advanced renal disease or anuria or when chronic obstruction is suspected, evaluation of the pelvicalyceal systems **independent of renal function is necessary**, because the contrast material intravenously injected for an IVP may be contraindicated or fail to visualize the kidneys. When a probable cause extrinsic to the urinary tract (like a pelvic mass) is known, **the sole issue is the presence or absence of obstruction**, because the likely cause and level of obstruction are usually not at issue.

Sonographic evaluation of the kidneys is independent of renal function and is especially useful when an IVP is contraindicated or renal function is poor. It demonstrates the renal contours, the pelvicalyceal systems, and the renal parenchyma; it is therefore a sensitive indicator of hydronephrosis and parenchymal scarring. Sometimes, but not reliably, the sonogram may also define proximal or distal ureteral dilatation, helping to reveal the level of an obstruction, but **usually it fails to define the cause or level**. A normal sonogram excludes all but very mild or early obstruction.

Once hydronephrosis has been confirmed, subsequent imaging focuses on the anatomic level or cause suggested by the initial IVP or sonogram.

(A) When intrinsic urinary tract lesions from the ureteropelvic junction to the urethra are suspected:

Step 2: Antegrade Pyelogram or Retrograde Pyelogram

The antegrade pyelogram visualizes obstructing lesions from above, revealing their level and possibly their cause. The renal pelvis is punctured percutaneously with a fine needle, guided by either fluoroscopy and/or sonography; urine is aspirated for culture and/or cytology, contrast material is injected, and the opacified urinary tract is radiographed. Subsequently, a percutaneous nephrostomy catheter can be placed to decompress the upper urinary tract. When a tumor obstructs the ureter, a stent can be placed percutaneously to bypass the obstruction.

The retrograde pyelogram visualizes lesions from below; retrograde pyelography is a relatively invasive technique that applies when more conventional methods fail. During cystoscopy, a catheter is placed in one or both ureters, and contrast material is injected, filling the ureters, until an obstruction is reached. A retrograde study may be therapeutic, because some obstructing ureteral calculi can be removed with various "basket" instruments during the study, and stents can sometimes be placed, relieving obstruction; furthermore, ureteral or bladder tumors can be biopsied.

The efficacy of computed tomography (CT) and the availability of antegrade pyelography have reduced the need for retrograde pyelography.

(B) When extrinsic compression of the ureters or bladder is suspected:

Step 2: Computed Tomography or Pelvic Sonography

"Enhanced CT" (CT with intravenous contrast material) images the opacified kidneys, ureters, and bladder in the transverse plane. Because this study defines the entire retroperitoneum and pelvis, it is usually the exam of choice to reveal space-occupying lesions that **extrinsically compress the ureters**, like neoplastic pelvic masses or adenopathy.

However, because sonography delivers no ionizing radiation, it may be the study of choice in females of childbearing age or in children, especially when a pelvic mass is strongly suspected (by virtue of other radiographic findings or clinical palpation).

(C) When urethral obstruction is suspected:

Step 2: Voiding Cystourethrogram

Under fluoroscopy the bladder is catheterized and filled with contrast material. After the catheter is removed the patient voids, filling the urethra and defining posterior urethral lesions like valves in male children and posttraumatic or postinflammatory strictures in adults. Reflux of contrast material from the bladder into the ureters is sought. Persistent reflux can cause calyceal widening that is sometimes difficult to differentiate from true obstructive uropathy; in this circumstance, a nuclear diuretic renogram may be conclusive (see **ADDITIONAL COMMENTS**).

SUMMARY AND CONCLUSIONS

1. A calculus is the most common cause of acute ureteral obstruction. Many stones are detected on plain abdominal films.
2. When acute obstruction with no known probable cause extrinsic to the urinary tract is suspected, an IVP is usually best, because it frequently defines the cause and/or anatomic level of obstruction. **A normal IVP ends the workup.**
3. When **chronic obstruction** is suspected, or in the presence of **anuria or chronic renal disease**, sonography is best, because it easily confirms or excludes pelvicalyceal widening **and examines the kidneys independent of renal function**. When acute obstructive uropathy with a known probable cause extrinsic to the urinary tract is suspected, the sonogram is ideal for confirming hydronephrosis.
4. When sonography or the IVP identify pelvicalyceal widening but not its cause, further imaging usually follows. Antegrade pyelography defines the lesion from above. Retrograde pyelography studies the lesion from below, can be therapeutic in terms of ureteral stone removal or stent placement, and provides information from the accompanying cystoscopy. Contrast-enhanced CT is unsurpassed for demonstrating extrinsic ureteral compression. Pelvic sonography may be appropriate

when a pelvic mass compressing the ureters is clinically suspected. A VCUG examines the posterior urethra and checks for vesicoureteral reflux.

ADDITIONAL COMMENTS

- When dilated pelvicalyceal systems have been demonstrated and an intrinsic obstruction is suspected but cannot be confirmed, **a nuclear diuretic renogram can differentiate dilated systems without obstruction from subtle intrinsic obstruction (usually at the ureteropelvic or ureterovesicular junction)**. Tc-99m-DTPA is injected intravenously, and the kidneys are imaged. An intravenous dose of furosemide is delivered to produce a rapid diuresis. Drainage from the collecting systems is quantitated by computer. Prolonged drainage ("washout") correlates well with significant obstruction.
- An IVP may be therapeutic in that the diuretic effect of intravenous contrast material sometimes helps a calculus pass from the ureter to the bladder during the study.
- The Whitaker test (pressure/flow study) is a more invasive test performed after percutaneous nephrostomy to clarify the presence or absence of a ureteropelvic junction (UPJ) obstruction. The renal pelvis is infused with saline through a needle or catheter at gradually increasing rates, while pressure in the renal pelvis is measured. UPJ obstruction is suggested if the pressure rises unduly, since the obstruction limits drainage.
- The nuclear renal scan is an excellent method of assessing glomerular and tubular function, even when function is too poor for visualization by an IVP. A nuclear study is particularly important when nephrectomy is contemplated, to assess contralateral function or determine whether enough function remains in the affected kidney to justify salvage.

- Radiographic contrast material in renal failure is controversial because of possible nephrotoxicity (see Chapter 16, Renal Failure); such cases should be discussed with the radiologist.

SUGGESTED ADDITIONAL READING

Davidson AJ. Radiology of the Kidney. Philadelphia, 1985, Saunders.

Dunnick NR, McCallum RW, Sandler CM. Textbook of Uroradiology. Baltimore, 1991, Williams & Wilkins.

Freeman LM, Lutzker LG. The kidneys. In Freeman LM, ed. Freeman and Johnson's Clinical Radionuclide Imaging, 3rd ed. Orlando, Florida, 1984, Grune & Stratton, pp 725-834.

19

Scrotal Lesions

INTRODUCTION

Scrotal lesions present as swelling—usually acute and painful, or chronic and asymptomatic. The differential diagnosis of acute swelling includes ischemia (from torsion of the spermatic cord) and epididymitis or epididymo-orchitis. The differential diagnosis of chronic swelling includes malignant or benign neoplasm, hydrocele, spermatocele, scrotal hernia, chronic epididymitis, abscess, and chronic ("missed") torsion. **Some of these processes require immediate surgical intervention; in acute ischemia, for example, viability of the testicle declines sharply after only 6 hours.**

On clinical grounds one cannot differentiate between surgical and nonsurgical scrotal disease; in fact, the clinical diagnosis in patients with acute scrotal pain is incorrect in up to 50% of patients.[1] Therefore, testicular imaging is crucial.

Applicable techniques include nuclear imaging, sonography or ultrasound (US), and color Doppler US. For the acutely painful scrotum, the chosen exam often depends on which is available **on an emergency basis**.

Costs: scrotal US, $179; nuclear scrotal scan, $132.

PLAN AND RATIONALE

Acute painful swelling, without previous trauma:

When color Doppler sonography (US) is **available on an emergency basis:**

Step 1: Color Doppler Sonography

After acoustical gel is applied, the transducer is placed on the scrotum, and high-resolution images of the testes and other scrotal contents are produced. The inguinal canal and abdomen can also be examined. Conventional US supplies strictly anatomic information, but **color Doppler US also provides an excellent assessment of blood flow to the testes.** Acute ischemia of the testis, caused by torsion of the spermatic cord (called "testicular torsion"), is clearly identified, and any underlying morphologic lesions are also revealed. Hyperemic states like epididymitis-orchitis can be accurately diagnosed. The workup of acute scrotal pain almost invariably ends with color Doppler US.

Prior to the refinement of color Doppler US, nuclear imaging was the "gold standard" for evaluation of the acute scrotum. With more widespread availability of color Doppler US and sonographic expertise, this modality has become competitive with nuclear imaging.[2,3] Also, sonography provides simultaneous high-resolution morphologic images and delivers no ionizing radiation.

Despite these obvious advantages, the highly operator-dependent nature of Doppler sonography and the great variability in equipment quality somewhat limit its application. **Therefore, although color Doppler US may**

eventually replace nuclear imaging everywhere as the initial study of choice in this setting, nuclear imaging remains the usual first exam in many centers.

Where color Doppler sonography (US) is **unavailable on an** *emergency basis:*

Step 1: Nuclear Scan

Nuclear scrotal scanning is available virtually everywhere; equipment and technique are highly standardized. A bolus of technetium-99m-pertechnetate is injected intravenously, and serial images of the scrotum are rapidly generated. **This sequence reveals perfusion of the testes as the bolus of radioactivity passes through the scrotal vessels—a "radionuclide angiogram." "Static" images, which reflect the presence or absence of hyperemia, are then obtained. The contralateral asymptomatic testis serves as a control.**

Acute ischemia of the testis, caused by torsion of the spermatic cord, is called "testicular torsion." This condition will appear as **decreased perfusion** on the nuclear scan.[1,4] In striking contrast, inflammatory lesions like epididymo-orchitis will produce **increased perfusion**. The findings are less clear-cut in testicular abscess or in torsion more than 1 day old ("missed torsion"). Also, an unsuspected testicular tumor occasionally presents as acute, painful swelling, caused by tumor hemorrhage or accompanying epididymitis-orchitis; in such unusual cases the nuclear findings may be confusing.

When the nuclear scan is definitive, as it usually is in acute torsion or epididymo-orchitis, the imaging workup ends. When the nuclear scan is equivocal, US may be helpful.[4] (See above, **Where color Doppler sonography is available on an emergency basis**).

Acute painful swelling, after trauma:

Step 1: Sonogram

Sonography is the best initial imaging study after acute scrotal trauma.[5] Intrascrotal injury, including hematoma (intra- or extratesticular), hematocele, and epididymal injury, are readily demonstrated. If color Doppler US has been performed, there is no need for a nuclear study, but if the sonogram was a conventional (non-Doppler) procedure and posttraumatic acute ischemia is suspected, then a nuclear scan may be required (see above, *Acute painful swelling, without previous trauma*).

Chronic, painless swelling:

Step 1: Sonogram

The primary diagnostic consideration in a patient with a painless, swollen scrotum is tumor. Sonography can clearly show whether a scrotal mass is intra- or extratesticular. **A solid intratesticular lesion is presumed to be malignant until proven otherwise.** Scrotal lesions with a fluid component, like complicated and uncomplicated hydroceles and spermatoceles, hernias, chronic epididymitis, and abscess, can usually be characterized. The nuclear scan is generally not helpful in chronic painless swelling.

SUMMARY AND CONCLUSIONS

1. **Testicular torsion is a diagnostic emergency, because surgery within 6 hours of torsion can save an ischemic testis.**
2. The nuclear scan is sensitive and specific for establishing or excluding acute testicular torsion; the accuracy

of US with color Doppler is comparable. The costs of these procedures are similar. Thus the choice often depends on which is available on an emergency basis.

3. US is an excellent follow-up in those unusual acute cases when nuclear scanning is equivocal. Often the underlying process is an abscess or a "missed torsion."

4. US is appropriate for posttraumatic testicular pain and swelling. Color Doppler US should be performed if possible, because ischemia sometimes follows testicular trauma, in which case an evaluation of perfusion is vital. Conventional US may require a follow-up nuclear study to rule out posttraumatic testicular ischemia.

5. US is appropriate for chronic scrotal swelling. Characterization of a lesion as intra- or extratesticular is important; solid intratesticular lesions are considered malignant until proven otherwise.

ADDITIONAL COMMENTS

- Torsion of the appendix of the testis usually presents with milder symptoms than spermatic cord torsion and acute inflammatory disease. Because its nuclear findings are identical with those of acute inflammatory disease, torsion of the testicular appendix can be confused with epididymitis. Failure to recognize torsion of the testicular appendix has little practical importance, because the testis and fertility are not at risk and surgery is not required.

- US is the best method for screening the clinically normal scrotum for occult disease—for example, in the search for a primary testicular tumor in the patient with metastatic disease or as a harbor for metastasis in patients with hematologic neoplasms or lymphoma.

REFERENCES

1. Riley TW, Mosbaugh PG, Coles JL, et al. Use of radioisotope scan in evaluation of intrascrotal lesions. J Urol 1976; 116:472-474.
2. Middleton WD, Siegal BA, Melson GL, et al. Acute scrotal disorders: prospective comparison of color Doppler US and testicular scintigraphy. Radiology 1990; 177:177-181.
3. Burks DD, Markey BJ, Burkhard TK, et al. Suspected testicular torsion and ischemia: evaluation with color Doppler US. Radiology 1990; 175:815-821.
4. Mueller DL, Amundson GM, Rubin SZ, et al. Acute scrotal abnormalities in children: diagnosis by combined sonography and scintigraphy. AJR 1988; 150:643-646.
5. Tumeh SS, Benson CB, Richie JP. Acute diseases of the scrotum. Semin US CT MR 1991; 12(2):115-130.

SUGGESTED ADDITIONAL READING

Benson CB. The role of US in diagnosis and staging of testicular cancer. Semin Urol 1988; 6:189-202.

Cramer BM, Schlegel EA, Thueroff JW. MR imaging in the differential diagnosis of scrotal and testicular disease. RadioGraphics 1991; 11:9-21.

Dunnick NR, McCallum R, Sandler C. Textbook of Uroradiology. Baltimore, 1991, Williams & Wilkins.

Stoller ML, Kogan BA, Hricak H. Spermatic cord torsion: diagnostic limitations. Pediatrics 1985; 76:929-933.

20

Adnexal Mass

INTRODUCTION

An adnexal mass can present with pelvic pain, nausea, anorexia, a palpable mass, and vaginal bleeding. The differential diagnosis is quite extensive and is different for pre- and postmenopausal women. In the premenopausal female, a serum beta human chorionic gonadotropin (bHCG) level should be determined; if the bHCG is positive, ectopic pregnancy should be excluded (see Chapter 21).

Ultrasound (US or sonography) is the established procedure of choice when an adnexal mass is suspected. It can establish the presence or absence of a mass; its size, shape, and contour; its origin and relationship to other structures; and the presence of ascites and/or adenopathy. Both transabdominal ultrasound (TAS) and transvaginal ultrasound (TVS) play a role in the workup. Magnetic resonance imaging (MR) may further characterize certain masses.

Costs: pelvic US, $184; abdominal US, $201; transvaginal US, $187; pelvic MR, $811.

PLAN AND RATIONALE

If an adnexal mass is suspected and the bHCG is negative:

Step 1: Transabdominal/Transvaginal Ultrasound

For TAS, a hand-held transducer moves across the skin of the lower abdomen and pelvis; images are generated instantly (in "real time") and recorded on film. Complete evaluation of the adnexa requires a full bladder. TVS requires that a probe containing a small transducer be placed within the vagina; a full bladder is unnecessary.

TAS can demonstrate the uterus, cul-de-sac, and ovaries in most patients. Large masses are easily visualized, and often their origin is defined. **If the adnexa are incompletely seen, if the bladder is insufficiently full, or if a mass is seen and clarification of its echotexture, origin, or extent is needed, TVS is appropriate.** TVS more accurately evaluates the uterus and adnexa, unless the ovary is especially high and lateral in position.

Many masses develop in the adnexal region, most commonly functional ovarian cyst, parovarian cyst, ectopic pregnancy, teratoma, endometrioma, tubo-ovarian abscess, hydrosalpinx/pyosalpinx, and ovarian tumor. The majority are benign ovarian lesions. The likelihood of an ovarian mass representing a malignant neoplasm increases with age, especially in the postmenopausal woman.

Certain ovarian masses can be fully characterized by US. A functional ovarian cyst has increased transmission of sound waves, a thin wall, and size variation during the menstrual cycle; a benign teratoma or dermoid cyst can have areas of cyst formation, fat, and coarse calcification.

Unfortunately, the majority of adnexal masses are nonspecific in appearance, containing partly solid and partly cystic components. Even the origin of large lesions may be unclear. **In the postmenopausal woman, any complex (partly cystic and partly solid) adnexal mass should be considered tumor, and laparoscopic staging is appropriate**. Postmenopausal ovarian cysts can develop and most are benign; the literature suggests that simple cysts under 6 cm in size can be safely followed sonographically.

In premenopausal women, most new complex adnexal masses without clinical evidence of infection or endometriosis should be laparoscoped for diagnosis and possible staging; if malignant neoplasm is discovered at laparoscopy, further surgical staging may be necessary. If tubo-ovarian abscess or endometriosis is suspected and has been treated with conservative pharmacologic therapy, US can be repeated after a suitable interval. Simple cysts can be followed with US, usually at a different point in the menstrual cycle.

If ultrasound of the adnexa is inconclusive or suboptimal:

Step 2: Magnetic Resonance Imaging

The pelvis and adnexa, as well as local lymph nodes and ascitic fluid, are well visualized by MR. In the uncommon circumstance when US has been suboptimal or inconclusive, MR can accurately diagnose dermoids, uterine leiomyomas, endometriomas, and simple cysts. **However, in the absence of clear evidence of tumor extension or metastases, MR will not differentiate benign from malignant epithelial ovarian tumors.**

MR staging of suspected ovarian malignancy is not as accurate as laparoscopy, which can visualize smaller peritoneal implants. **Therefore MR has no current role in staging of ovarian cancer.**

SUMMARY AND CONCLUSIONS

1. TAS is the initial exam for a suspected adnexal mass. Supplementary TVS is often appropriate, usually when

visualization of the adnexa is limited or for further characterization of a mass. Although certain benign masses have distinct features, most ovarian lesions are not characteristically benign or malignant.

2. If TVS is equivocal or if visualization of the adnexa is limited, MR can define and characterize a mass.

3. **If a suspicious or overtly malignant ovarian mass is found, imaging plays no role in staging, which is best accomplished laparoscopically or by further surgery.**

ADDITIONAL COMMENTS

• Occasionally, if a dermoid is suspected on US, CT without intravenous contrast material can definitively diagnose the lesion by demonstrating its fat and calcification. CT can also show large masses, local adenopathy, and ascites, although it may not reveal the exact site of origin of a pelvic mass. **CT is not as accurate as either MR or laparoscopic surgery for staging ovarian cancer, and it does not compare with TAS or TVS as an initial procedure.**

• Some recent studies utilizing TVS and Doppler waveforms suggest that the demonstration of low-resistance blood flow in an ovarian mass may be common in malignant neoplasms. However, these studies have shown that fast-growing benign lesions may have similar flow patterns, especially in premenopausal women.

SUGGESTED ADDITIONAL READING

1. Coleman BG. Transvaginal sonography of adnexal masses. Radiol Clin North Am 1992; 30:4.

2. Levine D, Gosink BB, Wolf SI, et al. Simple adnexal cysts: the natural history in postmenopausal women. Radiology 1992; 184:653–659.

3. Mitchell DG. Benign disease of the uterus and ovaries: applications of magnetic resonance imaging Radiol Clin North Am 1992; 30:777.

4. Outwater E, Kressel HY Evaluation of gynecologic malignancy by magnetic resonance imaging. Radiol Clin North Am 1992; 30:789.

5. Schiller VL. Doppler ultrasound of the pelvis. Radiol Clin North Am 1992; 30:735.

6. Sutton CL, McKinney CD, Jones JE, et al. Ovarian masses revisited: radiologic and pathologic correlation. RadioGraphics 1992; 12:853.

21

Ectopic Pregnancy

INTRODUCTION

Ectopic pregnancy (EP) is a serious, potentially life-threatening, first trimester complication that occurs in 1.4% of all pregnancies. Its incidence is rising, because of the increased prevalence of risk factors, particularly pelvic inflammatory disease.[1] An EP, however, can occur in any woman.[1,2]

Although its presenting symptoms include pelvic pain (in particular, adnexal pain or cervical motion tenderness during a pelvic exam), an adnexal mass, vaginal bleeding, shoulder pain, syncope, hypotension, or shock, the presentation of EP is often relatively nonspecific. Transvaginal sonography (TVS) and transabdominal sonography (TAS) play an important diagnostic role.

Costs: TVS, $187; TAS, $184.

PLAN AND RATIONALE

At our institution, all women with suspected ectopic pregnancies are first evaluated by an obstetrician; if the patient is hypotensive and her condition unstable, laparoscopic surgery is performed. Such an urgent presentation is uncommon, and in almost all patients time permits determination of the serum beta human chorionic gonadotropin (bHCG) level; this test is crucial, because **a negative serum bHCG effectively excludes pregnancy (ectopic or intrauterine).**

If the bHCG is positive:

Step 1: Transvaginal Sonography

TVS is the test of choice for evaluating women with possible EP. The resolution of TVS is superior to that of TAS; intrauterine pregnancies and adnexal abnormalities are detected earlier and more accurately. However, TVS is more "operator dependent" than TAS.

If the quantitative **bHCG is over 1000 IU/liter** (Second International Standard), **a** *normal* **intrauterine pregnancy, if present, should be conclusively demonstrated by TVS.** If an **intrauterine** pregnancy is demonstrated, an EP is virtually excluded (rarely a "heterotopic" pregnancy exists—i.e., an intrauterine pregnancy coexists with an EP; see **ADDITIONAL COMMENTS**). If an intrauterine pregnancy is not found, indirect findings of EP may be present. However, an extrauterine embryo or/and a fetal heartbeat are the only direct findings of EP, and these are seen in the minority of cases.[2-4]

If the serum quantitative **bHCG is less than 1000 IU/liter,** even TVS will not confidently detect an intrauterine pregnancy. If the patient's condition is clinically stable, no intrauterine pregnancy is seen, and no other abnormalities are found in the pelvis, then one of three scenarios is likely: (1) there is a viable intrauterine pregnancy that is too early to be seen, (2) there is a nonviable fetus that is aborting, or (3) there is an early ectopic pregnancy that cannot be identified. **Careful clinical follow-up and serial quantitative serum bHCG are indicated.**

In a normal first trimester pregnancy, the serum bHCG usually doubles about every 2 days. If the fetus is aborting, the bHCG level should decrease, whereas the bHCG level in an EP should increase but less than expected in a normal pregnancy. **Once the bHCG level approaches 1000, TVS should be repeated. However, the timing of the repeat exam(s) must be tailored to the individual patient; occasional EPs have been described in which the bHCG level does not increase or increases at the rate of a normal pregnancy.**

SUMMARY AND CONCLUSIONS

1. TVS is the test of choice for evaluating women with suspected EP. If the patient is clinically stable, a quantitative serum bHCG level followed by TVS is appropriate. **A negative serum bHCG effectively excludes a viable ectopic or intrauterine pregnancy.**

2. If the bHCG is over 1000, a normal intrauterine pregnancy should be demonstrated by TVS.

3. **An intrauterine pregnancy virtually excludes EP.** (See **ADDITIONAL COMMENTS** regarding heterotopic pregnancy.)

4. If an intrauterine pregnancy is not demonstrated and the bHCG is over 1000, the probability of EP rises; if there are indirect signs of EP, the probability increases further. Identification of an embryo and/or fetal heartbeat outside of the uterus is diagnostic of EP.

5. If no intrauterine pregnancy is identified, the serum bHCG is less than 1000, and no other abnormalities are identified in the pelvis, careful clinical follow-up and serial quantitative serum bHCGs are necessary. If the bHCG reaches 1000, TVS can be repeated.

ADDITIONAL COMMENTS

- If the bHCG is over 1800, an acceptable alternative to initial TVS is TAS. An intrauterine pregnancy should definitely be visible at this bHCG level. However, if no intrauterine pregnancy is identified, TVS is appropriate. Therefore, many authors recommend performing TVS as the initial imaging exam, regardless of the bHCG level.

- **If the serum bHCG is less than 1000, TVS is nonetheless appropriate.** Although the study is often normal and the results inconclusive, **EP may be discovered on TVS, despite the low bHCG.**[1,5-6]

- **A negative sonogram (TV and/or TA) never excludes EP if the bHCG is positive.**

- **TVS can miss an EP that is located in a high position, beyond the field of view of the TV probe.**[7] **Therefore, if TVS is negative and the bHCG level is over 1000, TAS should be performed immediately after TVS to help exclude this possibility.** Infrequently, an abnormality on TVS is incompletely seen (the TV probe has a more limited focal length than TA transducers)—for example, only part of an adnexal mass is seen—and TAS is needed for clarification.[3]

- Recent studies have shown that the use of color Doppler imaging during TVS increases the diagnostic accuracy for EP, particularly if the sonographic findings are equivocal.[2,4]

- If an intrauterine gestation is identified by sonography, the likelihood of an EP coexisting with the intrauterine gestation (a heterotopic pregnancy) is very low (incidence 1:4000 to 1:30,000). However, the incidence of heterotopic pregnancy is increasing. If an intrauterine gestation is identified and abnormalities are also detected in the pelvis (adnexal mass, free fluid) but no definite extrauterine embryo is found, the probability of a heterotopic pregnancy remains low. **However, caution should be used if the woman is undergoing assist-**

ed reproduction therapy, which places her at a much higher risk for heterotopic pregnancy[6]; and careful follow-up is mandatory.

- The higher the bHCG in a woman without evidence of an intrauterine pregnancy, the higher the probability of EP.[1]
- An uncommon cause of markedly elevated bHCG is molar pregnancy, which is usually readily diagnosed by TVS.

REFERENCES

1. Levi CS, Lyons EA, Dashefsky SM. The first trimester. In Rumack CM, Wilson SR, Charboneau JW, eds. Diagnostic Ultrasound. St Louis, 1991, Mosby, pp 711-716.
2. Filly RA. Ectopic pregnancy. In Callen PW. Ultrasonography in Obstetrics and Gynecology. Philadelphia, 1994, Saunders, pp 641-658.
3. Bohm-Velez M, Mendelson EB, Freimanis MG. Transvaginal sonography in evaluating ectopic pregnancy. Semin US CT MR 1990; 11:44-58.
4. Pellerito JS, Taylor KJW, Quedens-Case C, et al. Ectopic pregnancy: evaluation with endovaginal color flow imaging. Radiology 1992; 183:407-411.
5. Nyberg DA. Ectopic pregnancy. In Nyberg DA, Hill LM, Bohm-Velez M, Mendelson EB. Transvaginal Ultrasound. St Louis, 1992, Mosby, pp 105-129.
6. Fleischer A, Pennell RG, McKee MS, et al. Ectopic pregnancy: features at transvaginal sonography. Radiology 1990; 174:375-378.
7. Thorsen MK, Lawson TL, Aiman EJ, et al. Diagnosis of ectopic pregnancy: endovaginal vs. transabdominal sonography. AJR 1990; 155:307-310.

SUGGESTED ADDITIONAL READING

Coleman BG. Transvaginal sonography of adnexal masses. Radiol Clin North Am 1992; 30:677-687.

Rempen A. Vaginal sonography in ectopic pregnancy: a prospective evaluation. J Ultrasound Med 1988; 7:381-387.

Stabile I. Clinical and ultrasound aspects of ectopic pregnancy. In Chervenak FA, Isaacson GC, Campbell S. Ultrasound in Obstetrics and Gynecology. Boston, 1993, Little, Brown, pp 1621-1627.

22

Urinary Tract Infection/Pyelonephritis in Infants and Children

INTRODUCTION

Young children with documented urinary tract infection (UTI) should be imaged to identify those **with vesicoureteral reflux and/or a structural abnormality predisposing to urinary stasis.** These children are at risk for recurrent or chronic pyelonephritis and reflux nephropathy. Early diagnosis and treatment can prevent renal damage.

Before the imaging workup begins, positive urine cultures should be obtained **by bladder catheterization or suprapubic tap**. Patients with documented urinary tract infections should be on prophylactic antibiotics until reflux can be excluded; antibiotics will not interfere with subsequent imaging.

Sonography (ultrasound or US), the intravenous pyelogram (IVP), the voiding cystourethrogram (VCUG), and the renal scan play a diagnostic role.

Costs: US, $201; VCUG, $121; IVP, $168; nuclear renal scan, $257.

PLAN AND RATIONALE

Step 1a: Voiding Cystourethrogram

The bladder is catheterized and filled with contrast material, while the radiologist fluoroscopically observes the abdomen and pelvis for any reflux of contrast material into the ureters or the renal collecting systems. The patient must void during the study or reflux can be missed. The urethra is examined during voiding for posterior valves in male patients.

Step 1b: Sonography

Sonography is rapid, uncomplicated, noninvasive, and relatively inexpensive. It measures renal size and parenchymal thickness accurately, evaluates the pelvicalyceal systems for dilatation, and can detect a variety of other congenital anomalies like duplicated collecting systems, as well as cysts and tumors. The bladder is also examined for ureteroceles or distal ureteral dilatation.

Sonography, however, **cannot exclude reflux**. Also, some patients suffer from **both upper urinary tract anomalies and reflux.** Therefore, a VCUG is necessary regardless of whether the sonogram reveals upper urinary tract abnormalities.

If sonography and the VCUG are normal, the workup ends.

If sonography is normal and the VCUG reveals reflux into the ureters but not the renal collecting system, the workup ends.

An IVP is indicated to rule out coexistent proximal obstruction at the ureteropelvic junction if sonography reveals dilatation of one or both renal

collecting systems and (1) the VCUG reveals no vesicoureteral reflux, or (2) there is reflux into one or both ureters only, or (3) there is both ureteral and pelvicalyceal reflux but the pelvicalyceal dilatation is less than that defined by sonography.

Step 2: Intravenous Pyelogram

Urinary tract obstruction between the kidney and bladder is the likely cause of upper tract dilatation in the absence of reflux; also, obstruction and reflux can coexist. An IVP will usually define the site of any obstruction, as well as renal scarring, duplicated collecting systems, and ureteroceles.

Intravenously injected contrast material is concentrated and excreted by the kidneys, opacifying the urinary tract. **The exam is more accurate with a catheter continuously draining the bladder.**

After surgical repair of an obstructing lesion, renal function and the presence or absence of subtle residual obstruction are usually followed by a nuclear renal scan (see below, **Step 3: Diuretic Nuclear Renal Scan**).

If a GFR measurement is needed and/or for postsurgical follow-up:

Step 3: Diuretic Nuclear Renal Scan

Intravenously injected Tc-99m-diethylenetriaminepenta-acetic acid (DTPA) is concentrated and excreted by the kidneys. The study is digitized, so that the rate of DTPA accumulation can be translated accurately into a total glomerular filtration rate (GFR) and a differential GFR—in other words, **the estimated GFR for each individual kidney**. This baseline value allows the clinician to assess the efficacy of any medical or surgical intervention.

The drainage rate of radiopharmaceutical from the collecting systems can also be quantified to determine whether obstruction is present. This assessment is more accurate if the baseline study is immediately followed by intravenous furosemide (Lasix). In the presence of a dilated upper urinary tract and reflux, the diuretic nuclear scan can differentiate dilatation caused by reflux from that caused by obstruction. **The exam is more accurate with a catheter continuously draining the bladder.**

Many urologic surgeons use the nuclear diuretic renal scan to follow the results of corrective surgery for both reflux and obstructing anomalies, because it **evaluates renal function and the drainage rate of each pelvicalyceal system.**

SUMMARY AND CONCLUSIONS

1. Young children with proven UTIs may have reflux and/or obstructing anomalies; therefore, **they require both a VCUG and a sonogram. Regardless of sonographic findings, a VCUG is the definitive test for reflux.**
2. If sonography and a VCUG are normal, further imaging is unnecessary.
3. If the sonogram reveals dilatation of one or both of the renal collecting system(s), an IVP can determine whether the dilatation is actually secondary to an obstruction.
4. A nuclear scan is excellent for measuring the GFR and following the results of reparative surgery, in terms of both renal function and the presence of residual obstruction. Performed with Lasix, the nuclear study can differentiate obstruction from residual pelvicalyceal dilatation secondary to chronic reflux, previous infection, etc.

ADDITIONAL COMMENTS

- Documentation of urinary tract infection is mandatory, to avoid the expense and radiation of unnecessary imaging.
- Children whose reflux is treated medically with antibiotics require follow-up, usually by serial VCUGs. Serial nuclear GFRs are also sometimes used to ensure that subtle parenchymal injury is not developing; alternatively, serial sonograms can monitor renal growth, but impaired renal growth is a much later effect of injury than a falling GFR.
- In a few institutions a nuclear reflux study (sometimes called a nuclear cystogram) is used in lieu of follow-up VCUGs; this exam is a very sensitive indicator of reflux but does not compete with the initial VCUG, because its anatomic resolution is limited. When available, the nuclear reflux study is preferred over the VCUG for follow-up, because it delivers one-hundredth of the radiation dose to the pelvis. (The nuclear cystogram is not to be confused with the nuclear renal scan, which does not concern reflux and addresses renal function and pelvicalyceal drainage.)
- This chapter deals with the workup of the young child with a documented UTI. Older children, especially otherwise healthy females of prepubescent age (10 to 13 years old) with an initial UTI but only lower urinary tract signs, probably do not require a direct study to search for reflux. A sonogram to check for renal scar, impaired renal growth, and dilatation of the collecting systems is probably sufficient; a reflux study usually follows only if the sonogram is abnormal or the UTI recurs.
- The discovery of reflux in a young child should alert the family and primary care physician to **the possibility of reflux and undiagnosed UTI in siblings.** At the very least, siblings should be closely observed; a proper urine culture is prudent. If a nuclear reflux study (nuclear cys-

togram) is available, many authorities believe that it is appropriate in this context, because the discovery and treatment of reflux can prevent a lifetime of illness secondary to renal failure.

SUGGESTED ADDITIONAL READING

Ben-Ami T, Rozin M, Hertz M. Imaging of children with urinary tract infection: a tailored approach. Clin Radiol 1989; 40:64-67.

Berdon WE. Contemporary imaging approach to pediatric urologic problems. Radiol Clin North Am 1991; 29:605-617.

Lebowitz RL, Mandell J. Urinary tract infection in children: putting radiology in its place. Radiology 1987; 165:1-9.

Leonidas JC, McCauley RGK, Klauber GC, Fretzayas AM. Sonography as a substitute for excretory urography in children with urinary tract infection. AJR 1985; 144:815-819.

23

Prostate Carcinoma

INTRODUCTION

Prostate cancer is the most common cancer in males and the second leading cause of cancer death in American men. As the population ages, its incidence will certainly increase.

Surgical excision can cure carcinoma confined to the prostate. Unfortunately, only 30% to 35% of prostate cancer is diagnosed at this early stage; therefore, screening the population at risk is important.

The most effective and common screening tests are the digital rectal exam and the serum prostate specific antigen (PSA) level. **Imaging is most useful when either screening exam is abnormal**, to verify the presence of cancer and/or to stage a tumor.

The relative value of ultrasound-guided biopsy versus random (unguided) prostate biopsy is controversial. Some studies have reported that ultrasound (US) guidance does not increase the positive biopsy yield. However, these studies are not conclusive, because the patients evaluated had such a high prebiopsy likelihood of prostatic cancer. With rare exception, guided biopsy is more accurate.

Costs: pelvic CT, enhanced, $407; transrectal US, $224; transrectal US with prostate biopsy, $474; endorectal MR, $957.

PLAN AND RATIONALE

Step 1: Digital Rectal Exam and PSA

A digital rectal exam should be performed yearly in men over the age of 50 and as a part of each previous routine physical exam. A PSA level should be obtained annually in males after age 50.

On rectal exam the size, texture, and contour of the prostate is evaluated. A well-defined, hard nodule is most suspicious. However, the digital exam tends to underestimate the volume and invasiveness of prostate cancer **and cannot differentiate prostate cancer from benign lesions like cysts, calculi, or even at times benign prostatic hypertrophy (BPH).** Therefore, if any abnormality is detected, a PSA determination is appropriate.

PSA is a glycoprotein **produced solely by the prostate;** a high PSA level (>4 ng/ml) raises the possibility of prostatic cancer. The higher the PSA (>10 ng/ml), the greater the likelihood of prostatic cancer and invasion or metastases. However, **PSA levels can also be elevated by BPH, trauma, or prostatitis.**

If the rectal exam is normal and the PSA is below 4 ng/ml, the workup ends. If the rectal exam is normal and the PSA level is moderately elevated (4 to 10 ng/ml), the PSA level can be rechecked in 2 to 4 months. If the repeat PSA level has not fallen below 4 ng/ml, US with the possibility of biopsy is appropriate.

If a nodule is palpated, biopsy is warranted, regardless of the PSA. Occasionally a digital rectal exam can guide the biopsy, but ultrasound guidance is more accurate and therefore generally preferred.

If the PSA is greater than 10 ng/ml yet the rectal exam is normal, transrectal US is appropriate, with the possibility of biopsy.

Step 2: Transrectal Ultrasound (Sonography), With or Without Guided Biopsy

A US probe is inserted into the rectum and images of the prostate and seminal vesicles are generated. Transrectal biopsy, both core and aspiration, is feasible through the probe. Patients are treated with prophylactic oral antibiotics before and after the biopsy. The procedure is moderately uncomfortable, but not painful, and is safe; significant bleeding and infection are rare.

The majority of cancers arise in the peripheral zone of the prostate and usually appear as ill-defined areas that reflect ultrasound poorly (hypoechoic). The likelihood of a hypoechoic peripheral lesion representing cancer is about 25% to 30%. Certain sonographic appearances warrant biopsy: a hypoechoic peripheral lesion, an asymmetric peripheral zone with inhomogeneous ultrasound reflection, a focal capsular bulge, and a capsular/pericapsular irregularity. **A normal US does not rule out cancer; over 40% of cancers greater than 5 mm can be missed.**

If the biopsy is positive, staging with magnetic resonance imaging (MR) is effective. If the biopsy is negative or inconclusive in the presence of a markedly elevated PSA, the biopsy can be repeated or MR can follow directly.

If US is normal in the absence of a palpable nodule, random or "quadrant biopsy" of the prostate may identify the responsible lesion.

Step 3: Magnetic Resonance Imaging, with an Endorectal Coil, if Available

After a positive biopsy, staging is necessary for prognosis and treatment. The most important staging factors are direct extension of tumor through the prostatic capsule, into the periprostatic fat and neurovascular structures, and metastases to pelvic lymph nodes.

Conventional MR with a "surface body coil" can accurately evaluate the local pelvic nodes for metastases. Moreover, MR with a body coil is more effective than computed tomography (CT) or US for evaluation of cancer spread through the capsule into the periprostatic fat and neurovascular bundle.

MR performed with an endorectal coil more accurately depicts prostatic zonal anatomy and evaluates the capsule, periprostatic fat, seminal vesicles, and neurovascular structures for cancer invasion. The availability of endorectal coils is limited; if unavailable, MR with a body coil only is worthwhile.

SUMMARY AND CONCLUSIONS

1. **A digital rectal exam and a PSA level are the most important annual screening tests for prostate cancer, especially for men over age 50.**
2. If the rectal exam and PSA are normal, the workup ends.
3. **Transrectal US is appropriate when a nodule is palpated or when the PSA levels are markedly elevated, with or without a nodule.** Guided biopsy through the US probe is generally more accurate than random biopsy.
4. MR with an endorectal surface coil, if available, is the most accurate imaging method for prostate cancer staging, because it best visualizes local tumor invasion/infiltration. MR with a conventional body surface coil effectively evaluates local pelvic nodes and can demonstrate local tumor spread more effectively than CT or US.

ADDITIONAL COMMENTS

- "Random" (unguided) prostate biopsy has some proponents, mainly urologists. If the pretest likelihood of cancer is high, it follows that both imaging-guided and random biopsy methods will be effective. Random biopsy involves tissue sampling from standard areas or "coordinates" within the prostate.
- Transrectal US has been used for staging of prostate cancer, but it is limited in its ability to define capsular involvement and extension, as well as nodal involvement.
- CT with intravenous contrast material has also been used to stage prostate cancer; CT poorly defines the primary tumor as well as capsular involvement and extension. However, nodal involvement by tumor can be established with a high level of confidence.
- Osseous metastases are common in prostate cancer and are accurately demonstrated by a bone scan (see Chapter 44). The majority of metastases are "hot" on bone scans and are radiographically dense or blastic.

SUGGESTED ADDITIONAL READING

Heiken JP, Forman HP, Brown JJ. Neoplasms of the bladder, prostate and testis. Radiol Clin North Am 1994; 32:81-98.

Lee F, Littrup PJ, Torp-Petersen ST, et al. Prostate cancer: comparison of transrectal US and digital rectal examination for screening. Radiology 1988; 168:389-394.

Rifkin MD. US of the prostate gland In Syllabus: Special Course on Ultrasound. Radiological Society of North America, December 1-6, 1991.

24

Infertility

INTRODUCTION

Infertility is the inability of a couple to conceive a child after a year of unprotected intercourse. Infertility is on the rise, affecting at least 15% of couples. Multiple factors are often responsible. Imaging plays a role in both diagnosis and management.

A complete discussion of the infertility workup is beyond the scope of this book, but the basic tests usually include semen analysis, tests of ovulation, hormone levels, serial transvaginal sonography (TVS) of the ovaries, and hysterosalpingography (HSG).[1,2] Magnetic resonance imaging (MR), endorectal ultrasound (EUS), and scrotal ultrasound (US) play a secondary role.

No sequential approach is provided here, because the imaging workup of infertility is tailored to individual circumstances.

Costs: TVS, $187; HSG, $226; pelvic MR, $811; testicular/scrotal US, $179; EUS, $484.

PLAN AND RATIONALE

(A) Radiological testing of infertile patients

1. Basic workup of the infertile woman

To evaluate ovulation: transvaginal ultrasound

Transvaginal ultrasound, also called transvaginal sonography (TVS), effectively evaluates spontaneous ovulation. TVS is preferable to transabdominal sonography (TAS) because its resolution is superior and because the procedure is often more comfortable (the bladder is full for TAS but empty for TVS).

Serial TVS monitors the development of ovarian follicles. Normally, at least one follicle per cycle enlarges to 17 to 25 mm and then ruptures.[3,4] Evidence of ovulation includes collapse of the mature follicle, development of a corpus luteum, and appearance of free fluid in the pelvis.[5] Sonographic evidence of ovulation can be correlated with increasing serum estradiol levels to determine the exact timing of ovultion.[4,6] The absence of ovarian follicles, rupture of small follicles, or abnormally enlarging follicles is apparent.[5,7]

TVS also detects complications of pelvic inflammatory disease that may cause infertility, like hydrosalpinx and tubo-ovarian abscess.[5]

To investigate fallopian tube patency and image the uterine cavity: hysterosalpingography (HSG)

HSG should be performed several days after the end of menses. The cervix is cannulated, and water-soluble contrast material is introduced into the uterus under fluoroscopy. Fallopian tube patency is confirmed when the contrast material spills out of the fimbriated end of each fallopian tube into the peritoneal cavity. Anomalies of the uterus and fallopian tube can be demonstrated; if congenital uterine abnormalities are suspected, magnetic resonance imaging may be warranted (see below).

HSG is less invasive than hysteroscopy and laparoscopy; these should be performed later in the workup, if needed.[1]

2. Further workup of the infertile woman

To stage fibroids before surgery: magnetic resonance imaging

Fibroids may be responsible for infertility, but other causes should be excluded in the woman with fibroids, especially if uterine-sparing surgery to remove fibroids is contemplated. Although US is a good screening test for fibroids and HSG will detect some fibroids (particularly those that are submucosal), **MR is the test of choice for preoperative planning.**[8]

To evaluate suspected or definite congenital uterine anomalies: magnetic resonance imaging

Congenital uterine anomalies are a rare cause of infertility, but when HSG or US detects them, MR is warranted because it accurately characterizes anomalies **and eliminates the need for laparoscopy.**[7,9] Unlike HSG (and more accurately than US), MR defines the external contour of the uterus.

MR can accurately differentiate between a bicornuate and a septate (or subseptate) uterus; the latter correlates strongly with fetal loss and infertility, whereas the former is not related to infertility in most cases.

3. To image the infertile man, in selected circumstances

To image infertile men with suspected obstruction and/or congenital lesions of the seminal tract: endorectal ultrasound

Imaging is limited in the evaluation of infertile men, despite the fact that males are responsible for 50% of infertility. However, if the volume of semen is reduced and retrograde ejaculation has been excluded, or if the volume of semen is normal and the sperm count is reduced (or nil) and an obstruction and/or congenital anomaly of the seminal tract is suspected, endorectal ultrasound (EUS) has a role. A transducer is placed in the rectum; abnormalities of the seminal vesicles, vas deferens, and ejaculatory ducts are detected.

To image suspected varicoceles: scrotal ultrasound

Varicoceles are abnormally dilated veins of the pampiniform plexus, most often affecting the left hemiscrotum. They are probably due to incompetent valves in the spermatic vein. Varicoceles are very common, and their relationship to infertility is controversial.[3]

Ultrasound confirms palpable varicoceles and detects varicoceles that are not detectable on physical exam.

(B) Imaging in the management of infertility

1. The infertile woman

To monitor follicle development in women undergoing ovulation induction: transvaginal sonography

Serial TVS is more accurate than basal body temperature monitoring or hormonal testing for following follicle development in women undergoing biochemical ovulation induction.[10] This knowledge determines the optimal time for insemination (natural or artificial).

To aspirate follicles for in vitro fertilization (IVF): transvaginal sonography

Women to undergo IVF usually have ovulation biochemically induced to optimize ova collection. The best way to aspirate ovarian follicles is under TVS guidance. When mature follicles are present, the vagina is cleaned, and a needle is guided through the TVS probe into the ovary. All follicles greater than 1 cm are aspirated.[7,10] The transvaginal approach is less invasive than laparoscopy and can be an outpatient procedure. New techniques have reported TVS guidance of gamete or embryo transfer into the fallopian tube, through a transcervical catheter, avoiding laparoscopy (and general anesthesia).

To recanalize an occluded fallopian tube: fluoroscopically or US-guided procedures

Several authors have recently successfully recanalized occluded fallopian tubes with a fluoroscopically or ultrasound-guided catheter technique (particularly if the obstruction is proximal [close to the uterus]), as an alternative to microsurgical reanastomosis.[11] The exact role of these procedures is presently undefined.

2. The infertile man

To treat a varicocele: angiographic occlusion

While the relationship of varicoceles to infertility is controversial, the sperm count of men who undergo repair of varicoceles does increase. An alternative to surgical ligation is angiographic occlusion; the femoral vein is punctured and a catheter is selectively inserted into the spermatic vein. A variety of techniques to occlude the spermatic vein and decompress the varicocele have been described.

SUMMARY AND CONCLUSIONS

1. The basic radiologic workup of infertile women includes serial TVS to evaluate ovulation and HSG to check fallopian tube patency and image the uterine cavity.
2. Additional testing of infertile women, if appropriate, includes preoperative MR to stage fibroids and MR to evaluate suspected congenital uterine anomalies.
3. In general, imaging of infertile men is not indicated. In selected instances, endorectal US can evaluate suspected obstruction and/or congenital anomalies of the seminal tract, and scrotal ultrasound can find or confirm suspected varicoceles.
4. TVS effectively monitors follicular development in women undergoing ovulation induction and can guide follicular aspiration for in vitro fertilization.

ADDITIONAL COMMENTS

- In spite of a thorough workup, the cause of infertility remains obscure in 10% to 15% of couples.[2]
- HSG is not foolproof—a fallopian tube may appear falsely occluded because of spasm or may appear patent although functionally occluded—i.e., an adjacent adhesion or endometrial deposit interferes with fallopian tube function.[1,4]
- Although US can detect large endometrial deposits and MR is the most sensitive imaging test for endometriosis, **laparoscopy remains the test of choice**. Small

lesions that no imaging technique can demonstrate are visualized directly. The role of MR in evaluating abnormalities of the seminal tract is unclear.

• If the prolactin level is elevated, imaging of the pituitary is indicated (see Chapter 41). If a hormonally active tumor is suspected, imaging of the adrenals (see Chapter 63), ovaries (see Chapter 20), or testicles (see Chapter 19) may be appropriate.

REFERENCES

1. Blackwell RE. The infertility workup and diagnosis. J Reprod Med 1989;34:81-85.
2. Lobo RA. Unexplained infertility. J Reprod Med 1989; 34:241-248.
3. Shane JM. Evaluation and treatment of infertility. Clin Symp 1993;45:1-32.
4. Fleischer AC, Herbert CM III, Hill GA, Kepple DM. Transvaginal sonography: applications in infertility. Semin US CT MR 1990; 11:71-81.
5. Itskovitz J, Boldes R, Levron J, Thaler I. Transvaginal ultrasonography in the diagnosis and treatment of infertility. J Clin Ultrasound 1990; 18:248-256.
6. Fleischer AC, Kepple DM, Vasquez J. Conventional and color doppler transvaginal sonography in gynecologic infertility: current clinical applications. Radiol Clin North Am 1992; 30:693-702.
7. Krysiewcz S. Infertility in women: diagnostic evaluation with hystero-salpingography and other imaging techniques. AJR 1992; 159:253-261.
8. Abbitt PL, Watson L, Howards S. Abnormalities of the seminal tract causing infertility: diagnosis with endorectal sonography. AJR 1991; 157:337-339.
9. Woodward PJ, Wagner BJ, Farley TE. MR imaging in the evaluation of female infertility. RadioGraphics 1993; 13:293-310.
10. Wiseman DA, Taylor PJ. Infertility. In Rumack CM, Wilson SR, Charboneau JW, eds. Diagnostic Ultrasound, vol. 2. St Louis, 1991, Mosby, pp 983-1005.
11. Hovsepian DM, Bonn J, Eschelman DJ, et al. Fallopian tube recanalization in an unrestricted patient population. Radiology 1994; 190:137-140.
12. Winfield AC, Fleischer AC, Moore DE. Diagnostic imaging of fertility disorders. Curr Probl Diagn Radiol 1990; 19:9-38.

SUGGESTED ADDITIONAL READING

Gonen Y, Blanker J, Casper RF. Transvaginal ultrasonographically guided follicular aspiration: a comparative study with laparoscopically guided follicular aspiration. J Clin Ultrasound 1990; 18:257-261.

Kuligowska E, Baker CE, Oates RD. Male infertility: role of transrectal US in diagnosis and management. Radiology 1992; 185:353-360.

Part III
CHEST

25

Solitary Pulmonary Nodule

INTRODUCTION

The solitary pulmonary nodule (SPN) is a round or ovoid lung lesion less than 3 cm in diameter, usually identified first on a chest film. Although some SPNs are malignant, in most age groups the majority are benign—commonly granulomas, hamartomas, or less commonly benign bronchial adenomas. Because **benign SPNs do not require surgery, the goal of imaging is to differentiate benign from possibly malignant SPNs.** This differentiation depends primarily on the presence or absence of calcification in the lesion and its growth rate.

This chapter concerns the evaluation of a solitary lung lesion with no obvious central (hilar or mediastinal) mass on the initial chest film. Noncalcified adenopathy or a central mass suggests malignancy, and the subsequent workup focuses on establishing a tissue diagnosis and the extent of disease by biopsy and computed tomography (CT). This chapter also assumes that other indicators of malignancy, like positive sputum cytology, are absent.

Although factors like patient age and history (e.g., prior malignancy, tuberculosis), influence the decision-making process in any given case, the nodule's appearance is critical. If the nodule remains suspicious for malignancy after adequate imaging and noninvasive clinical investigation, guided biopsy may provide tissue with minimal morbidity at far less expense than thoracotomy (see Chapter 61, Percutaneous Invasive Guided Biopsy).

Costs: PA and lateral chest films, $59; PA, lateral, and oblique chest films, $129; chest CT, $429; chest lesion biopsy, fluoroscopically guided, $493; chest lesion biopsy, CT guided, $854.

PLAN AND RATIONALE

Step 1: Chest Radiograph

After nodule detection with standard PA and lateral films, supplementary oblique or apical lordotic films may be required to prove that the nodule is truly intrapulmonary. Sometimes, at the discretion of the radiologist, additional films are exposed with lead markers on skin lesions or the nipples, to prove that these confusing "pseudonodules" are extrapulmonary.

Certain characteristic patterns of calcification virtually assure benignity, and such calcifications may be obvious on chest films. When calcifications characteristic of benignity are identified, the workup ends, but when calcifications are absent or ambiguous, **every attempt must be made to obtain previous films, to establish whether the lesion has grown. Although the lesion's margins, by themselves, are an unreliable indicator of benignity, a radiographically smooth nodule unchanged in size for 2 years can confidently be considered benign, ending the imaging workup. Conversely, growth of any nodule is suspicious for malignancy, regardless of its morphology. When no old films are available, computed tomography (CT) is mandatory.**

Step 2: Computed Tomography

CT will confirm the presence of the nodule, map its exact location, and often reveal additional nodules unsuspected on the original chest film (additional nodules may suggest alternative diagnoses such as metastases and therefore affect planning for biopsy or surgical resection). Moreover, CT clearly defines the mediastinum, hila, and pleura, where it may detect unsuspected disease. When probable adenopathy or a mass is identified in any of these sites, the diagnostic focus may shift from the SPN itself to these areas.

Although morphologic criteria like margins and shape are suggestive, the presence or absence of calcification is far more reliable; certain patterns of calcification are highly characteristic of benignity. **When these patterns are present, the workup ends.** However, when calcification is not grossly visible, the nodule can be biopsied (see **Step 3: Percutaneous Biopsy,** below) or analyzed further with a CT "phantom." The choice usually depends on the availability of CT phantom studies.

Where computed tomography "phantom" studies are available:

Step 2a: Computed Tomography "Phantom" Study

The presence of calcium that is not grossly visible may be inferred by an analysis of nodule density with the help of a radiologic "phantom." The phantom is a mechanical model of a nodule—sufficiently dense to simulate a benign, not grossly calcified nodule—in a human thorax. The patient and the phantom are scanned sequentially, and a computer compares the density of the patient's nodule to that of the phantom. If the patient's nodule is denser (i.e., calcified) and there are no other CT criteria of malignancy, then the SPN is very likely benign. Otherwise, the lesion is "indeterminate."

Lesions considered benign on the CT phantom study are usually followed by chest films for 2 additional years— every 6 months for 1 year and then 12 months later— because the CT diagnosis is considered by most authorities to be **highly likely** rather than **absolutely certain**; in other words, the index of suspicion is too low to warrant biopsy but high enough to require radiographic follow-up. Nonetheless, 2 additional years without growth ends the workup.

Indeterminate lesions require tissue diagnosis, because they may be malignant. Imaging-guided biopsy is frequently possible, at much lower cost than thoracotomy.

Step 3: Percutaneous Needle Biopsy

Percutaneous needle biopsy, a minimally invasive technique with proven efficacy, is often preferred for tissue diagnosis (see Chapter 61, Percutaneous Invasive Guided Biopsy). Under fluoroscopic or CT guidance, the biopsy needle is advanced through the skin and into the nodule. The study usually provides material suitable for cytology; therefore, it requires the cooperation of an expert cytologist. Depending on the location of the lesion and the biopsy technique, sufficient tissue for histology is sometimes obtained.

The procedure is well tolerated by most patients. The most common complication is pneumothorax, which can usually be treated conservatively. Each potential case for percutaneous needle biopsy should be discussed with the interventional radiologist, because in some situations open lung biopsy may be preferred.

SUMMARY AND CONCLUSIONS

1. Standard frontal and lateral chest films are sometimes supplemented with additional views to confirm the presence of a nodule and to identify calcification. If calcification characteristic of benignity is identified, the workup ends.

2. If no characteristic calcifications are seen, previous chest films must be sought, to establish the SPN's growth rate. **A nodule that has not changed in size for at least 2 years is considered benign. Growth of any nodule is worrisome for malignancy, despite its configuration.**

3. CT can establish whether the nodule is truly solitary and whether there is unsuspected disease in the mediastinum, hila, or pleura. CT can often characterize nodules as **almost certainly benign** or **indeterminate** on the basis of gross calcification or density analysis with a phantom (when gross calcification is absent).

4. SPNs that are benign by CT phantom criteria should be followed radiographically for 2 additional years, to achieve an even higher level of certainty. No growth after these 2 years ends the follow-up.

5. Indeterminate SPNs require tissue diagnosis. Usually percutaneous needle biopsy under radiologic guidance is preferred to diagnostic thoracotomy. Although the technique may provide tissue for histology as well as cytology, it requires an expert cytopathologist. Each potential case should be discussed individually with the interventional and/or thoracic radiologist.

ADDITIONAL COMMENTS

- When sputum cytology is positive and the chest film is normal, chest CT and bronchoscopy are appropriate, but **a thorough ear, nose, and throat examination should precede these studies, because the abnormal cytology may originate from malignant lesions of the nose, oropharynx, nasopharynx, mouth, trachea, or upper esophagus.**

- Positive sputum cytology establishes the presence of malignancy but does not localize a lesion itself. Cytology is more likely negative when the lesion is an isolated, malignant, peripheral nodule.

- Although bronchoscopy is an established and pivotal tool for evaluating chest malignancy, it is often fruitless in the evaluation of a peripheral nodule with no central mass/adenopathy.

- CT has supplanted conventional tomography in the evaluation of the solitary pulmonary nodule.

- Magnetic resonance imaging has no role as yet in the workup of the SPN.

- Positron emission tomography (PET), a sophisticated nuclear imaging technique that requires a cyclotron and a special camera to detect positrons, has demonstrated far greater uptake of F-18 fluorodeoxyglucose in malignant SPNs than in benign SPNs. The sensitivity of PET for this purpose is very high, with an acceptable specificity. The cost of PET, however, is much higher than CT, and the technique is available in only a few dozen major medical centers.

- This section has addressed the evaluation of a peripheral nodule with no central mass on the initial chest films. In the presence of central disease, the workup focuses on the central disease rather than on the nodule itself. Sputum cytology, bronchoscopy, transbronchial biopsy, and mediastinoscopy play key roles in establishing a pathologic diagnosis. CT is the established noninvasive imaging technique to stage the presumed neoplasm, but

MR is more sensitive for invasion of the chest wall and perhaps the central soft tissues—heart, trachea, and esophagus.

SUGGESTED ADDITIONAL READING

Gupta NC, Frank AR, Dewan NA, et al. Solitary pulmonary nodules: detection of malignancy with PET with 2-[F-18]-fluoro-2-deoxy-D-glucose. Radiology 1992; 184:441-444.

Patz EF, Lowe VJ, Hoffman, JM, Paine SS, Burrowes P, Coleman RE, Goodman PC. Focal pulmonary abnormalities: evaluation with F-18 fluorodeoxyglucose PET scanning. Radiology 1993; 188:487-490.

Swensen SJ, Harms GF, Morin Rl, Myers JL. CT evaluation of solitary pulmonary nodules: value of 185-HU reference phantom. AJR 1991; 156:925-929.

Webb WR. Radiologic evaluation of the solitary pulmonary nodule. AJR 1990; 154:701-708.

Zerhouni EA, Stifik FP, Siegelman SS, et al. CT of the pulmonary nodule: a cooperative study. Radiology 1986; 160:319-327.

26

Mediastinal Mass

INTRODUCTION

Most patients are asymptomatic when a mediastinal mass is detected. If mediastinal disease is suspected clinically or a mediastinal mass is incidentally noted on a chest film, additional diagnostic imaging can confirm or exclude a lesion, suggest a specific diagnosis, or at least characterize a lesion sufficiently to guide further testing or therapy.

Computed tomography (CT) and magnetic resonance imaging (MR) have made evaluation of the mediastinum safe and noninvasive. These techniques generate a cross sectional anatomic display—transverse for both CT and MR, transverse, sagittal, and coronal for MR. Limited tissue characterization is possible—fat is differentiated from other tissues—but usually neither CT nor MR can separate benign from malignant masses solely by their appearance.

Nuclear studies target specific organs or disease states; in the mediastinum, substernal goiter is defined by radioactive iodine (I-131) or technetium-99m-pertechnetate, whereas lymphomas and some inflammatory nodes are localized by gallium-67 (Ga-67) citrate. Radiolabeled leukocytes can confirm that a mass contains pus.

A barium swallow evaluates the esophagus and gastroesophageal junction, and endoscopic ultrasound (EUS) plays an auxiliary role.

Although imaging has replaced diagnostic thoracotomy in

many cases, it has not eliminated the need for histologic diagnosis; needle biopsy or mediastinoscopy is often necessary.

Costs: chest US, $128; echocardiogram, $316; nuclear labeled leukocyte scan, $505; chest CT, unenhanced, $429; chest CT, enhanced, $498; chest MR, $798; gallium scan of chest, SPECT, $745; I-131 mediastinal scan, $124; barium swallow, $105; EUS, $484.

PLAN AND RATIONALE

(A) Suspected substernal goiter:

Step 1: Nuclear Substernal Goiter Scan

Mediastinal extension of thyroid tissue accounts for 10% of all mediastinal masses. Nuclear scanning with radioactive iodine (I-131) or Tc-99m pertechnetate can confirm the presence of a substernal goiter. I-131 is trapped by thyroid tissue and organified, as the first step in thyroid hormone synthesis; Tc-99m pertechnetate is trapped but not organified. The nuclear scan is noninvasive, simple, highly sensitive, and 100% specific. If the scan is positive, substernal goiter is proven; if the study is negative, substernal thyroid tissue is excluded, and CT is appropriate to characterize the mass and study the remainder of the chest.

The nuclear scan should precede CT, because the intravenous iodinated contrast material sometimes required for CT may interfere with nuclear imaging for 2 to 3 weeks.

Step 2: Computed Tomography

CT characterizes the location, effect on adjacent structures, radiographic density, size, and contour of a mediastinal mass. The lung parenchyma is studied for possibly associated lesions, like nodules, and the hila, thoracic inlet, and chest wall are also visualized.

When the unenhanced study is not definitive, enhanced CT (with intravenous contrast material) may help, especially to differentiate vascular from nonvascular masses.

(B) Dysphagia (also see Chapter 13):

Step 1: Barium Swallow

The esophagus is best studied by a barium swallow. Fluoroscopy while the patient drinks a suspension of barium reveals abnormalities of the lumen and wall. Conditions like peptic stricture, hiatus hernia, or achalasia, which can appear as a "mass" on the chest film, are easily diagnosed.

When an **intraluminal** abnormality likely represents extension of **extraluminal** disease or when **extrinsic compression** is present, CT is appropriate. (See above, under **Step 2: Suspected Substernal Goiter.**) However, when biopsy is indicated, endoscopic guidance is preferable to CT guidance.

Endoscopic ultrasound is the preferred technique for evaluating possible extension of intraluminal lesions through the esophageal wall. This new study involves placement of a tiny ultrasound transducer into the distal esophagus by the endoscopist. The procedure is best performed as a cooperative effort by an endoscopist and a radiologist experienced in ultrasound. The exam defines all layers of the esophageal wall, **revealing the extent of any intramural or extramural extension by tumor or inflammation.** The resolution of endoscopic ultrasound is far superior to that of CT, but its availability is limited, and indications for the exam have not been fully defined.

(C) All other situations: Computed tomography or magnetic resonance imaging:

CT is the best initial study for mediastinal masses (see above, under **Suspected Substernal Goiter**). However, MR provides the anatomic information of combined unenhanced and enhanced CT, without contrast material or radiation.

MR is particularly valuable for differentiating vascular from nonvascular masses and for the study of tumor encroachment on—or displacement of—blood vessels. Furthermore, it is somewhat superior to CT for evaluating chest wall invasion by tumor. MR is clearly superior in the evaluation of **posterior** mediastinal masses that abut the bony spine, since the relationship of the mass to the spinal column and spinal canal is shown. **Nonetheless, these advantages are counterbalanced by MR's reduced ability to define lesions in the lung parenchyma, like nodules—an essential requirement of any imaging technique that is the primary study for mediastinal masses. Also, MR is more costly than CT.** Thus MR is a specialized follow-up technique that should be ordered to answer specific questions, after consultation with the radiologist.

A normal chest CT or MR excludes any mediastinal mass and ends the imaging workup. **If a lesion is identified, its characteristics determine the next step:**

Fatty Lesion:

Fat is characteristic on both CT and MR, which can classify the lesion as lipomatosis, lipoma, or omental hernia, ending the workup.

Nonfatty Soft Tissue Mass:

A conclusive diagnosis usually cannot be reached with high confidence by imaging alone. Tissue can be obtained by imaging-guided biopsy, mediastinoscopy, or surgery, depending on the lesion's location and characteristics.

Transthoracic needle biopsy can confirm mediastinal invasion by bronchogenic carcinoma and sample mediastinal lymph nodes. This procedure is much less invasive and much less expensive than mediastinoscopy or transbronchial biopsy and may become a first step in the staging of lung cancer. The role of transthoracic needle biopsy in the staging of noncarcinomatous mediastinal masses is not as clear.

Suspected Substernal Goiter:

Because it is less expensive and more specific, the nuclear scan should **precede** CT when mediastinal thyroid tissue is suspected, but if CT has already been completed, a nuclear scan can confirm the diagnosis; 3 weeks between the two studies will be necessary if contrast material has been administered for the CT. (See above, under ***SUSPECTED SUBSTERNAL GOITER***).

Vascular Lesion:

Step 2: Angiography or Magnetic Resonance Imaging

Angiography of suspected vascular mediastinal lesions has been, to some extent, replaced by MR because **MR can confirm that a mediastinal mass is vascular with much lower risk and at lower cost than**

angiography. However, if the patient is very ill, or if other conditions—like MR-incompatible life-support systems **or a pacemaker**—preclude MR, then angiography is appropriate. Depending on whether the lesion is considered arterial or venous, a catheter is introduced into the appropriate mediastinal vessels and contrast material injected.

Cystic Lesion:

Step 2: Ultrasound, if technically feasible

Sonography can confirm that fluid-density lesions are cysts, if they are favorably located. However, ultrasound cannot penetrate bone or aerated lung, and because the mediastinum is bounded by the ribs and sternum anteriorly, the lungs laterally, and the spine posteriorly, the effort is often futile. If a cyst is probably pericardial, a sonogram of the heart (echocardiogram) may help. Sonography is particularly helpful in evaluating suspected cystic mediastinal lesions in young children.

Step 3: Guided Cyst Puncture

When the diagnosis cannot be made by imaging, or in selected circumstances where mediastinal cysts are believed to be responsible for the patient's symptoms, percutaneous CT- or ultrasound-guided cyst puncture may be feasible.

Lymphadenopathy:

Enlarged nodes and their distribution are clearly demonstrated by CT. However, neither CT nor

MR can differentiate benign from malignant lymph node enlargement. Furthermore, diseased nodes of normal size usually will be missed. A nuclear scan with Ga-67–citrate (see below) may be helpful in cases of suspected lymphoma or sarcoid.

If lymphoma or sarcoid are suspected and specific information regarding activity or staging is required:

Step 2: Gallium-67 Citrate

A Ga-67 citrate nuclear scan can confirm that mediastinal masses, particularly adenopathy, result from lymphoma or sarcoid. In lymphoma the study is useful for confirmation, **staging, and differentiating active disease from posttherapy fibrosis**; in sarcoid, the study determines **activity of the disease**. The radionuclide is injected intravenously, and images are generated at 1, 2, and sometimes 3 days. The exam is sensitive and noninvasive, but like most nuclear studies its specificity is relatively low.

Abscess, Mediastinitis:

A nuclear scan with In–111-labeled autologous leukocytes can be definitive.

Step 2: Labeled Leukocyte Study

A 20 ml sample of the patient's blood is drawn and the leukocytes are labeled with In–111-oxine; the cells are then injected intravenously, and images are generated 24 hours later; the sensitivity and specificity of the exam for detecting localized pus collections are high, and the study is noninvasive.

SUMMARY AND CONCLUSIONS

1. CT is the best initial study for evaluating mediastinal masses; it defines and differentiates them from normal structures. **CT also examines the lung parenchyma, a critically important function in patients who may harbor a chest neoplasm.** CT may require contrast material ("enhancement") in some cases. **For the mediastinum itself, excluding the lungs, MR is the best imaging modality, but it is considered a secondary study here, because it is more costly than CT and evaluates the lung parenchyma poorly. MR is a valuable adjunctive exam that should be reserved to resolve questions unanswered by CT.**

2. The nuclear thyroid scan is effective when a substernal goiter is suspected. The thyroid scan should precede CT, because the iodine in radiographic contrast material interferes with the thyroid scan.

3. For dysphagia, a barium swallow is the first exam. If an esophageal carcinoma is found, CT usually follows for staging. When available, the new technique of endoscopic ultrasound can reveal the extent of transluminal/extraluminal extension of subtle benign and malignant lesions. Endoscopic biopsy may obtain tissue.

4. **The choice of follow-up studies after CT depends on the lesion's characteristics.** Angiography, labeled autologous leukocytes, Ga-67 citrate, MR, and rarely sonography may be appropriate.

ADDITIONAL COMMENTS

- Currently, MR of the chest is degraded by the motion artifact of breathing, but newer MR software/hardware is rapidly overcoming this disadvantage. **If MR proves**

as effective as CT for the detection of associated
lung parenchymal lesions, like nodules, and if the
cost of the procedure falls, it may replace CT as
the primary study for mediastinal masses.

• Standard chest films have a preliminary role in evaluating the mediastinum. They help in interpreting other
studies and are routinely obtained in many radiology
departments along with CT, barium swallow, nuclear
thyroid scan, angiography, etc. **Also, once the diagnosis and extent of disease have been established,
chest films are often helpful in following the
course of disease and therapy.**

SUGGESTED ADDITIONAL READING

Aronberg DJ, Glazer HS, Sagel SS. MRI and CT of the mediastinum:
comparisons, controversies, and pitfalls. Radiol Clin North Am
1985; 23:439-448.

Cohen AM. Magnetic resonance imaging of the thorax. Radiol Clin
North Am 1984; 22:829-846.

Feigin DS, Padua EM. Mediastinal masses: a system for diagnosis based
on computed tomography. J CAT 1986; 10:11-21.

Naidich DP, Zerhouni EA, Siegelman SS. Computed Tomography of
the Thorax. New York, 1993, Raven Press.

von Schulthess GK, McMurdo K, Tscholakoff D, et al. Mediastinal
masses: MR imaging. Radiology 1986; 158:289-296.

27

Pulmonary Embolism

INTRODUCTION

Pulmonary embolism is a common clinical consideration whose real incidence, clinical manifestations, and natural history are poorly understood. The "treatment" of pulmonary embolism is anticoagulation, a sometimes hazardous therapy. Anticoagulation does not treat pulmonary embolism per se; it prevents further thrombus formation and subsequent embolism. Thus a diagnosis of pulmonary embolism raises the likelihood of future pulmonary emboli, and avoidance of that likelihood is the benefit that clinicians balance against the risks of anticoagulation.

The chest film, nuclear lung scan, and pulmonary angiogram apply. As an ancillary study, Doppler ultrasound (US) can detect deep venous thrombosis in the legs.

Costs: chest films, PA and lateral, $59; ventilation and perfusion lung scan, $442; pulmonary angiogram, $1546; Doppler US, $287.

PLAN AND RATIONALE

Step 1: Chest Radiograph

The chest film in patients with suspected pulmonary embolism is virtually always normal or nonspecific.

Suggestive findings like an elevated hemidiaphragm, a small collection of pleural fluid, patches of discoid or plate-like atelectasis, and right ventricular enlargement have numerous causes. Thus a more definitive study is required.

The chest film is nonetheless necessary because it excludes other causes of symptoms, like rib fracture, pneumothorax, etc. Moreover, a chest film is required for accurate lung scan interpretation.

Step 2: Nuclear Lung Scan (Ventilation/Perfusion or V/Q Scan)

Perfusion:

For the perfusion scan, technetium-99m-tagged macroaggregated albumin (MAA) particles are injected intravenously. Too large to pass through the pulmonary capillary bed, these protein particles lodge in the pulmonary microcirculation, producing hundreds of thousands of radioactive microemboli, whose distribution correlates with pulmonary blood flow. **Thus nonradioactive areas indicate poor perfusion.** Poorly perfused areas can result from emboli or decreased blood flow from other causes, including pulmonary vasospasm. **Because pulmonary vasospasm occurs wherever local alveolar hypoxia exists, any condition that decreases ventilation may decrease perfusion as well. Accordingly, for an intelligent interpretation of an abnormal perfusion lung scan, one must also perform a ventilation scan, to see if the areas of poor perfusion coincide with areas of poor ventilation.**

Ventilation:

Techniques of performing the ventilation scan vary. Most centers use xenon-133. The patient breathes a xenon/oxygen mixture from a fixed-volume reservoir for about 3 minutes, during which serial images reveal gradual alveolar filling, until the lungs are in equilibrium with the reservoir. This "wash-in" portion of the study reveals areas of hypoventilation, which fill slowly or not at all. During subsequent ventilation with room air, serial "wash-out" images reveal air trapping. A limitation of the xenon-133 technique is that it provides images in one projection only, typically posterior.

A few centers in the United States use Tc-99m in gaseous form, either Technegas or Pertechnegas. The chief advantage of these two agents is that they provide images in multiple projections.

Both xenon-133 and the Technegas/Pertechnegas systems can establish whether areas of poor ventilation coincide with areas of poor perfusion. Congruent areas of poor ventilation and perfusion are called a "match."

The custom of reporting lung scans in terms of **probabilities** as opposed to **certainties** is discouraging to some clinicians, and the issue of whether angiography should directly follow a chest film is sometimes raised. Invariably, **a lung scan should precede angiography,** because (1) some lung scans are, in fact, definitively normal (not "low probability"), and (2) even an "indeterminate" lung scan usually directs the angiographer to a questionable area, shortening a subsequent angiographic procedure.

The following general guidelines apply to ventilation/perfusion scans:

1. **A normal perfusion study excludes pulmonary embolism.** Despite anecdotes to the contrary, there is no well-documented case of a **completely normal high-quality** perfusion lung scan followed in less than 12 hours by angiographic, surgical, or postmortem evidence of a significant pulmonary embolism.

2. A definite perfusion deficit indicates that blood flow is reduced with absolute certainty. Acute embolus is **highly probable** where there is a perfusion deficit, normal ventilation, and a normal radiograph, unless the area is very small. This combination of findings is sufficient for anticoagulation. (Other causes of decreased blood flow can occur, like old emboli, arterial hypoplasia, or neoplastic compression of a central blood vessel; thus the term "highly probable" is applied in lieu of "certain".) **Angiography for definitive confirmation of acute embolus may be justified if anticoagulation is contraindicated or if clinical evidence favors another cause of reduced perfusion.**

3. **Where perfusion and ventilation deficits coincide and the chest film shows no parenchymal disease, the probability of pulmonary embolus is low**, because the poor ventilation is sufficient cause for decreased perfusion. (The ventilation abnormality typically results from focal air trapping caused by obstructive airway disease or bronchial obstruction from mucous plugging.) **However, matching ventilation and perfusion deficits reported as "low probability" do not completely exclude superimposed emboli, and about 18% of such low-probability scans will have associated emboli.** If the clinical need for virtual certainty is compelling, then angiography is appropriate.

4. The matching of multiple areas of poor perfusion and ventilation is often imprecise, and the scan becomes "indeterminate"; in some instances the term "intermediate" is used. Both of these literally mean that the study has not satisfactorily answered the question of whether an embolus exists. **Because the risk of embolus (variously described as 30% to 70%)**

in these studies is higher than in a low-probability scan, the decision to use angiography rests with the referring clinician.

5. Any sizable radiographic lesion usually produces abnormal ventilation and resultant alveolar hypoxia; the alveolar hypoxia causes pulmonary vasoconstriction and therefore a perfusion deficit. **Thus a radiographic lesion usually produces matching ventilation and perfusion deficits, but the scan is "indeterminate," not "low probability," because the radiographic density itself could represent various lesions (pulmonary infarct, pneumonia, etc.), and the imager has no means of differentiating between them.**

Step 3: Pulmonary Angiogram

Angiography is reserved for patients whose ventilation/perfusion scans are nondiagnostic or are seriously discordant with clinical suspicion.

Pulmonary angiography involves insertion of a catheter, introduced through a peripheral vein, into the pulmonary arterial tree. Contrast material injected during rapid filming opacifies the pulmonary circulation. Morbidity may result from arrhythmias as the catheter passes through the right side of the heart or from the elevation of already high pulmonary arterial pressure. Relative contraindications to pulmonary angiography are left bundle branch block and marked pulmonary artery hypertension. The mortality rate of the study is 0.5% to 1%. False-positive and false-negative pulmonary angiograms are very uncommon.

If the angiogram clearly reveals emboli and anticoagulation is contraindicated, the angiographer can place a filter in the inferior vena cava to prevent thrombi in the pelvis and legs from reaching the lungs.

SUMMARY AND CONCLUSIONS

1. A chest film is always first, to exclude other causes of symptoms and to assist in lung scan interpretation.
2. Invariably a ventilation/perfusion lung scan should precede angiography.
3. A completely negative scan excludes embolus.
4. If the scan is strongly positive ("high probability"), decreased pulmonary blood flow is certain and **acute embolus is likely**; angiography is appropriate only if anticoagulation is contraindicated or if rare causes of decreased blood flow or old emboli are suspected. If old emboli are likely, a repeat scan in 2 to 3 days is less invasive than angiography and may solve the problem. (New emboli frequently evolve in 2 to 3 days, whereas older emboli usually remain stable.)
5. "Low-probability" scans are associated with emboli in about 15% of cases. If virtual certainty is necessary, angiography is appropriate.
6. Although an abnormal radiograph is often accompanied by an "indeterminate" scan, the scan should be performed nonetheless, to help guide any subsequent angiogram. Moreover, despite the radiographic lesion, in some cases the scan can be "low-" or "high-probability."

ADDITIONAL COMMENTS

- Some investigators believe that after a chest film, ultrasound of the lower extremities—a Doppler study—is appropriate because Doppler is excellent for detection of deep venous thrombi (DVTs). They reason that since the goal of anticoagulation is not really to dissolve pulmonary emboli but to prevent later catastrophic emboli, detection and treatment of DVTs would seem to accomplish that goal. The problem with this approach is that it simply does not address the issues of chest pain and dyspnea, the common presenting symptoms of pulmonary emboli, and after DVT detection and treatment the clinician is left with the unexplained chest symptoms. Therefore we advocate the chest film, lung scan, and—when necessary—an angiogram, focusing on the original chest problem. When clinical suspicion is at odds with the lung scan (except when the lung scan is **completely normal**), and when the scan is indeterminate, then **Doppler studies can reinfore a clinical decision to perform or omit angiography.** Also, if pulmonary emboli are proven, then lower extremity Doppler may be appropriate as a baseline and to define the status of any thrombi in the legs.

- A sudden marked drop in systemic PO_2 usually does not indicate pulmonary embolus. An embolus causes decreased pulmonary arterial flow, usually in an area of good ventilation. Unless the embolus is massive, straining the right side of the heart or compromising an already diseased pulmonary arterial bed, loss of part of the pulmonary circulation should not cause a marked drop in systemic PO_2. The frequently observed drop in PO2 is usually mild or moderate, and, in fact, its cause has never been clearly explained. Sudden endobronchial obstruction, on the other hand, results in poorly ventilated alveoli that may remain transiently well perfused; this combination produces a functional right-to-left shunt, with blood returning to the left side of the heart unoxygenated. Many documented cases of sudden drastic fall in PO_2 have been associated with this phenomenon, usually because of mucous plugging or aspiration.

- Sudden hemoptysis, frank and copious, without a radiographic parenchymal infiltrate, is not characteristic of fresh pulmonary embolus. The mechanism of hemoptysis after embolus is pulmonary infarction or a hybrid state known as "congestive atelectasis" in which alveoli are filled with blood or bloody fluid, secondary to capillary disruption or, at least, massive increase in capillary permeability. This situation requires hours to evolve and is almost invariably visible radiographically, because radiographs of the lung are excellent for the demonstration of even small quantities of intraalveolar fluid. Thus sudden frank hemoptysis in the absence of a parenchymal radiographic abnormality and without hours of previous symptoms is uncharacteristic of embolus and usually implies a bleeding lesion in the tracheobronchial tree—neoplastic, inflammatory, or traumatic (post aspiration). A bronchoscopist is usually more helpful than the nuclear imager.

- Lung scanning is safe. The Tc-99m-labeled protein aggregates are themselves microemboli, and in the normal lung they transiently occlude about 1:1,500 arterioles and one in many thousands of capillaries. Lung scanning is therefore safe in the normal lung, but when the pulmonary vascular bed has been decimated by very advanced lung disease, especially extensive carcinomatosis, chronic obstructive airway disease, or advanced pulmonary endarterial obliteration, the safety factor is smaller. In these situations, the nuclear physician should be consulted, so that the option of reducing the scanning dose of Tc-99m-MAA can be considered.

- A related issue is the safety of lung scanning in the presence of known right-to-left intracardiac shunts, because some of the Tc-99m-MAA particles injected intravenously will proceed to the left side of the heart and then to the cerebral capillary bed, in proportion to brain blood flow. Shunts of less than 10% are considered insignificant in this regard, but with larger shunts the option of reducing the scanning dose might be considered. Few human data on this problem exist, because few shunt patients require lung scans. Animal data, however, suggest a very wide safety margin.

• Although standard pulmonary angiography is far superior to any competitive imaging techniques for defining emboli, newer unconventional angiographic methods, using MR and CT, are gaining ground. MR angiography (MRA) produces exquisite blood vessel images, often without the need for contrast material, and ultra-fast "spiral CT" scanners can reveal detail of even the coronary arteries. However, a number of technical difficulties remain with both techniques, and for the next 3 to 5 years neither is likely to replace the conventional pulmonary angiogram at the clinical level.

SUGGESTED ADDITIONAL READING

Biello DR, Mattar AG, McKnight RC. Ventilation-perfusion studies in suspected pulmonary embolism. AJR 1979; 133:1033-1037.

Moser KM, Fedullo PF, LittleJohn JK, et al. Frequent asymptomatic pulmonary embolism in patients with deep venous thrombosis. JAMA 271; 3:223-225.

Needleman L. Peripheral venous US. In Curriculum: Syllabus of Ultrasound. Radiological Society of North America, December 1-6, 1991.

Palmer EL, Scott JA, Strauss HW Lung scanning. In Practical Nuclear Medicine. Philadelphia, 1992, Saunders.

Worsley DF, Alavi A, Palevsky HI. Role of radionuclide imaging in patients with suspected pulmonary embolism. Radiol Clin North Am 31:4; 849-858.

28

Aortic Injury in Blunt Chest Trauma

INTRODUCTION

Blunt chest trauma commonly results from the deceleration and direct impact sustained in motor vehicle accidents. One of the most immediate diagnostic concerns is rupture of the thoracic aorta. Most victims of aortic rupture die at the crash site; survival of those who reach the hospital depends on **prompt** diagnosis and treatment. Plain films, angiography, and computed tomography (CT) play a role.

When injury is massive or vital signs are unstable, delay of surgery for imaging is inappropriate.

Costs: chest film, frontal only, $34; CT, enhanced, $498; thoracic angiogram, $1278.

PLAN AND RATIONALE

Step 1: Plain Radiography

The portable anteroposterior (AP) film of the injured supine patient's chest is often diagnostically limited. The AP supine position exaggerates the apparent width of the mediastinum, one of the crucial signs of aortic laceration. The posterior-anterior (PA) film more accurately evaluates the mediastinum, reducing the number of false positive interpretations, and should be obtained whenever possible. **A normal AP or PA film effectively excludes aortic injury and ends the imaging workup.**

If the original AP film is abnormal and a PA film is unfeasible, or if the PA film is abnormal, angiography is necessary:

Step 2: Angiography

A thoracic aortogram is the definitive study for diagnosing aortic rupture. A catheter is introduced into the ascending aorta, via percutaneous femoral artery puncture, contrast material is injected, and the opacified thoracic aorta and its major branches are evaluated. **The angiogram, normal or abnormal, ends the workup.**

If the AP or PA film is equivocal, computed tomography with intravenous contrast material (dynamic "contrast-enhanced CT") of the thorax may be used to further evaluate the mediastinum:

Step 2: Computed Tomography with Intravenous Contrast Enhancement

The role of contrast-enhanced CT remains controversial, and many specific indications for the exam have not been fully defined. However, **like a normal plain chest film, a normal CT effectively excludes aortic laceration**, ending the workup. **Thus the real value of CT is to exclude mediastinal hematoma and/or aortic contour abnormalities in the large number of plain chest films that are equivocal, avoiding some angiograms.**

If CT is equivocal or clearly reveals blood in the mediastinum, angiography follows to determine whether aortic rupture is the cause.

SUMMARY AND CONCLUSIONS

1. An immediate plain chest film, PA erect when possible, is the initial study in blunt thoracic trauma. A normal AP or PA film effectively excludes aortic rupture.
2. Angiography follows the initial **abnormal** AP or PA film.
3. If the AP or PA film is **equivocal**, the mediastinum can be further evaluated by contrast-enhanced CT.
4. **A normal CT ends the workup**, but if CT reveals blood in the mediastinum and/or aortic contour abnormalities, angiography is necessary for clarification.

ADDITIONAL COMMENTS

- One potential drawback of CT is that the contrast material required for the study adds to the contrast material of angiography; the combined contrast material burden is well tolerated by most patients but may be a problem for those with impaired renal function.
- A very small percentage of patients with aortic rupture survive undiagnosed and untreated; they form chronic pseudoaneurysms, which may later undergo spontaneous rupture. These pseudoaneurysms may also present as asymptomatic mediastinal masses.
- Magnetic resonance imaging can define mediastinal vascular anatomy but currently has no role in the evaluation of acute blunt thoracic trauma.
- Many multiple trauma patients undergo CT for evaluation of the head, cervical spine, or abdomen (see Chapters 31, 32, and 11). A few images of the lower

thorax, when viewed with "lung window settings," can identify an unsuspected pneumothorax. (The initial supine chest film can miss sizable pneumothoraces.)

- Plain films of the clavicles, ribs, sternum, scapula, and thoracic spine may detect chest wall injury undetected by a portable supine chest film. CT may further improve the evaluation of these areas. Chest wall hematoma, often difficult to differentiate from pleural fluid or lung contusion on plain chest films, will be characterized by CT. However, immediate, emergency chest CT is generally not indicated in these cases.

SUGGESTED ADDITIONAL READING

Ben-Menachem Y. Angiography in trauma: a work-atlas. Philadelphia, 1981, Saunders.

Goodman PC. CT of chest trauma. In Federle MP, Brant-Zawadski M, eds. Computed Tomography in the Evaluation of Trauma, 2nd ed. Baltimore, 1986, Williams & Wilkins, pp 168-180.

Marnocha KE, Maglinte DDT. Plain film criteria for excluding aortic rupture in blunt chest trauma. AJR 1985;144:19-21.

Mirvis SE, Pais SO, Gens DR. Thoracic aortic rupture: advantages of intraarterial digital subtraction angiography. AJR 1986;146:987-991.

Schwab CW, Lawson RB, Lind JF, Garland LW. Aortic injury: comparison of supine and upright portable chest films to evaluate the widened mediastinum. Ann Emerg Med 1984;13:896-899.

Tocino IM, Miller MH, Frederick PR, Bahr AL, Thomas F. CT detection of occult pneumothorax in head trauma. AJR 1985;143:987-990.

29

Aortic Dissection

INTRODUCTION

Dissection is the most common aortic catastrophe, occurring more often than aortic aneurysm rupture. Most patients have the predisposing factor of hypertension. Many of the clinical signs and symptoms of dissection are nonspecific, complicating the diagnosis. Chest pain is most frequent, radiating to various areas, depending on the type and site of dissection. Other supportive findings include pulse deficit, aortic insufficiency murmur, stroke, or peripheral neuropathy. Dissection is often rapidly fatal if untreated, yet current medical and surgical therapy has increased both short- and long-term survival.

According to the Stanford classification, any dissection involving the ascending aorta is a type A, whereas any other is type B. Type A can cause acute aortic insufficiency, cardiac tamponade, or myocardial infarction and is usually treated surgically. Type B can often be treated pharmacologically, with control of blood pressure.

The chest film, computed tomography without contrast material (unenhanced CT), computed tomography with intravenous contrast material (enhanced CT), magnetic resonance imaging (MR), and aortography play a role in the workup.

Costs: chest CT, enhanced and unenhanced, $608; chest MR, $798; thoracic and abdominal aortography, $2057; chest films, PA and lateral, $59; transesophageal ultrasound of the aorta, $484.

PLAN AND RATIONALE

Step 1: Chest Radiograph

The chest radiograph can sometimes diagnose aortic dissection. Most of the findings are nonspecific and include widening of the superior mediastium or aorta, medial displacement of intimal calcifications, and disparity in size of the ascending and descending aorta. However, the chest radiograph is often normal **and cannot exclude dissection.**

If the patient has NO documented contraindication to intravenous contrast material:

Step 2: Computed Tomography Without and With Intravenous Contrast Material

CT unenhanced and then enhanced can establish the diagnosis of dissection in the vast majority of cases by demonstrating two or more "channels" in the aorta separated by an intimal flap. CT also clearly defines the mediastium, pleural spaces, and pericardium.

In type B dissection, the scan is extended into the abdomen, to follow the extent of the tear.

If aortic dissection is demonstrated, the imaging workup usually ends. However, if the surgeon requires an angiographic "road map" before surgery, aortography is effective.

If the patient has a proven contraindication to intravenous contrast material:

Step 2: Magnetic Resonance Imaging, Without Contrast Material

Magnetic resonance imaging (MR) of the aorta is possible with current hardware and cardiac gating software. The accuracy of MR is comparable to CT. However, **MR is limited to hemodynamically stable patients**, since it is incompatible with most electronic life-support devices. **In fact, a pacemaker is an absolute contraindication to MR.**

MR may play a significant role in the follow-up of patients with chronic dissection.

If aortic dissection is demonstrated, the imaging workup usually ends.

Step 3: Aortography

The role of aortography is controversial, since CT and MR are extremely accurate. Many surgeons will operate from CT or MR only, yet others consider arteriography essential for preoperative planning.

A catheter is introduced by transcutaneous femoral artery puncture and threaded retrograde up the aorta. Contrast material is injected as rapid-sequence films are exposed.

The aortogram can demonstrate the extent of the dissection, aortic insufficiency, and coronary artery or branch vessel extension of the dissection.

SUMMARY AND CONCLUSIONS

1. A chest radiograph is the initial exam. Findings are usually nonspecific.

2. The most cost-effective study for aortic dissection is CT, usually both unenhanced and enhanced.
3. If contrast material is contraindicated and the patient is hemodynamically stable, MR is as effective as CT. **A pacemaker is an absolute contraindication to MR.** MR is considered a "second echelon" test, because it is more expensive.
4. The role of aortography remains controversial and depends on the preferences of the vascular surgeon.

ADDITIONAL COMMENTS

- Transesophageal ultrasound (US) can accurately demonstrate dissection of the arch and descending aorta. An ultrasound transducer is introduced along with a nasogastric tube, and images are displayed on a television screen. Bedside availability of this modality is its major advantage. Unfortunately, the ascending aorta and great vessels are not well seen, and dissection below the diaphragm (aortic hiatus) is not visible. Moreover, the examination is highly operator dependent and is not widely available. Most patients require sedation, and esophageal perforation is a rare complication.
- "Spiral" or "helical" CT can scan patients faster, with superior resolution, decreased motion artifact, and better vascular opacification. Moreover, the images can be reconstructed in the coronal and sagittal planes, like those of MR. Spiral CT is no more expensive than conventional CT and, because of decreased scanning times, may be less expensive in the future. The current availability of these scanners is limited.

SUGGESTED ADDITIONAL READING

Demos TC, Posniak HV, Marsan RE. CT of aortic dissection. Semin Roentgenol 1989; 24:22-37.

Petasnick JP. Radiologic evaluation of aortic dissection. Radiology 1991; 180:297-230.

Stanford W, Rooholamini SA, Galvin JR. Ultrafast computed tomography in the diagnosis of aortic aneurysms and dissections. J Thorac Imaging 1990; 5:32-39.

Thomas EA, Dubbins PA. Duplex ultrasound of the abdominal aorta—a neglected tool in aortic dissection. Clin Radiol 1990; 42:330-334.

Part IV

CENTRAL NERVOUS SYSTEM

30

Cerebral Metastases

INTRODUCTION

Throughout most of the 1980s computed tomography (CT) was the modality of choice for the detection of cerebral metastases. Lately, however, for this purpose magnetic resonance imaging (MR) has proven superior even to CT with intravenous contrast material (enhanced CT).[1,2] Furthermore, MR performed with intravenous contrast material (enhanced MR) is especially sensitivie for detection of leptomeningeal carcinomatosis.[3,4] Finally, MR is extremely sensitive to the presence of CNS bleeding and defines hemorrhagic metastases missed by CT.[5]

Costs: brain CT, enhanced, $396; brain MR, enhanced, $1073; brain MR, enhanced and unenhanced, $1478.

PLAN AND RATIONALE

Where MR is routinely available:

Step 1: Magnetic Resonance Imaging

A normal MR, enhanced and unenhanced, excludes cerebral metastases. The details of MR imaging are best left to the radiologist (or neuroradiologist), but for those readers with a particular interest in technical specifics, axial precontrast T2-weighted images, with pre- and postcontrast axial T1-weighted images, are appropriate.

Where MR is not routinely available:

Step 1: Computed Tomography

Although it is less sensitive than MR, contrast-enhanced CT remains an effective screen for cerebral metastases. **CT without intravenous contrast material (unenhanced CT) should be avoided, since it is much less sensitive;** it should be performed as a metastatic screen only if even the less toxic nonionic contrast materials cannot be tolerated.

SUMMARY AND CONCLUSIONS

1. **MR is the modality of choice for the detection of cerebral metastases.**
2. Contrast-enhanced CT is not as sensitive as MR for cerebral metastatic screening, and if performed as a second choice it will inevitably miss some lesions.
3. If CT is the primary screen, in the absence of MR, every attempt should be made to augment the sensitivity of the exam with intravenous contrast material. **If no contrast material is used, the sensitivity of the study declines severely.**

ADDITIONAL COMMENTS

- The radionuclide brain scan has no role in this workup.
- MR has no known risks and uses no ionizing radiation.

REFERENCES

1. Sze G, Milano E, Johnson C, Heier L. Detection of brain metastasis: comparison of contrast-enhanced MR with unenhanced MR and enhanced CT. AJNR 1990; 11: 785-791.
2. Davis PC, Hudgins PA, Peterman SB, Hoffman JC. Diagnosis of cerebral metastases: double-dose delayed CT vs. contrast-enhanced MR imaging. AJNR 1991; 12:293-300.
3. Sze G, Soletsky S, Bronen R, Krol G. MR imaging of the cranial meninges with emphasis on contrast enhancement and meningeal carcinomatosis. AJNR 1989; 10: 965-975.
4. Yuh WTC, Engelken JD, Muhonen MG, Mayr NA, Fisher DJ, Ehrhardt JC. Experience with high-dose gadolinium MR imaging in the evaluation of brain metastases. AJNR 1992; 13:335-345.
5. Atlas SW, Grossman RI, Gomori JM, Hackney DB, Goldberg HI, Zimmerman RA, Bilaniuk LT. Hemorrhagic intracranial malignant neoplasms: spin-echo MR imaging. Radiology 1987; 164:71-77.

31

Acute Head Trauma

INTRODUCTION

Computed tomography without intravenous contrast material (unenhanced CT) has long been the primary diagnostic imaging modality for the evaluation of acute head trauma. The study clearly and rapidly defines lesions that may require immediate surgical intervention, like depressed fractures, extracerebral blood collections, and intracerebral hematomas.[1,2] Although magnetic resonance (MR) imaging is superior to CT in many CNS applications, MR's inability to detect fractures and subarachnoid hemorrhage, the requirement for special MR-compatible life-support equipment, and MR's long scanning times preclude it as a first-line test in the acute head trauma setting.

Costs: head CT, unenhanced, $287; head MR, unenhanced, $845.

PLAN AND RATIONALE

Step 1: Computed Tomography, Unenhanced

The images are electronically adjusted to reveal details of brain parenchyma, the subdural spaces, and bone—in the technical jargon of radiology three "window settings." In almost all cases, CT alone is sufficiently diagnostic to end the imaging workup. However, if the clinical status is unexplained by a normal CT, then MR should follow.

Step 2: Magnetic Resonance Imaging

MR defines a small number of important acute CNS injuries, notably brain stem hemorrhagic and nonhemorrhagic contusions and diffuse axonal injuries, that CT can miss. Moreover, in the **subacute** and **chronic** setting MR is invaluable; chronic nonhemorrhagic and hemorrhagic contusions, diffuse axonal injuries, and small subdural hematomas are better delineated MR than by CT.[3-5]

SUMMARY

1. CT is the modality of choice for the evaluation of acute head injury and almost always ends the imaging workup. **The study is performed without contrast material.**
2. **MR is inappropriate as a first-line study in the setting of acute head trauma** but is sometimes indicated as a follow-up to normal CT when clinical symptomology remains unexplained; brain stem contusions and axonal injuries are better defined by MR than CT.
3. In the **subacute** and **chronic** setting MR is invaluable; it is superior for nonhemorrhagic and hemorrhagic contusions, diffuse axonal injuries, and small subdural hematomas.

ADDITIONAL COMMENTS

- Cervical spine injury may accompany closed head trauma (see Chapter 32).

- **Plain skull films have no role in the evaluation of head trauma.**
- Angiography defines vascular injuries that result from trauma.

REFERENCES

1. Dublin AB, French BN, Rennick JM. Computed tomography in head trauma. Radiology 1977; 122:365-369.
2. Koo AH, LaRoque RL. Evaluation of head trauma by computed tomography. Radiology 1977; 123:345-350.
3. Zimmerman RA, Bilaniuk LT, Hackney DB, Goldberg HI, Grossman RI. Head injury: early results of comparing CT and high-field MR. AJNR 1986; 7:757-764.
4. Gentry LR, Godersky JC, Thompson BH, Dunn VD. Prospective comparative study of intermediate-field MR and CT in the evaluation of closed head trauma. AJNR 1988; 9:91-100.
5. Hesselink JR, Dowd CF, Healy ME, Hajek P, Baker LL, Luerssen TG. MR imaging of brain contusions: a comparative study with CT. AJNR 1988; 9:269-278.

32

Acute Spine Trauma

INTRODUCTION

The potentially injured spine must be imaged with the patient immobilized to prevent damage to the spinal cord. Plain films, computed tomography (CT), and magnetic resonance imaging (MR) are utilized.

Costs: cervical spine plain films, $106; thoracic spine plain films, $66; lumbar spine plain films, $108; cervical spine CT, unenhanced, $471; thoracic spine CT, unenhanced, $441; lumbar spine CT, unenhanced, $467; cervical spine MR, unenhanced, $915; thoracic spine MR, unenhanced, $763; lumbar spine MR, unenhanced, $849.

PLAN AND RATIONALE

Cervical spine:

Step 1: Plain Radiographs

A lateral plain film is the first step.

If a fracture is demonstrated, CT is next in the evaluation (see **Step 2a, Computed Tomography,** below).

If no fracture is defined by the initial lateral film, additional plain films are appropriate: anteroposterior (AP), "swimmer's," oblique, and open-mouth views.(The patient's neck is immobilized by a special collar during positioning for these films, to prevent spinal injury.)

If a fracture is detected by any of these additional views, CT is next (see **Step 2a, Computed Tomography,** below).

If the additional views are normal and there is **focal pain** without other related neurologic signs or symptoms, views in **flexion and extension**, with the immobilizing collar removed, are an essential next step. (Flexion and extension views may identify ligamentous injury that can induce instability of the cervical spine, and, if undetected, cause major cervical cord injury later.)

If the additional views are normal and there is no focal pain, yet symptoms or signs suggest spinal cord trauma, MR is next (see **Step 2b, Magnetic Resonance Imaging,** below).

In the comatose patient, who cannot cooperate for additional views after the initial lateral film or communicate symptoms, **MR can exclude spinal cord injury** (see **Step 2b, Magnetic Resonance Imaging,** below).

Thoracic and lumbar spine:

Step 1: Plain Radiographs

Anteroposterior (AP) and lateral films are the first step.

If the initial films are normal and there are no significant symptoms or signs of spine trauma, the workup ends.

If there are significant symptoms or signs of spine trauma, despite normal initial plain films, MR is appropriate to exclude injury to the spinal cord itself or an adjacent traumatic lesion, like hematoma encroaching upon the cord (see **Step 2b, Magnetic Resonance Imaging,** below).

If the initial AP and lateral films reveal a fracture or are equivocal, CT is appropriate (see **Step 2a, Computed Tomography,** below).

Step 2a: Computed Tomography

CT displays the bony spine in exquisite detail in the axial projection.[1,2] Fracture fragments and their relationship to the spinal cord and nerve roots are well defined, and fractures missed by plain films are sometimes detected. Images can be "reformatted" in the sagittal and coronal projections, augmenting their diagnostic value. The study is rapid and for spine trauma imaging requires no intravenous contrast material.

If CT is abnormal and explains the patients symptoms/signs, then the workup ends. If CT is normal despite clear symptoms of spinal injury or if CT findings do not explain the patient's signs/symptoms, MR should follow (see **Step 2b, Magnetic Resonance Imaging,** below).

Step 2b: Magnetic Resonance Imaging

The multiplanar imaging capability of MR and its **direct** visualization of the spinal cord, ligaments, and CSF allow it to define the relationship of fracture fragments to the thecal sac and spinal cord, the presence of spinal cord compression, ligamentous injuries, disk herniation, epidural hematoma, and nonhemorrhagic and hemorrhagic spinal cord contusion. **With the sole exception of fractures, virtually all significant spinal injures are better defined by MR than by CT.**[3-6] Nonetheless, MR is not appropriate as a first-line study because of CT's superiority for fracture detection.

SUMMARY AND CONCLUSIONS

1. Plain films are the initial study.
2. CT is the appropriate second examination if plain films are equivocal or a fracture requires further study.

MR is the appropriate second study if initial plain films are normal yet signs or symptoms of significant spinal cord injury persist.

3. In the comotose patient who cannot cooperate for additional views of the cervical spine, MR can exclude spinal cord injury.

ADDITIONAL COMMENTS

- Conventional tomography (polytomography) has been superseded by CT, except for the specialized study of some odontoid fractures.
- Conventional CT requires patient immobility for several minutes to obtain an adequate scan. If the patient is uncooperative, general anesthesia may be necessary. Newer "spiral" or "helical" scanners can create high-resolution images in less than 1 second.

REFERENCES

1. Brandt-Zawadski M, Miller EM, Federle MP. CT in the evaluation of spine trauma. AJR 1981; 136:369-375.
2. Post MDJ, Green BA. The use of computed tomography in spinal trauma. Radiol Clin North Am 1983; 21:327-375.
3. McArdle CB, Crofford MJ, Mirfakhraee M, Amparo EG, Calhoun JS. Surface coil MR of spinal trauma: preliminary experience. AJNR 1986; 7:885-893.
4. Tarr RW, Drolshagen LF, Kerner TC, Allen JH, Partain CL, James AE Jr. MR imaging of recent spinal trauma. JCAT 1987; 11:412-417.
5. Kulkarni MV, McArdle CB, Kopanicky D, Miner M, Cotler HB, Lee KF, Harris JH. Acute spinal cord injury: MR imaging at 1.5T. Radiology 1987; 164:837-843.
6. Mirvis SE, Geisler FH, Jelinek JJ, Joslyn JN, Gellad F. Acute cervical spine trauma: evaluation with 1.5-T MR imaging. Radiology 1988; 166:807-816.

33

Normal Pressure
Hydrocephalus

INTRODUCTION

Although uncommon, normal pressure hydrocephalus
(NPH) is of considerable importance and interest, because
it is one of the few treatable causes of dementia. The hall-
marks of NPH are large ventricles and abnormal CSF
migration. Paradoxically, some cases of NPH are associated with normal ventricles.

Two possible causes explain the usual ventricular dilatation of NPH: (1) obstruction to CSF flow at the level of
the basal cisterns or arachnoid villi from previous inflammatory disease or subarachnoid hemorrhage and (2)
ischemic damage to the periventricular white matter with
decreased ventricular wall tensile strength. Magnetic resonance imaging (MR) produces superb images of the ventricles, easily confirming or excluding ventricular enlargement, **but a conclusive diagnosis of NPH requires
analysis of CSF flow.** In some cases MR can reveal a relatively specific abnormality in CSF flow that is characteristic of NPH, but in other cases reliable analysis of CSF
migration requires a gamma cisternogram.

Costs: head MR, unenhanced, $845; gamma cis-
ternogram, including lumbar puncture, $499.

PLAN AND RATIONALE

Step 1: Magnetic Resonance Imaging

MR is the best initial study in suspected NPH to confirm the presence of hydrocephalus and **to exclude other causes of neurologic symptoms**. NPH typically produces large ventricles and compressed sulci, but in some cases the ventricles and sulci are both enlarged, mimicking the appearance of atrophy. Moreover, because some cases of NPH are associated with ventricles of normal size, MR cannot firmly exclude the diagnosis.

MR can detect changes in CSF "signal" that relate to CSF flow rates. Normally, bright signal is detected in the ventricles on T2-weighted images, because of CSF. The CSF flow void sign (CFVS) seen in the aqueduct of Sylvius and the third and fourth ventricles results from rapid and/or turbulent CSF flow.[1,2] Although the CFVS can also be present in normal individuals and in patents with acute communicating hydrocephalus or atrophy, a **pattern of exaggerated CFVS is compatible with NPH in the appropriate clinical context.**[3] **In these cases a positive MR ends the workup**. Patients with an increased CFVS and the clinical criteria of NPH benefit from placement of a ventriculoperitoneal shunt.[4]

However, cerebral atrophy cannot be differentiated from extraventricular obstructive hydrocephalus based only on the CVFS.[5]

If MR demonstrates hydrocephalus but the CFVS is not exaggerated or if the ventricles are normal in size and clinical findings strongly suggest NPH, then a gamma cisternogram is appropriate. If MR is normal and the initial clinical index of suspicion is relatively low, the workup usually ends.

Step 2: Gamma Cisternogram

Gamma cisternography involves installation of a radio-pharmaceutical into the subarachnoid space by lumbar puncture. Indium-111-diethylenetriamine penta-acetic acid (In-111-DTPA) is used, because its half-life permits 72 hours of imaging, it is nontoxic, and it is not absorbed from the CSF. Images at 24, 48, and even 72 hours define ventricular filling and emptying as well as CSF migration over the cerebral convexities. Normal lateral ventricles may fill transiently at 24 hours but should be essentially clear of radiopharmaceutical at 48 hours, whereas continued ventricular radioactivity at 48 hours and afterward indicates NPH. Failure of radiopharmaceutical to migrate normally over the convexities is confirmatory.

A normal gamma cisternogram excludes NPH.

SUMMARY AND CONCLUSIONS

1. MR is the appropriate screening exam for NPH, to confirm hydrocephalus and exclude other causes of symptoms.
2. MR can sometimes diagnose NPH, by means of the CFVS, ending the workup.
3. Some cases of NPH are associated with ventricles of normal size. If there is strong clinical suspicion of NPH, a normal MR should be followed by a gamma cisternogram. If the initial clinical index of suspicion is low, a normal MR usually ends the workup.
4. If MR reveals large ventricles without an underlying lesion and a nonspecific CFVS, a gamma cisternogram can confirm or exclude NPH. The gamma cisternogram requires lumbar puncture and takes at least 48 hours to complete.

ADDITIONAL COMMENTS

- A CT cisternogram can be performed with intrathecal injection of nonionic contrast material. The contrast material follows CSF flow. This examination is cumbersome and costly relative to the gamma cisternogram and has no clear-cut advantages.

REFERENCES

1. Sherman JL, Citrin CM. Magnetic resonance demonstration of normal CSF flow. AJNR 1986; 7:3-6.
2. Sherman JL, Citrin CM, Bonen BJ, Gangarosa RE. MR demonstration of altered cerebrospinal fluid flow by obstructive lesions. AJNR 1986; 7:571-579.
3. Bradley WG Jr, Kurtman KE, Burgoyne B. Flowing cerebrospinal fluid in normal and hydrocephalic states: appearance on MR images. Radiology 1986; 159:611-616.
4. Bradley WG Jr., Whittmore AR, Kortman KE, Wantanabe AS, Homyar M, Teresi LM, Davis SJ. Marked cerebrospinal fluid void: indicator of successful shunt in patients with suspected normal pressure hydrocephalus. Radiology 1991; 178:459-466.
5. Sherman JR, Citrin CM, Gangarosa RE, Bowen BJ. The MR appearance of CSF flow in patients with ventriculomegaly. AJR 1987; 148:193-199.

34

Cerebrospinal Fluid Leak

INTRODUCTION

When a posttraumatic or postsurgical cerebrospinal fluid (CSF) leak is suspected, imaging focuses on proving that a CSF leak exists and detecting the bony discontinuity through which CSF escapes. Meningitis may occur if the leak is not spontaneously or surgically closed.

In patients with a **suspected but unconfirmed CSF leak**, a screening procedure is indicated. In patients with a **proven CSF leak through an unknown site**, a high-resolution technique to define anatomy is appropriate. The nuclear gamma cisternogram and the computed tomography (CT) cisternogram apply.

Costs: CT cisternogram, including LP, $645; gamma cisternogram, including LP, $499.

PLAN AND RATIONALE

When a CSF leak is suspected but no specific site is known:

Step 1: Gamma Cisternogram

The gamma cisternogram is a sensitive screen for leaking CSF. Tc-99m-diethylenetriamine penta-acetic acid (DTPA) is injected intrathecally via lumbar puncture. Over the next 24 hours, images of the head and neck can reveal passage of radioactive CSF outside of its normal confines. This technique can detect CSF leaks in many sites, including the middle ear, nose, and pharynx, yet the study can detect only leaks that are active.[1] Occasionally, cotton pledgets placed in the nasopharynx are later assayed in a sensitive radiation counter to confirm radioactive CSF in the nose.

When the approximate site of a CSF leak is known:

Step 1: Computed Tomography Cisternogram

Several milliliters of nonionic contrast material are injected intrathecally via lumbar puncture. The patient is usually positioned prone, head down, for several minutes and then scanned, but the exam can be "customized," so that the suspected leakage site is dependent. The resolution of CT cisternography is exquisite, but, like the gamma cisternogram, it can detect only active leaks. The study detects contrast material beyond the normal confines of the CSF—for example, in the sinuses below the leakage site—and the bony defect through which the leak occurs may also be defined.[2-4]

SUMMARY

1. A gamma cisternogram is the initial screening study for a suspected but unconfirmed CSF leak.
2. When the approximate site of a CSF leak is known, a CT cisternogram can often identify its precise location, as a "road map" for surgical repair.

ADDITIONAL COMMENTS

- Magnetic resonance imaging (MR) demonstrates the central nervous system and its coverings in exquisite detail. CSF is particularly well demonstrated, because of its high signal intensity on T2-weighted images. However, MR does not adequately display the bony anatomy of the paranasal sinuses and skull base; therefore, **bony discontinuities through which CSF can leak will not be detected.**
- CSF leaks are often intermittent, and multiple examinations may be necessary to "catch" an on-going leak. **Sometimes no leak is demonstrated, even in the presence of overwhelming clinical evidence.**

REFERENCES

1. Staab EV. Radionuclide cisternography. In Freeman LM, ed. Freeman and Johnson's Clinical Radionuclide Imaging, 3rd ed. Orlando, Florida, 1984, Grune & Stratton, pp 679-723.
2. DeLaPaz R, Brant-Zawadzki M, Rowe LD. CT of maxillofacial injury. In Federle MP, Brant-Zawadzki M, eds. Computed Tomography in the Evaluation of Trauma, 2nd ed. Baltimore, 1986, Williams & Wilkins, pp 64-107.
3. Manelfe C, Cellerier P, Sobel D, Prevost C, Bonaf Ç A. Cerebrospinal fluid rhinorrhea: evaluation with metrizamide cisternography. AJR 1982; 138:471-476.
4. Morris RE, Hasso AN, Thompson JR, Hinshaw DB Jr, Vu H. Traumatic dural tears: CT diagnosis using metrizamide. Radiology 1984; 152:443-446.

35

Encephalitis

INTRODUCTION

The differentiation of encephalitis from lesions that may, in unusual circumstances, mimic encephalitis (hemorrhage, abscess, or tumor) is important, **because their management differs radically**.

Current techniques do not differentiate herpes encephalitis from other acute encephalitides. Three techniques apply: magnetic resonance imaging with intravenous contrast material (enhanced MR), computed tomography with intravenous contrast material (enhanced CT), and the nuclear brain scan.

Costs: brain MR, enhanced, $1073; head CT, enhanced, $396; nuclear brain scan, SPECT, $531.

PLAN AND RATIONALE

Where magnetic resonance imaging is feasible and available:

Step 1: Magnetic Resonance Imaging

Enhanced MR is the modality of choice for the evaluation of suspected encephalitis,[1,2] **but MR is not feasible in the presence of certain life-support systems.**

In herpes encephalitis, subtle areas of hyperintense signal on T2-weighted images are evident in the temporal lobes as early as 2 days after the onset of symptoms.[2] The temporal lobes are better defined by MR than by CT, because MR produces multiplanar images and is not affected by temporal bone artifacts that degrade CT. MR's sensitivity is augmented by the intravenous administration of contrast material. **A normal or abnormal MR ends the imaging workup for encephalitis.**

Where magnetic resonance imaging is not feasible or is unavailable:

Step 1: Computed Tomography

Enhanced CT can diagnose encephalitis. In herpes encephalitis, characteristic hypodense lesions that enhance after the intravenous injection of contrast material are visualized in the temporal lobes.[3-5] **However, a normal CT does not exclude encephalitis.** If CT is normal or equivocal and herpes encephalitis is suspected on clinical grounds, a nuclear brain scan can be helpful.[6,7]

Step 2: Nuclear Brain Scan

Brain scanning was classically performed after a peripheral intravenous bolus injection of a radiolabeled small molecule, usually the renal agent diethylenetriamine penta-acetic acid (DTPA). These molecules cross an injured blood–brain barrier, accumulating in damaged brain tissue, which is then visualized against a background of normal surrounding brain. The DTPA brain scan was nonspecific and far less sensitive than MR or CT; moreover, it generated morphologically crude images.[7]

In recent years technetium-99m-hexamethylpropyle-neamine oxime (Tc-99m-HMPAO) has become **the agent of choice for nuclear brain imaging**. This newer pharmaceutical is **lipid soluble and enters the normal brain**; combined with the technology of single photon emission computed tomography (SPECT), the study provides good anatomic detail and high sensitivity.

Tc-99m-HMPAO-SPECT reveals **increased radioactivity at the site of encephalitis.** Although HMPAO-SPECT may be competitive in sensitivity with MR and CT, **MR and CT are far superior**, because they are more specific and much better in terms of spatial resolution.

A positive nuclear scan, preceded by a negative or borderline CT, is very strong evidence for encephalitis.[8]

SUMMARY AND CONCLUSIONS

1. MR is the procedure of choice for encephalitis.
2. When MR is unfeasible or unavailable, contrast-enhanced CT is appropriate. Although CT is less effective than MR for visualizing the temporal lobes, which are the site of most findings in herpes encephalitis, a positive CT ends the imaging workup. **A normal CT does not exclude encephalitis, and a nuclear brain scan is recommended when CT is normal and imaging confirmation of presumptive encephalitis is necessary.** Furthermore, a nuclear brain scan is an appropriate follow-up to an equivocal or borderline CT.
3. **Both CT and the nuclear scan can be normal in the presence of encephalitis; if institution of therapy depends on a firm diagnosis, transfer to a facility with MR imaging should be seriously considered.**

REFERENCES

1. Zimmerman RA, Bilaniuk LT, Sze G. Intracranial infection. In Brandt-Zawadzki M, Norman D, eds. Magnetic Resonance Imaging of the Central Nervous System. New York, 1987, Raven Press, pp 235-257.
2. Schroth G, Kretzschmar K, Gawehn J, Voigt K. Advantage of magnetic resonance imaging in the diagnosis of cerebral infections. Neuroradiology 1987; 29:120-126.
3. Herman TE, Cleveland RH, Kushner DC, Taveras JM. CT of neonatal herpes encephalitis. AJNR 1985; 6:773-775.
4. Benator RM, Magill LH, Gerald B, Igarashi M, Fitch SJ. Herpes simplex encephalitis: CT findings in the neonate and young infant. AJNR 1985; 6:539-543.
5. Zimmerman RD, Russell EJ, Leeds NE, Kaufman D. CT in the early diagnosis of herpes simplex encephalitis. AJR 1980; 134:61-66.
6. Kim EE, Deland FH, Mantebello J. Sensitivity of radionuclide brain scan and computed tomography in early detection of viral meningoencephalitis. Radiology 1979; 132:425-429.
7. Holmes RA. Conventional brain imaging. In Freeman LM, ed. Freeman and Johnson's Clinical Radionuclide Imaging, 3rd ed. Orlando, Florida, 1984, Grune & Stratton, pp 611-663
8. Meyer, MA. Focal high uptake of HMPAO in brain perfusion studies: a clue in the diagnosis of encephalitis. J Nucl Med 1990; 31:1094-1098.

36

New Onset Seizures

INTRODUCTION

The patient with seizures of new onset may have a surgical lesion, so cranial imaging is appropriate. Two techniques apply to screening this population: magnetic resonance imaging without and with intravenous contrast material (unenhanced and enhanced MR) and computed tomography with intravenous contrast material (enhanced CT). MR better detects small lesions and is unaffected by artifacts that degrade CT.[1] Cerebral angiography is useful to further characterize some lesions.

Costs: brain MR, unenhanced, $845; brain MR, enhanced and unenhanced, $1418; head CT, enhanced, $396; cerebral angiography, complete "four-vessel study," $3496; nuclear brain scan, SPECT, $531.

PLAN AND RATIONALE

Where MR is available:

Step 1: Magnetic Resonance Imaging

Because of its superior spatial resolution and multiplanar imaging capacity, **MR is the study of choice for evaluation of the patient with seizures of new onset.**[2,3]

Intravenous contrast material is usually **not** required but should be reserved for selected cases to better define abnormalities seen on the unenhanced study.[4]

Where MR is not available:

Step 1: Computed Tomography With Intravenous Contrast Material

For maximum sensitivity, enhanced CT is performed. Although CT exquisitely defines intracranial anatomy, it is less sensitive than MR.[2]

If a vascular lesion detected by CT or MR requires further study:

Step 2: Cerebral Angiography

Because both CT and MR can image the cerebral vasculature, angiography is indicated only when a vascular lesion needs further characterization for pre-interventional/surgical planning. The angiogram involves injection of contrast material directly into blood vessels of the head or neck, through a catheter threaded retrograde up the aorta, introduced via percutaneous femoral arterial puncture.

SUMMARY AND CONCLUSIONS

1. MR is the best initial imaging method for screening the patient with seizures of new onset.
2. Enhanced CT is an adequate screen where MR is not available.
3. If both MR and CT are unavailable in a community, the patient should be referred elsewhere, since **no**

combination of other tests can detect or characterize intracranial lesions nearly as well.

4. Angiography can better characterize a vascular lesion detected by CT or MR.

ADDITIONAL COMMENTS

• **Plain skull films have no value in the evaluation of patients with new onset seizures.**

• Positron emission tomography (PET) and SPECT nuclear brain scanning have a place in the study of certain seizure patients; PET technology is limited to a few large research centers, whereas SPECT is fairly widespread. The goal of these techniques is to define hypermetabolic areas of brain that are suitable for stereotaxic or surgical ablation. If successful, ablation may eliminate seizures and a lifetime of medication. **These methods are usually applied to the study of chronic, intractable epilepsy, rather than adults with new onset seizures** (see Chapter 37).

• A surgical lesion is unlikely in patients under 30 years old with a normal neurologic exam and typical primary, idiopathic, generalized seizures; however, many clinicians choose to exclude a surgical lesion before committing the patient to anticonvulsant therapy.

REFERENCES

1. Bloom RJ, Vinuela F, Fox AJ, Blume WT, Girvin J, Kaufman JCE. Computed tomography in temporal lobe epilepsy. JCAT 1984; 8(3):401–405.
2. Schîrner W, Meencke HJ, Felix R. Temporal-lobe epilepsy: comparison of CT and MR imaging. AJR 1987; 149:1231–1239.
3. Triulzi F, Franceshi M, Fazio F, Del Maschio A. Nonrefractory temporal lobe epilepsy: 1.5-T MR imaging. Radiology 1988; 166:181–185.
4. Elster AD, Mirza W. MR imaging in chronic partial epilepsy: role of contrast enhancement. AJNR 1991; 12:165–170.

37

Chronic, Intractable Epilepsy

Chronic, intractable epilepsy most frequently results from a temporal lobe condition called mesial temporal sclerosis, which occurs in the body of the hippocampus.[1,2] Mesial temporal sclerosis is often associated with a subtle change in local brain volume and also with abnormal metabolism—increased blood flow during a seizure (ictally) and decreased blood flow between seizures (interictally). Magnetic resonance imaging without and with intravenous contrast material (unenhanced and enhanced MR) is the best method to detect the volumetric changes, and nuclear brain scanning best evaluates the brain's metabolic status. Neoplasms and vascular malformations less commonly cause seizures in this population; for the latter, angiography is definitive.

Costs: brain MR, unenhanced, $845; brain MR, unenhanced and enhanced, $1418; nuclear brain scan, SPECT, $531; cerebral angiography, complete "four-vessel study," $3496.

PLAN AND RATIONALE

Step 1: Magnetic Resonance Imaging, Initially Without Contrast Material

MR is the modality of choice for the initial evaluation of chronic intractable epilepsy,[1-3] because it effectively studies the temporal lobes for mesial temporal sclerosis and also excludes neoplasms and vascular malformations. MR is superior to CT in this regard because of its multiplanar imaging capability, superior spatial resolution, and freedom from temporal bone artifacts.[1] Intravenous contrast material is **sometimes** used to better characterize an abnormality detected on the unenhanced study.[4]

Hippocampal volume measurements derived from three-dimensional MR are extremely useful.[5] Some neuroradiologists believe that abnormal hippocampal volume measurements are sufficiently specific to end the workup, but most believe that one or more additional signs, like associated white matter atrophy, increased "signal" on T2-weighted images, and increased volume of the ipsilateral temporal ventricular horn are also necessary. **A small percentage of patients with chronic intractable epilepsy will have a normal MR. In these cases, nuclear brain scanning may define metabolically abnormal foci that are morphologically normal.**

If MR reveals a vascular malformation that requires better definition before intervention, angiography is appropriate.

If MR is normal:

Step 2: Nuclear Brain Scanning

Technetium-99m-hexamethylpropyleneamine oxime (Tc-99m-HMPAO) is the agent of of choice for brain imaging. This pharmaceutical is lipid soluble and enters the normal brain; combined with the technology of **s**ingle **p**hoton **e**mission **c**omputed **t**omography (SPECT), the study provides good anatomic detail and high sensitivity for locally altered blood flow.

For appropriate study of intractable epilepsy, close coordination between the clinical and nuclear imaging services is mandatory. Patients should be scanned interictally and **also immediately after a seizure.** The injection of radiopharmaceutical **within a minute or two of a seizure is mandatory, so that images reflect the status of brain blood flow during seizure activity;** only in this way can hypeperfused foci—usually in the temporal lobe—be defined. Such close coordination usually means that the patient remains in the nuclear medicine department, under supervision and monitoring, until seizure activity begins, at which time the radiopharmaceutical is injected. Most nuclear imagers believe that unless this procedure is followed, the scan will be of little value. **Therefore consultation with the nuclear medicine physician is essential before a Tc-99m-HMPAO-SPECT study for chronic seizures is ordered.**

If a normal MR is followed by a normal Tc-99m-HMPAO-SPECT scan, the workup stops, unless the patient is close to a positron emission tomography (PET) center.

If a normal MR is followed by a positive Tc-99m-HMPAO-SPECT study, then further imaging is unnecessary, and neurosurgical consultation is appropriate. A normal MR and an equivocal Tc-99m-HMPAO-SPECT study can be managed clinically, rescanned at a later date, or referred to a PET center.

When MR is normal, Tc-99m-HMPAO is normal or equivocal, and PET is available:

Step 3: Positron Emission Tomography

PET is a specialized form of nuclear imaging that requires cyclotron-produced isotopes and a positron camera to image their emissions. Currently, PET systems are limited to a few dozen large research-oriented medical centers. The advantage of PET imaging is that isotopes of the major elements of life—oxygen, nitrogen, etc.—can be produced and their biodistribution imaged. The major disadvantage is the cost of the cyclotron-PET center and the large number of skilled personal required to support it. Moreover, many cyclotron-produced isotopes have half-lives measured in seconds or minutes.

Despite its disadvantages, PET is applicable to the problem of chronic, intractable epilepsy. Interictal hypometabolism and ictal hypermetabolism have been documented in seizure foci by PET imaging, using the isotope fluorine-18, in the form of fluorodeoxyglucose; these studies are usually considered sufficient to justify sterotactic ablation or surgery.[6]

When MR reveals a neoplasm or vascular malformation that requires intervention:

Step 2: Angiography

Angiography is appropriate to determine the vascular supply of vascular malformations and provide a "road map" for surgical or angiographic intervention. The study involves injection of contrast material into blood vessels of the head or neck, through a catheter that has been threaded retrograde up the aorta, introduced via percutaneous femoral arterial puncture.

SUMMARY AND CONCLUSIONS

1. **MR is the modality of choice for the initial evaluation of chronic intractable epilepsy. In many cases MR is sufficient to end the imaging workup.**

2. A normal MR should be followed by a nuclear Tc-99m-HMPAO-SPECT study.

3. Usually, a normal MR and a normal Tc-99m-HMPAO-SPECT end the workup, but PET studies can rarely be positive when both of these are not. PET is available only in large medical centers.

4. Angiography can further characterize vascular lesions detected by MR.

5. Although CT is effective for many intracranial lesions, it is poorly suited to study of the temporal lobes, the site of mesial temporal sclerosis. **Therefore, if only CT is available, the patient should be referred elsewhere.**

REFERENCES

1. Triulzi F, Franceschi M, Fazio F, Del Maschio A. Nonrefractory temporal lobe epilepsy: 1.5-T MR imaging. Radiology 1988; 166:181-185.
2. Bronen RA, Cheung G, Charles JT, Kim JH, Spencer DD, Spencer SS, Sze G, McCarthy G. Imaging findings in hippocampal sclerosis: correlation with pathology. AJNR 1991; 12:933-940.
3. Jackson GD, Berkovic SF, Duncan JS, Connelly A. Optimizing the diagnosis of hippocampal sclerosis using MR imaging. AJNR 1993; 14:753-762.
4. Elster AD, Mirza W. MR imaging in chronic partial epilepsy: role of contrast enhancement. AJNR 1991; 12:165-170.
5. Jack CR, Sharbrough FW, Twomey CK, Cascino GD, Hirschorn KA, Marsh WR, Zinsmeister AR, Scheithauer B. Temporal lobe seizures: lateralization with MR volume measurements of the hippocampal formation. Radiology 1990; 175:423-429.
6. Fisher RS, Frost JJ. Epilepsy. J Nucl Med. 1991; 32:651-659.

38

Aneurysms and Arteriovenous Malformations

INTRODUCTION

Aneurysms and arteriovenous malformations (AVMs) are common anomalies of the central nervous system. Both often present acutely: aneurysms with headache, cranial nerve palsies, and subarachnoid hemorrhage; AVMs, with seizures or intracerebral hematomas. Computed tomography with and without intravenous contrast material (enhanced and unenhanced CT), magnetic resonance imaging with intravenous contrast material (enhanced MR), magnetic resonance angiography (MRA), and conventional angiography effectively study aneurysms and AVMs.

Costs: head CT, enhanced and unenhanced, $476; MR, unenhanced, $845; MR angiography, excluding standard MR, $849; conventional cerebral angiography, complete "four-vessel study," $3496.

PLAN AND RATIONALE

For the acutely ill patient with possible subarachnoid hemorrhage or intracerebral hematoma:

Step 1: Computed Tomography

CT is the initial study of choice for the assessment of aneurysms and AVMs that present acutely, because their presenting complications—subarachnoid hemorrhage and intracerebral hematoma—are clearly demonstrated. CT is compatible with virtually all life-support systems, and scanning times are sufficiently short that the study is almost always feasible.

In addition to detecting hemorrhage or hematoma, enhanced CT can often detect the AVM or aneurysm itself.

When CT detects an AVM or aneurysm that may be amenable to endovascular and/or neurosurgical therapy, angiography is required.

For the elective evaluation of suspected AVMs and aneurysms:

Step 1: Magnetic Resonance Imaging and Magnetic Resonance Angiography

Unenhanced MR can detect aneurysms with and without thrombus.[1] Sophisticated new software has permitted MR to visualize blood vessels, without the need for arterial catheterization; this technology, MRA, is completely noninvasive and has replaced conventional cerebral angiography to some extent. MRA can demonstrate aneurysms as small as 3 mm; however, some smaller lesions may be missed.[2]

The arterial supply and venous drainage of AVM's are seen without intravenous contrast material.[3] MRA is capable of demonstrating much of the arterial supply and venous drainage, although small arterial feeders may escape detection.[4]

Although CT can also detect AVMs and aneurysms before they have bled, MR is more sensitive and specific. **Therefore CT does not compete with MR as a screening study in the nonacute patient.**

If MR detects an aneurysm or AVM that explains the patient's symptoms, the workup ends unless the lesion is possibly amenable to neurosurgical and/or endovascular treatment, in which case angiography is required (see **Step 2: Angiography,** below). Moreover, if there are unexplained symptoms that likely result from a very small AVM or aneurysm that has escaped detection by MR, angiography is the definitive study.

Step 2: Angiography

Angiography is the definitive study for the evaluation of aneurysms and AVMs, but it requires transfemoral puncture and passsage of a catheter up the aorta, catheterization of the great vessels of the neck, and injection of contrast material. Thus angiography is too invasive and expensive to compete with MR as a screening study in the non-emergency setting.

Angiography can demonstrate the AVM or aneurysm, its arterial and venous connections, as well as the parent vessel.

SUMMARY AND CONCLUSIONS

1. **CT is the initial study of choice in the emergency evaluation of aneurysms and AVMs, because the hemorrhagic consequences of these lesions are clearly identified.**
2. CT can also identify some AVMs and aneurysms that have not bled, but CT is less sensitive and specific than MR for this purpose.

3. MR (with MRA) is the imaging modality of choice in the nonemergency evaluation of suspected aneurysms and AVMs. Sometimes a normal MR will be followed by conventional angiography to seek very subtle vascular lesions that MR and MRA might have missed.

4. Angiography is the definitive study for AVMs and aneurysms; it is too invasive to compete with MR as a screening exam, but it is currently required prior to endovascular or neurosurgical treatment.

ADDITIONAL COMMENTS

- Many vascular lesions in the brain are amenable to endovascular therapy by an interventional neuroradiologist. The feeding vessel(s) of a lesion can be catheterized by the transfemoral arterial route (without a craniotomy) and various forms of thrombotic therapy instituted, involving intravascular balloons, Gelfoam, or other materials.

REFERENCES

1. Atlas SW, Grossman RI, Goldberg HI, Hackney DB, Bilaniuk LT, Zimmerman RA. Partially thrombosed giant intracranial aneurysms: correlation of MR and pathologic findings. Radiology 1987; 162:111-114.

2. Masaryk TJ, Modic MT, Ross JS, Ruggieri PM, Laub GA, Lenz GW, Haacke EM, Selman WR, Wiznitzer M, Harik SI. Intracranial circulation: preliminary clinical results with three-dimensional (volume) MR angiography. Radiology 1989; 171:793-799.

3. Kucharczyk W, Lemme-Pleghos L, Uske A, Brant-Zawadzki M, Dooms G, Norman D. Intracranial vascular malformations: MR and CT imaging. Radiology 1985; 156:383-389.

4. Huston J, Rufenacht DA, Ehman RL, Wiebers DO. Intracranial aneurysms and vascular malformations: comparison of time-of-flight and phase-contrast MR angiography. Radiology 1991; 181:721-730.

39

Spinal Cord Compression from Metastases

INTRODUCTION

Spinal cord compression from metastases can progress rapidly to profound and irreversible neurologic damage.[1] Imaging can define the level, extent, and cause of the compression.

Spinal cord studies are often requested on an emergency basis, reinforcing the need for rapid, accurate diagnosis. Several techniques apply: myelography, computed tomography with intrathecal contrast material (CT myelography), and magnetic resonance imaging without intravenous contrast material (unenhanced MR). The choice may depend on availability, particularly in an emergency.

Costs: cervical MR, unenhanced, $915; thoracic MR, unenhanced, $763; lumbar MR, unenhanced, $849; cervical CT myelography, $1246; thoracic CT myelography, $1237; lumbar CT myelography, $1135.

PLAN AND RATIONALE

Where magnetic resonance imaging is available:

Step 1: Magnetic Resonance Imaging

MR is the examination of choice for evaluating suspected spinal cord compression.[2] It images the spine in multiple planes, clearly defining the cerebrospinal fluid, spinal cord, nerve roots, intervertebral disks, and vertebral bodies. The location and extent of lesions and their relationship to the spinal cord and dura are well delineated. MR is noninvasive and better tolerated than myelography.[3] Although usually not required, intravenous contrast material can augment lesion conspicuity.[4]

Where emergency magnetic resonance imaging is unavailable:

Step 1: Computed Tomography Myelography

CT myelography is an acceptable alternative if MR is unavailable. The technique is almost as sensitive as MR for defining the cause of spinal cord compression.[3] Contrast material is injected into the lumbar subarachnoid space, and the patient is positioned head down. The contrast material usually flows beyond the level of an obstruction, defining its superior extent.[5] **CT without intrathecal contrast material is usually insufficient.**

Where magnetic resonance imaging and computed tomography are unavailable or unfeasible:

Step 1: Plain Film Myelography

In some hospitals emergency MR and CT are unavailable; moreover, these studies may be unfeasible because of massive patient obesity or metal "hardware" from spinal surgery.

Before the advent of CT and MR, conventional myelography was the standard study for spinal cord compression.[5] Contrast material is injected into the lumbar subarachnoid space, and the patient is placed head down, so that the contrast material migrates craniad. Although the study can reveal spinal cord compression, the offending lesion itself is inferred, and the superior extent of the block may not be visualized at all.[5-7] In some instances, a separate cervical puncture may be necessary to determine the superior extent of the block. **Clearly, myelography is inferior to MR or CT myelography.**

SUMMARY AND CONCLUSIONS

1. **MR is the modality of choice for evaluating suspected spinal cord compression from metastatic tumor.**
2. If MR is unavailable, CT myelography is an acceptable alternative.
3. If MR and CT are unavailable or unfeasible, conventional plain film myelography can define the level of a spinal cord compression, but the study is clearly inferior to MR or CT myelography.

REFERENCES

1. Gilbert RW, Kim JH, Posner JB. Epidural spinal cord compression from metastatic tumor: diagnosis and treatment. Ann Neurol 1978; 3:40–51.
2. Smoker WRK, Godersky JC, Knutzon RK, Keyes WD, Norman D, Bergman W. The role of MR imaging in evaluating metastatic spinal disease. AJR 1987; 149:1241–1248.
3. Carmody RF, Yang PJ, Seeley GW, Seeger JF, Unger EC, Johnson JE. Spinal cord compression due to metastatic disease: diagnosis with MR imaging versus myelography. Radiology 1989; 173:225–229.

4. Sze G, Krol G, Zimmerman RD, Deck MDF. Malignant extradural spinal tumors: MR imaging with Gd-DTPA. Radiology 1988; 167:217-223.
5. Fink IJ, Garra BS, Zabell A, Doppman JL. Computed tomography with metrizamide myelography to define the extent of spinal canal block due to tumor. JCAT 1984; 8:1072-1075.
6. Dublin AB, McGahan JP, Reid MH. The value of computed tomographic metrizamide myelography in the neuroradiological evaluation of the spine. Radiology 1977; 146:79-86.
7. Kelly WM, Badami P, Dillon W. Epidural block: myelographic evaluation with a single-puncture technique using metrizamide. Radiology 1984; 151:417-419.

40

Demyelinating Disease

INTRODUCTION

Traditionally, multiple sclerosis (MS) has been a clinical diagnosis. The previous role of neuroimaging was to exclude other diseases that might simulate MS, but **magnetic resonance imaging with and without intravenous contrast material (enhanced and unenhanced MR) is now capable of confirming the diagnosis of MS since it excludes other diseases.**[1]

Costs: brain MR, unenhanced, $845; brain MR, enhanced and unenhanced, $1418.

PLAN AND RATIONALE

Step 1: Magnetic Resonance Imaging

MR has replaced computed tomography (CT) as the modality of choice for the evaluation of MS and other demyelinating disease.[2,3] The multiplanar imaging capability of MR demonstrates lesions that are specific for MS.[4,5] Intravenous contrast material increases both the sensitivity and the specificity of the study.[4] Lesions that are more conspicuous on the enhanced study sometimes correlate with specific symptoms.[6]

SUMMARY AND CONCLUSIONS

1. MR is the modality of choice for the evaluation of demyelinating disease.
2. CT can exclude other diseases that mimic MS, but CT is not recommended in the workup of MS, because a normal CT must be followed by MR, unnecessarily increasing the cost of the workup.

ADDITIONAL COMMENTS

- Special MR techniques like "fat suppression" may augment detection of optic nerve lesions in patients with optic neuritis, a common presenting symptom of MS.
- Demyelinating lesions of the spinal cord are visualized by MR but rarely by CT.

REFERENCES

1. Simon JH. Neuroimaging of multiple sclerosis. Radiol Clin North Am 1993; 3(2):229-246.
2. Gebarski SS, Gabrielsen TO, Gilman S, Knake JE, Latack JT, Aisen AM. The initial diagnosis of multiple sclerosis: clinical impact of magnetic resonance imaging. Ann Neurol 1985; 17:469-474.
3. Kirshner HS, Tsai SI, Runge VM, Price AC. Magnetic resonance imaging and other techniques in the diagnosis of multiple sclerosis. Arch Neurol 1985; 42:859-863.
4. Gean-Marton AD, Vezina LG, Marton KI, Stimac GK, Peyser RG, Taveras JM, Davis KR. Abnormal corpus callosum: a sensitive and specific indicator of multiple sclerosis. Radiology 1991; 180:215-221.
5. Horowith AL, Kaplan RD, Grewe G, White RT, Salberg LM. The ovoid lesion: a new MR observation in patients with multiple sclerosis. AJNR 1989; 10:303-305.
6. Grossman RI, Gonzalez-Scarano F, Atlas SW, Galetta S, Silberberg DH. Multiple sclerosis: gadolinium enhancement in MR imaging. Radiology 1986; 161:721-725.

41

Sellar and Juxtasellar Lesions

INTRODUCTION

Sellar and juxtasellar lesions usually present with endocrine syndromes, like amenorrhea/galactorrhea, diabetes insipidus, and acromegaly, or with neurologic syndromes, like visual loss. The goal of imaging is to determine whether a significant lesion exists and, if so, to localize and characterize it for therapy. Magnetic resonance imaging with and without intravenous contrast material (enhanced and unenhanced MR), computed tomography with and without intravenous contrast material (enhanced and unenhanced CT), and angiography can play a role in the workup.

Costs: brain MR, unenhanced, $845; brain MR, enhanced and unenhanced, $1418; head CT, enhanced and unenhanced, $476; cerebral angiogram, complete "four-vessel study," $3496.

PLAN AND RATIONALE

Where magnetic resonance imaging is available:

Step 1: Magnetic Resonance Imaging

Magnetic resonance imaging (MR) is the modality of choice for the evaluation of sellar/juxtasellar lesions.[1-3]

The study is superior to computed tomography because of its multiplanar imaging capability, lack of bone-induced artifact, and superior spatial resolution. MR clearly delineates sellar/juxtasellar masses and their relationship to adjacent structures like the optic chiasm, hypothalamus, carotid arteries, and cavernous sinus. Studies with intravenous contrast material (contrast enhanced) better characterize pituitary macroadenomas and microadenomas.[4] **Very often a firm diagnosis is possible without surgery or biopsy.**

When bone destruction and calcifications must be further defined, CT can be helpful (see ***Where Magnetic Resonance Imaging is Not Available,* Step 1: Computed Tomography,** below). When vascular lesions require study before surgical or angiographic intervention, cerebral angiography is effective (see **Step 3: Angiography**, below).

Where magnetic resonance imaging is not available:

Step 1: Computed Tomography

CT with and without intravenous contrast material (unenhanced and enhanced) can evaluate most sellar and juxtasellar lesions.[5,6] Unenhanced CT will clearly reveal soft tissue abnormalities, cortical bone, and calcifications. Enhanced CT helps to characterize juxtasellar vascular masses like carotid artery aneurysms. The findings in some lesions, particularly meningiomas, are pathognomonic. **Normal CT excludes all but very small lesions, like isodense pituitary microadenomas. Frequently, a definite diagnosis is possible.**

CT is superior to MR in defining bone destruction and calcifications; nonetheless, these advantages do not fully compensate for its important weaknesses relative to MR. Thus **MR remains the examination of choice.**

If CT is normal, the workup usually ends, but if a lesion is nonetheless suspected on clinical grounds, then the patient should be referred to a facility that has MR. When vascular lesions require further study, cerebral angiography is necessary.

Step 2: Cerebral Angiography

Angiography is useful in the evaluation of vascular lesions, like aneurysms and arteriovenous malformations, and certain tumors, like meningiomas, before surgical resection. A catheter is threaded retrograde up the aorta following percutaneous femoral artery puncture, and the catheter tip is positioned in one of the great vessels of the neck. Contrast material is injected as serial films are exposed, revealing the vascular components of a lesion and the vascularity of adjacent brain. Some vascular lesions can be treated by "endovascular therapy," eliminating the need for neurologic surgery.

SUMMARY AND CONCLUSIONS

1. MR is the best initial study for suspected sellar/juxtasellar lesions.
2. If MR is unavailable, CT is a reasonable alternative, although CT is not as sensitive for small lesions.
3. CT may be a useful adjunct to MR in the evaluation of bone destruction and in the detection of calcification.
4. Angiography has limited **diagnostic** value but is helpful to further characterize vascular lesions, provide a presurgical "vascular road map," or be a part of endovascular therapy.

ADDITIONAL COMMENTS

- Coronal images with CT require hyperextension of the neck, which is uncomfortable and difficult for young children and the elderly. MR generates coronal images with the patient in a comfortable supine position, a critical advantage for these patients.
- Newer MR software—"gradient recall echo techniques"— increase the sensitivity of MR for calcification, eliminating the need for CT in most cases.

REFERENCES

1. Chakeres DW, Curtin A, Ford G. Magnetic resonance imaging of pituitary and parasellar abnormalities. Radiol Clin North Am 1989; 27:265-281.
2. Kucharczyk W, David DO, Kelly WM, Sze G, Norman D, Newton TH. Pituitary adenomas: high-resolution MR imaging at 1.5T. Radiology 1986; 161:761-765.
3. Sartor K, Karnaze MG, Winthrop JD, Gado M, Hodges FJ III. MR imaging in infra-, para- and retrosellar mass lesions. Neuroradiology 1987; 29:19-29.
4. Davis PC, Hoffman JC Jr, Malko JA, Tindall GT, Takei Y, Avruch L, Braun IF. Gadolinium-DTPA and MR imaging of pituitary adenoma: a preliminary report. AJNR 1987; 8:817-823.
5. Taylor S. High resolution computed tomography of the sella. Radiol Clin North Am 1982; 20:207-236.

42

Stroke

INTRODUCTION

Stroke is a major cause of morbidity and mortality in the developed world. The early diagnosis of stroke is critical, because early therapy can improve prognosis. Computed tomography without intravenous contrast material (unenhanced CT), magnetic resonance imaging with and without intravenous contrast material (enhanced and unenhanced MR), and angiography each play a role.

Costs: head CT, unenhanced, $287; brain MR, unenhanced, $845; brain MR, enhanced and unenhanced, $1418; cerebral angiogram, carotid catheterizations only, $3063.

PLAN AND RATIONALE

Step 1: Computed Tomography

CT is the modality of choice for the evaluation of acute stroke. The study can easily exclude lesions that simulate stroke, like tumor and abscess, and can often differentiate between ischemic and hemorrhagic infarction, usually by 24 hours after the onset of symptoms.[1] Intravenous contrast material is usually not required, since the majority of infarctions are evident without it.

When CT is decisive, the workup ends, but in some cases MR may be necessary.

Step 2: Magnetic Resonance Imaging

When CT fails to differentiate infarction from another disease process, when posterior fossa infarction is suspected, or when CT does not explain the patient's clinical findings, MR is appropriate. MR better visualizes the posterior fossa because it is not hampered by occipital bone artifacts that degrade CT. MR is more sensitive than CT for early infarction,[2,3] and the greater sensitivity of MR can be further augmented by intravenous injection of contrast material.[4,5]

Despite its advantages, MR is not always feasible in the acute setting, because most life-support systems are not MR compatible and the acutely ill patient often cannot tolerate the relatively long scanning times of most MR units.

When MR or CT reveals lesions that may be caused by carotid or vertebral artery disease or when MR directly visualizes vascular flow abnormalities and when interventional therapy is contemplated, angiography is next.

Step 3: Angiography

Angiography involves percutaneous femoral artery puncture, passage of a catheter up the aorta, and catheterization of one of the arteries of the neck. Contrast material is injected as serial films are exposed. The technique exquisitely demonstrates narrowed areas that restrict blood flow.

SUMMARY AND CONCLUSIONS

1. **CT is the modality of choice for the evaluation of stroke**.
2. In some cases MR is required after CT, particularly to better image the posterior fossa or detect early infarction.
3. Enhanced MR can detect stoke earlier that CT. However, MR is not always practical in the evaluation of acute stroke, because of relatively long scanning times and MR-incompatible life-support systems.
4. Angiography can demonstrate arterial narrowing in the neck that restricts blood flow to the brain.

ADDITIONAL COMMENTS

• The scanning times of newer MR units are markedly faster. Moreover, more and more life-support systems are MR compatible. **Therefore, if the cost of MR falls, it may well replace CT as the procedure of choice in acute stroke.**

REFERENCES

1. Inoue Y, Takemoto K, Miyamoto T, Yoshikawa N, Taniguchi S, Saiwai S, Nishimura Y, Komatsu T. Sequential computed tomography scans in acute cerebral infarction. Radiology 1980; 135:655-662.
2. Bryan RN, Levy LM, Whitlow WD, Killian JM, Preziosi TJ, Rosario JA. Diagnosis of acute cerebral infarction: comparison of CT and MR imaging. AJNR 1991; 12:611-620.
3. Yuh WTC, Crain MR, Loes DJ, Greene GM, Ryals TJ, Sato Y. MR imaging of cerebral ischemia: findings in the first 24 hours. AJNR 1991; 12:621-629.
4. Crain MR, Yu WTC, Greene GM, Loes DJ, Ryals TJ, Sato Y, Hart MN. Cerebral ischemia: evaluation with contrast-enhanced MR imaging. AJNR 1991; 12:631-639.
5. Elster AD, Moody DM. Early cerebral infarction: gadopentetate dimeglumine enhancement. Radiology 1990; 177:627-632.

Part V

MUSCULOSKELETAL

43

Osteomyelitis

INTRODUCTION

Plain radiographs, nuclear scans, computed tomography (CT), and magnetic resonance imaging (MR) can address two issues regarding bone inflammation: (1) Is acute osteomyelitis present in previously normal bone? (2) Is there active osteomyelitis in bone with previous disease?

Costs: plain bone films, variable cost according to area radiographed, $50 to $120; bone scan, without SPECT, $270; cervical MR, $915; thoracic MR, $763; lumbar MR, $849; upper extremity MR, $859; lower extremity MR, $935; nuclear WBC scan, $505; Ga-67 scan, SPECT, $745.

PLAN AND RATIONALE

(A) When acute osteomyelitis is suspected in previously normal bone:

Step 1: Plain Radiographs

In the presence of osteomyelitis, typical radiographic signs appear in about 1 week. Earlier, plain films are usually normal or nonspecific, and further imaging is needed. However, plain films should not be skipped during the first week, because they can exclude other causes of symptoms, like fracture, tumor, or radiopaque soft tissue foreign body, and sometimes they can be diagnostic of osteomyelitis during the first week.

When initial plain films are normal:

Step 2: Nuclear Bone Scan

The nuclear bone scan for osteomyelitis is a "three-phase" study, involving a peripheral intravenous bolus injection of Tc-99m-labeled methylene diphosphonate (MDP), rapid-sequence "flow" images of the area of interest, immediate "static" or "blood pool" images, and images of the entire skeleton after 1 to 2 hours. The bone scan in osteomyelitis usually becomes abnormal by 24 hours, **much earlier than plain films**.

MDP accumulates in the crystalline structure of bone, according to local bone blood flow, and areas of osteomyelitis almost always appear "hot." In the patient **without preexisting bone disease** (i.e., normal plain radiographs) a focal abnormality at the symptomatic site on a three-phase bone scan is quite specific.[1] Thus **a positive scan is diagnostic of osteomyelitis in the proper clinical context**—e.g., in the presence of fever, leukocytosis, and local pain. However, an abnormal bone scan in the presence of concomitant bone lesions—including old or recent trauma, primary or metastatic bone tumor, arthritis, metabolic bone disease, and Paget's disease—is nonspecific; further imaging is usually needed.

In patients over 3 years old, **a normal scan almost always excludes osteomyelitis and ends the workup**; rarely, if the patient has been scanned within a few hours of onset, the scan may be falsely negative because the infected bone has had insufficient time to react to the infection; a follow-up scan in 24 hours is usually conclusive. In patients under 3 years old, the bone scan is less sensitive, and in children under 3 months old, it is often falsely negative.

When the scan is negative in young children or nonspecific or equivocal in older children and adults, additional imaging may help.

*When the initial bone scan is negative in young children and nonspecific or equivocal in older children or adults and osteomyelitis **of the spine** is suspected:*

Step 3: Magnetic Resonance Imaging

MR produces "sectional" images that can be displayed in any plane; it excels in early detection of **bone marrow edema**, an early change in osteomyelitis. For this condition it is as sensitive and specific as the bone scan, especially in the spine, which has abundant red marrow.[6,7] (Some investigators suggest that MR could replace total body bone scanning as a screen, except that the present generation of MR scanners is limited to one or two anatomic areas per study. Furthermore, MR is more costly.)

Bony and soft tissue involvement, including sinus tracts and soft tissue abscesses, are clearly defined. **MR reveals the relationship of an infectious process to the subarachnoid space, the spinal cord, and nerve roots.**[8]

The specificity of MR falls in patients with preexisting bone disease—fracture, surgery, or neoplasm.

*When the initial bone scan is negative in young children or nonspecific or equivocal in older children and adults and **extraspinal** osteomyelitis is suspected:*

Step 3: White Blood Cell Scan (Labeled Autologous Leukocytes) or Gallium-67 Citrate Scan

A WBC scan involves harvesting leukocytes from a small sample of the patient's blood, labeling them with indium-111(In-111) oxine or technetium-99m-hydroxymethyl-propyleneamine oxime (Tc-99m-HMPAO), and injecting them intravenously.[2,3] The labeled cells accumulate in sites of purulent infection, especially in the appendicular skeleton. The study is highly specific for osteomyelitis and when positive ends the imaging workup. **Tc-99m-HMPAO is strongly favored over In-111-oxine**, because it produces images of much higher quality. Furthermore, the skeleton is imaged only 3 hours after Tc-99m-HMPAO injection, whereas an 18- to 24-hour interval between injection and imaging is required for In-111-oxine. In the setting of suspected osteomyelitis, an 18- to 24-hour delay is undesirable.

Gallium-67 accumulates in various inflammatory (and sometimes neoplastic) foci 2 to 3 days after intravenous injection. The mechanism of gallium accumulation has not been established but probably relates to its affinity for lactoferrin released by polymorphonuclear neutrophilic leukocytes. Gallium is less sensitive and specific for osteomyelitis than WBC scanning; however, gallium is a reasonable alternative when a WBC study is unavailable.

(B) When plain films reveal no acute osteomyelitis but there is significant bone disease (traumatic, postsurgical, neoplastic, or postinflammatory):

Step 2: White Blood Cell (WBC) Scan (Labeled Autologous Leukocytes) or Gallium-67 Citrate Scan

In the presence of preexisting bone abnormalities—surgical, traumatic, or neoplastic—**the bone scan will virtually always be abnormal but, unfortunately, nonspecific.** (The "three-phase" bone scan was designed to obviate this problem, because the "flow" portion of the study reflects perfusion; lesions that hyperperfuse are theoretically inflammatory, rather than traumatic, postsurgical, or neoplastic, but all-too-often the distinction between infections and noninfectious lesions blurs.) Thus **many nuclear imagers prefer to skip the bone scan when there is significant preexisting bone disease and proceed directly to WBC or gallium scans** (see above, *When the initial bone scan is negative in young children or nonspecific or equivocal in older children and adults and extraspinal osteomyelitis is suspected*).

A normal WBC or gallium scan in an area of radiographically abnormal bone excludes osteomyelitis with high degree of probability, especially in the appendicular skeleton. However, WBC or gallium accumulation, unless intense, may be nonspecific. **In such cases, it may be necessary to compare the WBC or gallium scan to a bone scan to determine for sure whether the abnormal accumulation is in bone or soft tissue.**

Step 3: Bone Scan

(See above, under "*When initial plain films are normal.*") The side-by-side comparison of plain films, a WBC or gallium study, and a bone scan is usually sufficient. **In very unusual cases, both WBC and gallium studies are appropriate to clarify equivocal situations. In practical terms, however, if conventional radiographs, a WBC scan, and a bone scan cannot solidify the diagnosis, many clinicians proceed directly to bone biopsy. Depending on the anatomic site, CT or MR may be required.**

Step 4: Computed Tomography or Magnetic Resonance Imaging

CT can accurately define sequestra, soft tissue abscesses, and bone destruction before surgery, and in some centers the biopsy itself is performed under CT guidance. MR is superior to CT in depicting the extent of bone marrow and soft tissue involvement, including sinus tracts and soft tissue abscesses, **but the technique is intrinsically unsuited to guided biopsy.** Each case should be discussed with the musculoskeletal radiologist before biopsy.

SUMMARY AND CONCLUSIONS

1. Plain radiographs are the first exam in the investigation of osteomyelitis; although 7 days usually pass before signs become manifest, the plain films exclude many other causes of symptoms and reveal any preexisting bone disease.
2. A Tc-99m-MDP bone scan is the most appropriate next exam when there is no preexisting bone disease.
3. A normal bone scan in patients over 3 years old usually ends the osteomyelitis workup. In patients under 3 or when new disease may be superimposed on old disease, further imaging may be required.
4. In the presence of preexisting bone disease, many imagers proceed directly from the plain films to a WBC study or MR. These studies are also often justified when the initial bone scan is normal in a patient under 3 years of age.
5. For suspected **osteomyelitis of the spine, MR is highly effective**. **Elsewhere, radiolabeled WBCs may clarify an abnormal but nonspecific bone scan in acute or chronic osteomyelitis** or may reveal osteomyelitis in very young patients with falsely negative bone scans. Tc-99m-HMPAO labeled cells

produce superior images that are generated within 3 hours of intravenous cell injection.

6. Gallium-67–citrate is a viable alternative if WBC scanning is not available. Uncommonly both studies are required.

7. When the exact extent of bony or soft tissue involvement must be known, MR or CT apply. **MR is superior for soft tissue definition but is intrinsically unsuited to biopsy guidance. CT defines bone disease quite well but is inferior to MR for soft tissue definition; however, CT biopsy guidance is highly effective.**

ADDITIONAL COMMENTS

- **MR is excellent for the detection of marrow edema in the long bones as well as in the spine.** However, its cost and limitation to one or two anatomic areas per study relegate MR to a secondary role. **If the cost of MR were lower and the entire skeleton could be scanned**, the study would compete effectively with total body bone scanning. A reduction in cost **without** the ability to image more than one anatomic area per study would leave MR behind bone scanning but probably position it ahead of WBC or gallium studies; such a development is expected by many investigators.

REFERENCES

1. Schauwacker DS. The scintigraphic diagnosis of osteomyelitis. AJR 1992; 158:9–18.
2. Neumann RD, Hoffer PB. Gallium-67 scintigraphy for detection of inflammation and tumors. In Freeman LM, ed. Freeman and Johnson's Clinical Radionuclide Imaging, 3rd ed. Orlando, Florida, 1984, Grune & Stratton, pp 1319–1364.
3. Pring DJ, Henderson RG, Keshavarzian A, Rivett AG, Krausz T,

Coombs RRH, Lavender JP. Indium-granulocyte scanning in the painful prosthetic joint. AJR 1986; 146:167-172.

4. Al-Sheikh A, Sfakianakis GN, Mnaymneh W, et al. Subacute and chronic bone infections: diagnosis using In-111, Ga-67 and Tc-99m MDP bone scintigraphy and radiography. Radiology 1985; 155:501-506.

5. O'Mara RE, Weber DA. The osseous system. In Freeman LM, ed. Freeman and Johnson's Clinical Radionuclide Imaging, 3rd ed. Orlando, Florida, 1984, Grune & Stratton, pp 1141-1239

6. Gold RH, Hawkins RA, Katz RD. Bacterial osteomyelitis: findings in plain radiography, CT, MR, and scintigraphy. AJR 1991; 157:365-370.

7. Tang JS, Gold RH, Bassett LW, Seeger LL. Musculoskeletal infection of the extremities: evaluation with MR imaging. Radiology 1988; 166:205-209.

8. Sharif HS. Role of MR imaging in the management of spinal infections. AJR 1992; 158:1333-1345.

9. Larcos G, Brown ML, Sutton RT. Diagnosis of osteomyelitis of the foot in diabetic patients: value of In-111 leukocyte scintigraphy. AJR 1991; 157:527-531.

10. Fletcher BD, Scoles PV, Nelson AD. Osteomyelitis in children: detection by magnetic resonance. Radiology 1984; 150:57-60.

11. McAfee JG. What is the best imaging method for imaging focal infections ? (editorial). J Nucl Med 1990; 31:413-416.

44

Skeletal Metastases

INTRODUCTION

Four imaging techniques can detect bone metastases: (1) conventional radiography, which largely reflects alterations in structure, (2) nuclear bone scanning, which largely reflects alterations in physiology, (3) computed tomography (CT), which provides more anatomic and morphologic information than plain radiographs and is more sensitive to changes in radiographic density, and (4) magnetic resonance imaging (MR), which reveals replacement of bone marrow by tumor.

The goal of imaging is to demonstrate metastatic lesions as early as possible or to exclude them with a high degree of confidence. Both the clinician and the imager should recall that **skeletal metastases are not necessarily painful or symptomatic.**

The majority of patients with metastases to bone have primary cancers of the prostate, breast, lung, kidney, or lymphoma. The rationale of **screening** for **unknown** skeletal metastases varies according to the site of the primary tumor: In prostate, the scan is useful at the time of initial diagnosis to help stage the disease and follow therapeutic response. In breast, since the likelihood of bone metastases is quite low early on, the value of early routine screening is controversial; some authors recommend studying every patient shortly after the initial diagnosis,[1] whereas others reserve the scan for stage III disease or bone pain.[2] (The incidence of bone metastases from breast cancer in stages I and II is only 2% and 6%, respectively; in stage III, 14%.) In lung, a positive bone scan means unresectable disease; if disease is unresectable on other grounds, the bone scan will not alter management and is superfluous, but if a lung cancer appears resectable, the bone scan is critical. In renal cell carcinoma, the bone scan is useful for initial staging. In lymphoma, the bone scan is valuable initially to help stage and later follow the disease.

The approach to patients without known skeletal metastases differs from that of patients with known metastases.

Costs: plain bone films, variable cost according to area radiographed, $50 to $120; bone scan, without SPECT, $270; bone scan, SPECT, $651; MR, unenhanced, variable cost according to area studied, $849 to $914; bone biopsy, fluoroscopically guided, "superficial" lesion, $331; bone biopsy, CT guided, "superficial lesion," $692; bone biopsy, fluoroscopically guided, "deep lesion," $549; bone biopsy, CT guided, "deep" lesion, $910.

PLAN AND RATIONALE

When no skeletal metastases are known:

Step 1: Bone Scan, Possibly With Single Photon Emission Computed Tomography

Bone scanning involves peripheral intravenous injection of technetium-99m methylene diphosphonate (Tc-99m-MDP). One to 2 hours later, the skeleton is scanned from head to foot. Most of the radiopharmaceutical accumulates in the crystalline structure of bone proportional to local bone blood flow. Skeletal metastases usually accumulate more radioactivity than adjacent normal bone and appear "hot." However, most other bone lesions—including old or recent trauma, primary benign or malignant neoplasm, acute or chronic osteomyelitis, inflammatory or degenerative arthritis, metabolic bone disease, and Paget's disease—also appear "hot." Thus **an abnormal bone scan is nonspecific.**[3]

In most malignancies, the bone scan is more sensitive than plain radiographs; neither is foolproof. Overall, about 30% of metastases detected by bone scans will be missed by bone radiographs; conversely, 2% of metastases detected by radiographs will be missed by scans.[3] The sensitivity of bone scanning is greatly enhanced by SPECT (single photon emission computed tomography), **especially for the all-important spine lesions**; unfortunately, SPECT virtually doubles the cost of a bone scan. Therefore many nuclear medicine practitioners perform a routine scan first and reserve SPECT for problems, particularly the study of symptomatic areas that are normal on the routine exam.

If the bone scan is normal and there is no bone pain, skeletal metastases are very likely absent, and the workup stops, but if there is bone pain in the presence of a normal scan, further imaging is appropriate.

If the bone scan is abnormal, revealing a "hot" lesion (or lesions), these can be considered metastatic in the proper clinical context, without further imaging. To a great extent this determination depends on the appearance and site(s) of the finding(s); for example, a focal vertebral pedicle lesion is much more likely to represent a metastasis than a focal rib lesion after trauma.

If the bone scan is abnormal, and findings are (1) atypical for metastatic disease, (2) consistent with a variety of conditions (like metastatic disease, benign degenerative change, or trauma), or (3) inconsistent with clinical status, follow-up radiographs are required for clarification.

Step 2: Skeletal Radiographs

If radiographs reveal benign lesions like degenerative arthritis that explain the bone scan findings, the imaging workup ends. If benign lesions are found that do not necessarily account for the bone scan findings, leaving the issue of bone metastases unresolved, the patient can be rescanned in 6 to 8 weeks to look for lesion growth (which would support a malignant etiology), proceed to biopsy,[3-5] or undergo MR imaging.

If radiographs reveal a lesion that explains pain in the presence of a normal scan, no further imaging is required, **but if both radiographs and the scan are normal in the presence of pain, MR is appropriate.**

Step 3: Magnetic Resonance Imaging

Conventional MR cannot directly image calcium; therefore, its use in bone imaging is limited. However, **normal bone marrow is beautifully demonstrated by MR and easily differentiated from tumor.** Because most metastatic disease of bone begins in the marrow space at least as early as it destroys the crystalline structure, MR is often helpful in confirming or excluding metastatic disease. Moreover, **MR is superior for defining soft tissue abnormalities (e.g., rotator cuff tear, disc protrusion, or ligamentous injury) that can cause pain in the presence of a normal bone scan.**

MR is particularly effective in back pain, because it demonstrates the spinal cord itself, nerve roots, and subarachnoid space; the status of these vital structures and spaces is determined along with the presence or absence of marrow replacement.

If MR is normal or reveals a nonbony cause of pain, the workup usually ends, but in occasional cases the cause of a bone scan abnormality remains unresolved, **even after radiographs and MR. In this event, biopsy is the sole remaining option.**

If MR reveals a probable metastatic lesion, the workup ends, unless definitive histology is required.

Step 4: Bone Biopsy

The area for biopsy is identified by bone scanning. Percutaneous biopsy under fluoroscopic or CT guidance (see Chapter 61, Percutaneous Invasive Guided Biopsy) with a large-bore biopsy needle is often feasible, but if the radiologist is not experienced with this technique, intra-operative biopsy is usually successful. Some aggressive nuclear medicine divisions can actually localize the lesion in the operating room with a portable radiation "probe."

When skeletal metastases are known:

Step 1: Skeletal Radiographs

When one or more bone metastases are already known, by means of previous imaging studies, confirmation of additional lesions in areas of new, worsening, or recurrent pain are sought most expeditiously with radiographs, because these are less expensive and simpler than a bone scan (unless the new suspected areas are so widespread that a scan would be simpler). **Positive, confirmatory radiographs need not be followed by a scan, since a search for additional asymptomatic lesions in a patient already known to have bone metastases often serves no purpose. However, negative radiographs in the face of persistent pain are followed by a scan.**

Step 2: Bone Scan

The bone scan may detect radiographically occult lesions. If both radiographs and a bone scan are negative, a follow-up scan in 6 to 8 weeks is often helpful. When it is crucial to establish the presence or absence of a lesion in a symptomatic site **and both the scan and radiographs are normal**, the remaining options are MR and biopsy (see above, *When no skeletal metastases are known,* **Steps 3 and 4**).

SUMMARY AND CONCLUSIONS

1. A nuclear scan is the best screen for metastases in the asymptomatic skeleton; it is more sensitive than radiographs, and it images the entire body. SPECT technology adds to the scan's sensitivity but almost doubles the cost and should be reserved for selected problems.
2. Normal or abnormal bone scans that are consistent with the patient's clinical status end the metastatic skeletal workup.
3. **When no metastases are known**, a **symptomatic** site is first studied by a bone scan, because the entire body is imaged; the study is much more sensitive than radiographs, and MR is more costly and is limited to one or two anatomic regions.
4. **A symptomatic site** that is normal on a scan and radiograph can be rescanned in 6 to 8 weeks; metastatic lesions may progress during that interval, declaring themselves on the second scan. Alternatively, MR is often definitive.
5. MR frequently defines marrow infiltration by tumor and often reveals soft tissue lesions causing apparent bone pain. MR is particularly effective for the spine and often avoids the need for biopsy.

6. **When metastases are known**, a new, painful site is probably best studied first by radiographs, because these are simpler and less expensive than a bone scan. Many times, however, the radiographs are normal, and a bone scan is also necessary. If **many** new, painful sites develop, the scan should come before radiographs, to ensure that all of the skeleton is covered.

ADDITIONAL COMMENTS

- In multiple myeloma of bone, the bone scan is often falsely negative. Plain radiographs are the best way to detect and follow the course of this disease, but when there is bone pain both radiographs and the scan are often necessary, because neither is extremely sensitive.

- Patients with follicular thyroid carcinoma may have bone metastases, and these lesions, like multiple myeloma, are usually missed by bone scans. Late in the disease, radiographs may be positive. **An iodine-131 total-body metastatic thyroid carcinoma search is the best diagnostic procedure.** This study requires careful preparation and therefore, patients with follicular thyroid carcinoma should be discussed individually with the nuclear medicine physician.

- Occasionally, a metastasis seen on a plain radiograph will be uncharacteristic of the primary cancer (e.g., a lytic lesion in a patient with prostate carcinoma). When this occurs, the possibility of a second primary should be considered. Often the most expedient way to resolve the question is bone biopsy.

- The "flare" phenomenon, an increase in lesion intensity on the bone scan following therapy, **accompanying clinical improvement** may rarely cause confusion. A follow-up scan in 2 to 3 months clarifies the situation.

- Some investigators speculate that MR could replace the total body bone scan as the primary skeletal screen for metastatic disease, except that the present generation of MR scanners is limited to one or two anatomic regions per study.

REFERENCES

1. McNeil BJ. Value of bone scanning in neoplastic disease. Semin Nucl Med 1984;14:277-286.
2. Haywood RB, Frazier TG. A reevaluation of bone scans in breast cancer. J Surg Oncol 1985; 28:111-113.
3. O'Mara RE, Weber DA. The osseous system. In Freeman LM, ed. Freeman and Johnson's Clinical Radionuclide Imaging, 3rd ed. Orlando, Florida, 1984, Grune & Stratton, pp 1141-1239.
4. Pagani JJ, Libshitz HI. Imaging bone metastases. Radiol Clin North Am 1982; 20: 545-560.
5. Kagan AR, Bassett LW, Steckel RJ, Gold RH. Radiologic contributions to cancer management. Bone metastases. AJR 1986; 147:305-312.

45

Fracture, Stress Fracture, "Shin Splints"

INTRODUCTION

The majority of serious fractures are detected by conventional radiographs. Sometimes, however, major fractures can be radiographically occult, requiring more sophisticated techniques for detection. Moreover, pain after sports-related injuries, although trivial compared to major trauma, often causes disability, necessitating further investigation. Effective techniques for the detection of skeletal injury include conventional radiography, bone scanning, computed tomography (CT), and magnetic resonance imaging (MR).

Costs: plain films, variable cost according to area radiographed, $50 to $120; MR, unenhanced, upper extremity, $849; MR lower extremity, unenhanced, $935; facial bones CT, unenhanced, $405; Skull CT, unenhanced, $287; pelvic CT, unenhanced, $372; bone scan, without SPECT, $270.

PLAN AND RATIONALE

Step 1: Conventional Radiograph

In virtually all cases where musculoskeletal pain, trauma,

or neurologic deficit suggest bony injury, radiographs are the appropriate first study.

A fracture or another cause of pain is often defined by radiographs, **but in the presence of continued pain and/or disability without a radiographic lesion, further imaging is appropriate.**

When fracture is clinically suspected but radiographs are normal and **when delay in definitive diagnosis is acceptable,** follow-up films in 10 to 14 days are the most practical and cost-effective option **for long tubular bones**. After this interval, tell-tale fracture healing is often manifested by periosteal reaction. Sometimes, however, rapid diagnosis is mandatory—for example, in serious trauma, with suspected fracture of the spine (see Chapter 32, Acute Spine Trauma) or when athletic training cannot easily be interrupted. In other cases follow-up films are not definitive or would image the site of interest ineffectively. Finally, in certain sites supplementary imaging is required to detect important additional fractures, even when conventional radiographs reveal a fracture. In these situations, a bone scan, MR, or CT can be decisive.

For fractures of the femoral neck in the elderly:

Step 2: Magnetic Resonance Imaging

MR produces "sectional" images that can be displayed in any plane. Although calcium is not directly detected, the bony cortex is seen as a "signal void" and the bone marrow is well seen; soft tissues are exquisitely defined.

Although the nuclear bone scan is highly sensitive for detection of fractures (see below: **"Where fracture in other sites or where stress fracture or stress injury are suspected"), nuclear findings may be delayed and nonspecific in elderly patients**, owing to physiologic differences and the higher incidence of preexisting bone/joint disease in this population. Theoretically, a follow-up bone scan in 3 or 4 days would be a viable option, but in view of the cost of hospitalization and the high morbidity and mortality associated with undiagnosed hip fracture in the elderly, MRI is a more appropriate follow-up to normal or equivocal plain radiographs when hip fracture is suspected.[1] **The precise anatomic extent of the fracture as well as associated soft tissue injuries are readily demonstrated, in addition to other radiographically occult injuries, like bone bruise or ligamentous/tendinous injury.**[2]

For most fractures other than the femoral neck (facial bones, spine, base of skull, pelvis, scapula, and calcaneus):

Step 2: Computed Tomography

CT detects fractures in these sites much more effectively than conventional films; moreover, for the skull and facial bones, CT is appropriate to define additional radiographically occult fractures, even when conventional films reveal one or more fractures. Each case should be discussed with the radiologist, since CT can be "customized" for a given anatomic area.

In the spine, conventional radiographs and CT may reveal no fracture, yet underlying injury to the spinal cord itself and supporting ligaments may exist (see Chapter 32, Acute Spine Trauma). Therefore, **if CT is equivocal or if CT is normal and fails to explain trauma-related cord symptoms, MR is appropriate.**

Step 3: Magnetic Resonance Imaging

MR clearly defines spinal cord compression, ligamentous injuries, disk herniation(s), epidural hematoma, and nonhemorrhagic and hemorrhagic spinal cord contusion. **With the sole exception of fractures, virtually all significant spinal injuries are better defined by MR than by CT. Nonetheless, MR should not precede CT, because of CT's superiority in fracture detection.**

For fractures elsewhere, or where stress injury or "shin splints" are suspected:

Step 2: Nuclear Bone Scan

In some sites where subtle fractures are suspected, CT is not helpful, **and MR, although sensitive and specific, is not cost effective.** Moreover, where stress remodeling, stress fracture, or "shin splints" are in question, a bone scan is usually diagnostic.[3-6]

The bones are scanned after intravenous injection of a technetium-99m-labeled phosphate compound, usually methylene diphosphonate (MDP). In the conventional scan, images of the skeleton are obtained after 1 to 2 hours. Single photon emission computed tomography (SPECT) technology increases the sensitivity and resolution of the study but almost doubles its cost; therefore, SPECT is reserved for solving problems in equivocal cases.

Tc-99m-MDP accumulates in bone according to several parameters, primarily bone blood flow and metabolism. Various conditions—trauma, inflammation, neoplasm, arthritis, etc.—can induce profound changes in isotope uptake. Because the scan patterns of these conditions overlap, the bone scan is not specific, but because it easily detects small changes in pharmaceutical uptake, it is highly sensitive. Thus **a normal scan excludes a traumatic bony lesion with very high probability; an abnor-**

mal scan indicates a lesion, type often unknown. In the patient with suspected neoplasm, this lack of specificity may be a diagnostic dilemma, but when ruling out fracture this lack of specificity is rarely perplexing; **the suspected injuries are usually in areas free of previous bone disease, and the issue is whether the site is normal or abnormal. For this purpose the bone scan excels.** Increased radiopharmaceutical uptake occurs within 1 day, even in minor, undisplaced cortical fractures.

Sports-related injuries—stress remodeling, stress fracture, periosteal avulsion, and subperiosteal hemorrhage ("shin splints")—are usually defined.[3-6] However, a stress injury scanned **very early in its development** is sometimes missed on a bone scan; rescanning in one week, if pain persists, is effective. MR is as sensitive as bone scanning for the detection of bony stress injuries, and MR findings parallel the course of nuclear findings, but MR is not recommended for detecting stress injuries because of its greater cost.

SUMMARY AND CONCLUSIONS

1. The plain radiograph is the best initial study when fracture, stress injury (remodeling or stress fracture), or "shin splints" are suspected.
2. If the initial radiographs are normal, follow-up films in 10 to 14 days are often helpful in long, tubular bones; by that time fracture healing is usually evident.
3. Where the sequelae of fracture could be life-threatening, or in certain specific anatomic regions, CT is extremely valuable—particularly for the facial bones, base of the skull, the pelvis, and the spine. Radiologic consultation is appropriate to "customize" the CT study. In the spine MR may also be necessary to visualize the spinal cord and soft tissues, depending on the clinical status.

4. If the lesion is not clarified by—or appropriately evaluated by—CT, a bone scan is usually definitive. In most anatomic regions and populations, a negative scan excludes fracture, stress injury, or "shin splints" with virtual certainty. A positive scan, in an area free of pre-existing bone disease, is diagnostic.

5. For suspected hip fracture in the elderly, the greater cost of MR is probably justified, assuming that initial radiographs are normal or equivocal. In this anatomic site and population, a bone scan can justifiably be skipped.

REFERENCES

1. Deutsch AL, Mink JH, Waxman AD. Occult fractures of the proximal femur: MR imaging. Radiology 1989; 170:113-116.
2. Berger PE, Ofstein RA, Jackson DW. MRI demonstration of radiographically occult fractures: what have we been missing? RadioGraphics 1989; 9(3): 407-436.
3. Holder LE, Matthews L. The nuclear physician and sports medicine. In Freeman L, Weissman H, eds. Nuclear Medicine Annual 1984. New York, 1984, Raven Press, pp 81-140.
4. Matin PM. Bone scintigraphy in the diagnosis and management of traumatic injury. Semin Nucl Med 1983; 12:104-122.
5. McBryde AM. Stress fractures in runners. Clin Sports Med 1985; 4:737-752.
6. Norfray JF, Schlacter L, Kernahan WT, Arenson DJ, Smith SD, Roth LF, Schlefman BS. Early confirmation of stress fractures in joggers. JAMA 1980; 243:1647-1649.
7. Daffner RH, Pavlov H. Stress fractures: current concepts. AJR 1992; 159:245-252.
8. Lee JK, Yao L. Stress fractures: MR imaging. Radiology 1988; 169:217-220.
9. Liberman CM, Hemingway DL. Scintigraphy of shin splints. Clin Nucl Med 1980; 5:31.
10. Michael RH, Holder LE. The soleus syndrome: a cause for medial tibial stress (shin splints). Am J Sports Med 1985; 13:87-94.
11. Mubarak SJ, Gould RN, Yu FL, et al. The medial tibial stress syndrome. Am J Sports Med 1982; 10:201-205.

46

Early Osteoporosis

INTRODUCTION

For women, risk factors for osteoporosis include post-menopausal status, oophorectomy, low body fat, and nul-liparity; for both men and women, risk factors include Caucasian or Asian origin, family history, small bones, low calcium intake, inactivity, poor calcium absorption, gluco-corticoid therapy, anticonvulsant therapy, hypoparathy-roidism, thyrotoxicosis, renal failure, advanced age, and heavy alcohol or tobacco use.

Osteoporosis is detectable on radiographs only when skeletal calcium loss reaches 30% to 45%. Therefore, radi-ographs are appropriate for **advanced** osteoporosis or its sequelae (e.g., compression fractures of the spine) but not for asymptomatic, **early** osteoporosis. Two different noninvasive methodologies have been developed for evaluation of early bone mineral loss: quantitative computed tomography (QCT) and absorptiometry of X-ray photons (DEXA) or gamma rays (DPA). All of these methods are generally termed "bone mineral analysis" or "bone densitometry."

Bone densitometry can identify individuals at high risk for fracture, so that therapy to augment bone mineral—or at least arrest bone mineral loss—can be instituted. Low bone mineral readings on DEXA correlate with increased fracture rates, although such a direct correlation has not been proved to date for QCT.

Costs: QCT, $217; DEXA, $132.

PLAN AND RATIONALE

The efficacies of QCT and absorptiometry are approximately equal. In the majority of locations, DEXA or DPA are more readily available and somewhat less expensive than QCT. Both DPA and DEXA are rapid and reliable, but DEXA is faster and more reliable than DPA, so that all manufacturers of DPA equipment have now switched to DEXA. The radiation dose delivered by DEXA is lower than that of QCT or DPA.

Step 1: Dual X-ray absorptiometry or, if unavailable, dual photon absorptiometry

DEXA and DPA measure the absorption of X-rays generated by a highly stable X-ray tube or gamma rays from a radioactive source as they pass through selected portions of the body, usually the lumbar spine or hip. Both techniques use a lower energy photon and a higher energy photon; absorption of the higher and lower energy photons by bone and soft tissue, respectively, is measured. Well-mineralized bone absorbs more energy than demineralized bone, and bone density can be quantitated after a correction is made for soft tissue absorption.

Both DEXA and DPA measure the conglomerate bone density of the spine and hip, without separating the measurements into trabecular and cortical bone. This disadvantage is more theoretical than practical. Degenerative change of the lumbar spine with osteophyte formation can reduce the accuracy of both techniques.

Usually, results are reported in absolute and relative terms, including a comparison of the patient's bone mineral to that of an age- and sex-matched group and a young normal (30-year-old) population. Comparison of the patient's bone mineral to the "fracture threshold" (i.e., the bone mineral at which fracture is likely) is usually included. Traditionally, both DEXA and DPA are performed **in nuclear medicine departments.**

Where DEXA or DPA are unavailable:

Step 1: Quantitative Computed Tomography

QCT is perfomed on a standard CT scanner but requires special software and materials of standardized density (called a "calibration phantom") that are scanned concurrently with the patient. The computer compares the density of the patient's spine or hip with that of the reference standards. Like DPA or DEXA, QCT results are reported in both absolute and relative terms. QCT of both the lumbar spine and the hip is possible, but hip measurement is considerably more complex; therefore, most often QCT is limited to the lumbar spine.

Unlike DPA, QCT can differentiate trabecular from cortical bone; in most institutions only trabecular values are reported. Trabecular density is theoretically more important, because trabecular bone turnover is more dynamic and is a better measurement of active demineralization. In practical terms, however, trabecular determinations have no proven advantage.

The radiation dose of QCT is higher than that of DEXA.

SUMMARY AND CONCLUSIONS

1. Standard radiographs are extremely insensitive for bone mineral loss and cannot screen for early osteoporosis.
2. DPA, DEXA, and QCT are effective for evaluating bone mineral density. DPA and DEXA are usually more readily available and less expensive than QCT.

3. DEXA is faster, more reliable, and more available than DPA. Therefore, DEXA is preferred.
4. Serial bone mineral determinations are appropriate to follow the course of bone loss or the reponse to therapy.

ADDITIONAL COMMENTS

- Historically, the treatment for osteoporosis has involved conservative, well-established therapies, including supplemental calcium and vitamin D, weight-bearing exercise, elimination of cigarettes and excessive alcohol, and estrogens. **However, no regimen was considered to reliably build bone mineral.** Recently, numerous reports have proven that oral diphosphonate therapy, originally developed for treatment of Paget's disease, unbalances the normal bone resorption–deposition cycle in favor of deposition, by inactivating osteoclasts; the therapy is very rarely associated with serious side effects. The deposition of bone mineral can be objectively measured **and also correlates with fewer fractures of the lumbar spine in clinical trials.** Similar results have been reported with calcitonin, which must be administered parenterally and is extremely expensive, about $4000 per patient per year.

SUGGESTED ADDITIONAL READING

Faulkner KG, Gluer, CC, Majumdar S, et al. Noninvasive measurements of bone mass, structure, and strength: current methods and experimental techniques. AJR 1991; 157:1229-1237.

Feyerabend AJ, Lear JL. Regional variations in bone mineral density as assessed with duel-energy photon absorptiometry and dual X-ray absorptiometry. Radiology 1993; 186:467.

Genant HK, Cann CE, Ettinger B, Gordon GS. Quantitative computed tomography of vertebral spongiosa: a sensitive method for detecting early bone loss after oophorectomy. Ann Intern Med 1982; 97:699-705.

Gillespy T III, Gillespy MP. Osteoporosis. Radiol Clin North Am 1991; 29:77-83.

Gluer C-C, Steiger P, Selvidge, R, et al. Comparative assessment of dual-photon absorptiometry and dual-energy radiography. Radiology 1990; 174:223-228.

Grampp S, Jergas M, Gluer C-C, et al. Radiologic diagnosis of osteo-porosis: current methods and perspectives. Radiol Clin North Am 1993; 31:1133-1145.

Lang P, Steiger P, Faulkner K, et al. Osteoporosis: current techniques and recent developments in quantitaive bone densitometry. Radiol Clin North Am 1991; 13:11.

Reinbold W, Genant HK, Reiser UJ, Harris ST, Ettinger B. Bone mineral content in early-postmenopausal and postmenopausal osteoporotic women: comparison of measurement methods. Radiology 1986; 160:469-478.

Riggs BL, Melton LJ. Involutional osteoporosis. N Engl J Med 1986; 314:1676-1686.

Silberstein EB, Schnur W. Cyclic oral phosphate and etidronate increase femoral and lumbar bone mineral density and reduce lum-bar spine fracture rate over three years. J Nucl Med 1992; 33:1.

47

Prosthesis Failure

INTRODUCTION

In our aging population, prosthetic hip and knee replacements abound. The long-term results of most prosthetic surgery are overwhelmingly favorable, but a significant number of patients develop complications, most often pain and/or limited mobility as a result of prosthetic loosening or infection. Imaging can detect and characterize such complications; the relevant techniques are plain films, arthrography, nuclear bone scanning, and infrequently other nuclear studies (indium-111-autologous leukocyte [WBC], gallium-67-citrate, and Tc-99m-sulfur colloid scans).

Costs: bone scan, without SPECT, $387; bone scan, with SPECT, $651; nuclear WBC scan, $505; knee films, $66; hip films, $69; hip arthrogram, $371; knee arthrogram, $330; gallium-67 scan, without SPECT, $358; gallium-67 scan, SPECT, $745; colloid marrow nuclear scan, $279.

PLAN AND RATIONALE

Step 1: Plain Radiographs

Plain radiographs are the best initial study for a painful hip or knee prosthesis. Plain films can reveal many causes of pain: heterotopic bone formation, methacrylate cement fracture, bone fracture, prosthesis fracture, gross prosthesis malpositioning (resulting from major loosening), dislocation, and extensive bone destruction (from major loosening or infection). Often, further imaging is not required, but additional studies are appropriate: (1) when loosening and/or infection is suspected despite a normal plain film, (2) when the cause of radiographic loosening must be characterized as infectious or mechanical, and (3) to clarify equivocal plain film interpretations—that is, "probable" or "possible" loosening.[1]

Step 2: Arthrography with Joint Aspiration

The joint space is entered percutaneously, fluid is aspirated, and contrast material is injected. The purposes of arthrography with joint aspiration are (1) to document the correct intraarticular location of the aspiration needle by injection of contrast material into the joint, (2) to obtain joint fluid for culture and gram stain, and (3) to diagnose loosening by filling any abnormal spaces created by loosening and/or infection with contrast material.

If loosening with infection is proven, the imaging workup stops. However, if loosening is documented and the joint aspirate is sterile, **infection is not necessarily excluded**; in fact, the sensitivity of joint fluid aspiration for infection is variable.[2-4] If the orthopedic surgeon requires a high presurgical confidence level regarding the presence or absence of infection, nuclear studies for infection can be helpful.

Uncommonly, both plain films and arthrography can miss loosening and/or infection. In the presence of pain, negative arthrography and plain films are followed by a nuclear bone scan.

When plain films and arthrography are negative, in the presence of pain:

Step 3a: Bone Scan

A technetium-99m (Tc-99m)-labeled phosphate compound, usually methylene diphosphonate (MDP), is injected intravenously; 1 to 2 hours later the entire skeleton is imaged. Additional selected high-resolution views may be obtained of any particular area of interest. Most of the MDP ultimately accumulates in the crystalline structure of bone, in proportion to bone perfusion, which, in turn, is a function of the bone's metabolic status. Almost all bone lesions—including old or recent trauma, acute or chronic osteomyelitis, inflammatory or degenerative arthritis, and metabolic bone disease—appear "hot," because these lesions increase bone metabolism and thus local blood flow to bone.

The bone scan is highly sensitive for detection of prosthesis loosening or infection, but an abnormal bone scan is nonspecific. Therefore the scan is useful for excluding significant inflammatory or mechanical disease, and a negative bone scan strongly reinforces negative plain films and arthrography. If all of these imaging procedures are normal, the workup for loosening and/or infection ends. However, if the scan is abnormal, revealing "hot" areas, then more specific nuclear studies may follow to establish whether infection is present, if the orthopedic surgeon requires that information before surgery (see **Step 3b**, below).

When previous studies are negative or equivocal for infection, despite clinical evidence of infection:

Step 3b: Labeled Autologous Leukocytes, Gallium-67 Citrate, or Tc-99m Sulfur Colloid

Various algorithms have been developed for using and interpreting these studies singly or in combination when joint/prosthesis infection is in question. Even among nuclear physicians the best combination is often a matter of dispute, and the choice usually depends on local availability and experience. Consultation with the nuclear imager at this point is mandatory.

SUMMARY AND CONCLUSIONS

1. A plain film is the best initial study for a painful prosthesis. The plain film may reveal major prosthesis problems (cement or bony fracture, marked prosthesis malposition, gross bone destruction, etc.), ending the imaging workup.
2. If plain films are normal, joint aspiration with arthrography is typically performed in all patients with suspected prosthesis loosening and/or infection. In many cases arthrography is appropriate even when the plain films reveal loosening, to help exclude infection.
3. An arthrogram that reveals loosening and infection ends the workup, but if only loosening is proven and infection remains suspect, further nuclear studies may then be appropriate. The nuclear physician should be consulted as to which study or combination of studies (labeled autologous leukocytes, gallium-67 citrate, or Tc-99m sulfur colloid) is appropriate.
4. Negative plain films, arthrography, and joint aspiration **in a symptomatic patient** are typically followed by a bone scan, because **in a few cases loosening is missed by both plain films and arthrography;** a normal bone scan ends the workup, but an abnormal

and nonspecific bone scan may require further nuclear studies (labeled autologous leukocytes, gallium-67 citrate, or Tc-99m sulfur colloid).

ADDITIONAL COMMENTS

- Computed tomography and magnetic resonance imaging have no clearly established role in the evaluation of the painful prosthesis.
- Increased uptake of bone-seeking radiopharmaceutical normally occurs for about 6 months after the insertion of a hip or knee prosthesis; therefore, bone scanning is not helpful until 6 months have passed after surgery.

REFERENCES

1. Rabin DN, Smith C, Kubica RA, et al. Problem prostheses: the radiologic evaluation of total joint replacement. RadioGraphics 1987; 7:1107-1127.
2. Hendrix RW, Anderson TM. Arthrographic and radiologic evaluation of prosthetic joints. Radiol Clin North Am 1981; 19:349-364.
3. Johnson JA,Christie MJ, Sandler MP, et al. Detection of occult infection following total joint arthroplasty using sequential technetium-99m HDP bone scintigraphy and Indium 111 WBC imaging. J Nucl Med 1988; 29:1347-1353.
4. Weiss PE, Mall JC, Hoffer PB, Murray WR, Rodrigo JJ, Genant HK. Tc99m methylene diphosphonate bone imaging in the evaluation of total hip prostheses. Radiology 1979; 133:727-729.
5. Gelman Ml, Coleman RE, Stevens PM, Davey BW. Radiology, radionuclide imaging, and arthrography in the evaluation of total hip and knee replacement. Radiology 1978; 128:677-682.
6. Williamson BRJ, McLaughlin RE, Wang GJ, Miller CW, Teates CD, Bray ST. Radionuclide imaging as a means of differentiating loosening and infection in patients with a painful total hip prosthesis. Radiology 1979; 133:723-725.
7. Schneider R, Abenavoli AM, Soudry M, Insall J. Failure of total condylar knee replacement: correlation of radiographic, clinical, and surgical findings. Radiology 1984; 152:309-315.
8. Weissman BN. Radiology of joint replacement surgery. Radiol Clin North Am 1990; 28(5):1111-1132.

48

The Physically Abused Child

INTRODUCTION

Dr. John Caffey described an association between subdural hematomas and skeletal injury in infants nearly 50 years ago[1]; since that time an immense body of literature has addressed the clinical and radiologic diagnosis of physical child abuse. Heightened physician awareness and improvements in imaging have facilitated the diagnosis.

Prompt identification of the "battered child" requires a high index of suspicion, especially when (1) a child (usually less than 6 years old) is brought by a caretaker to the physician with skeletal, central nervous system, soft tissue, or other injuries out of proportion to the reported history and (2) when physical findings include human bites, thermal burns, multiple soft tissue injuries in various stages of healing, unexplained seizures, or psychologic/emotional depression.

The radiographic skeletal survey, nuclear bone scan, chest film, abdominal film, computed tomography without intravenous contrast medium (unenhanced CT), and magnetic resonance imaging without intravenous contrast medium (unenhanced MR) can contribute to the workup.

Costs: radiographic skeletal survey, $175; bone scan, without SPECT, $270; head CT, unenhanced, $287;

brain MR, unenhanced, $845; chest films, PA and lateral, $59; abdominal films, $57.

PLAN AND RATIONALE

(A) When clinical suspicion of physical child abuse exists and the presentation does not suggest intracranial or thoracoabdominal injury:

Step 1: Radiographic Skeletal Survey

Skeletal injury is the most common radiologic finding in the "battered child"; therefore, complete evaluation of the bones is necessary. Skull (AP and lateral), chest (frontal and lateral), and lumbar spine (lateral) films are mandatory, as well as frontal views of the humeri, femora, forearms, tibias, hands, feet, and pelvis. Extra views may be requested by the radiologist. **A single image of the entire infant, the "babygram," is inadequate and therefore inappropriate. Furthermore, radiographic examination of only the suspected sites of injury decreases the sensitivity and specificity of the workup.**
Although solitary long bone fractures are common in abused children, they are not specific. However, some findings are highly suggestive, including fractures in various stages of repair, fractures at specific sites that are unlikely to be accidentally injured (e.g., posterior ribs, sternum, scapula, vertebrae, vertebral spinous processes), and certain metaphyseal fractures. In fact, because of their etiologic mechanism, avulsion of a metaphyseal fragment by the adherent periosteum following torsion on a long bone, metaphyseal fractures, called "corner" or "bucket handle fractures," are virtually diagnostic of physical abuse.[2] **Although far less specific (but more common) than multiple or metaphyseal fractures, soli-**

tary fractures of a long bone should be viewed with great suspicion in the nonambulating infant.

If the skeletal survey supports the impression of child abuse, the workup generally ends, unless injury to other organs is suspected. If the initial radiographs are equivocal or normal, then a bone scan may be appropriate.

Step 2: Bone Scan

Although most authorities recommend a skeletal survey as the first step in the workup, because of its universal availability on an emergency basis and superior specificity **the bone scan is more sensitive for subtle or occult injuries, especially of the ribs, spine, and long bone diaphyses.**[2] Moreover, the study may incidentally reveal soft tissue lesions like rhabdomyolysis and, because the bone-seeking radiopharmaceutical may accumulate in parenchymal hematomas or contusions, occasionally detects unsuspected thoracic, brain, or abdominal injuries.[3]

(B) When the clinical status suggests an acute intracranial injury (i.e., depressed mental status, focal neurologic deficit, or delayed mental development):

Step 1: Computed Tomography

Intracranial injury is the major cause of morbidity and mortality in physically abused children.

Unenhanced CT is the first study in the child with acute head injury and/or neurologic deficit. Depressed skull fractures, extracerebral fluid collections—subdural and epidural hematomas, subarachnoid hemorrhages—as well as parenchymal injuries, including edema, hemorrhage, contusion, and laceration, are readily detected. CT is more widely available than MR, less expensive,

and more technically feasible in the acute head trauma setting. Also, when CT of the thorax or abdomen is indicated, the study can easily continue to include these areas. If abnormalities detected by CT explain the acute neurologic signs and symptoms, the imaging workup ends. However, if clinical signs and symptoms are out of proportion to CT findings (e.g., normal or slightly abnormal CT in an obtunded battered infant), MR is indicated.[4]

Step 2: Magnetic Resonance Imaging

MR clearly defines a number of important acute CNS injuries—notably brain stem hemorrhagic and nonhemorrhagic contusions and diffuse axonal injuries—that CT can miss.

(C) When the clinical status suggests a chronic intracranial abnormalitiy:

Step 1: Magnetic Resonance Imaging

Children may present with impaired physical and/or mental development or other neurologic abnormalities years after trauma. MR should be the initial study in the **nonacute** head trauma setting because of its greater sensitivity for virtually all chronic CNS injuries, including hemorrhagic and nonhemorrhagic contusions, diffuse axonal injuries, and small subdural hematomas. MR is able to **estimate the age of hematomas**, which is especially important. (Subdural hematomas of various ages indicate repetitive intracranial injury.)

(D) When thoracic and/or abdominal injury is suspected:

Step 1: Chest and Abdominal Plain Films

About 3% of injuries in battered children evaluated radiographically involve the chest or abdomen.[3] **Standard chest films are necessary when chest trauma is suspected, regardless of whether a skeletal survey has preceded the chest/abdomen workup.** Although CT is more sensitive than plain radiography for the detection of most chest trauma, it is, in fact, rarely needed in the physically abused child. Most serious thoracic injury will be apparent on plain films; therefore, in all but the most unusual cases the workup ends with plain films. If abnormal findings require clarification, then CT of the thorax may be indicated; this circumstance is most uncommon and must be tailored by the radiologist.

Evaluation of the abdomen begins with plain supine and erect films. If the plain abdominal films are normal, CT or ultrasound may at times be needed; **their appropriateness depends entirely on the type of organ damage sought**. Moreover, a variety of other studies, including cystography and GI examinations, may be necessary. Extremely close consultation between the radiologist and clinician is mandatory, to avoid unnecessary delay, expense, and studies.

SUMMARY AND CONCLUSIONS

1. A skeletal survey is the initial examination in children suspected of suffering from physical abuse, except in the setting of **acute** head or thoracoabdominal trauma. Bone scanning is supplementary.
2. **CT is the primary exam in children with suspected acute intracranial injury**. If CT is inadequate to explain signs/symptoms or if CT findings require clarification, MR is appropriate.

3. MR is the initial exam in the stable child with a **chronic** neurologic deficit because of its superiority in defining virtually all chronic central nervous system injuries.
4. In suspected thoracoabdominal injury, plain films are first. CT can clarify suspected abnormalities on the chest radiograph, yet it is rarely used when the initial chest films for trauma are normal. If abdominal injury is suspected, follow-up CT, ultrasound, or other specialized organ-specific studies are often necessary.

ADDITIONAL COMMENTS

- Although skeletal findings like metaphyseal fractures of the "corner" or "bucket handle" type are virtually pathognomonic of battering, other findings like diaphyseal fracture and periosteal thickening are nonspecific. Such lesions should engender a high index of suspicion, but inaccurate and premature diagnosis—reached without correlating clinical and historical data—is a significant danger.
- Although skull fractures and **intracranial** injury correlate very poorly, the **rarity** of skull fractures in **accidental** head injury makes skull films crucial to the diagnosis of physical abuse.
- Subdural hematomas are common after battering, and an interhemispheric location supports a nonaccidental cause.[5]

REFERENCES

1. Caffey J. Multiple fractures in the long bones of infants suffering from chronic subdural hematoma. AJR 1946; 56:163-173.
2. Kleinman PK Diagnostic Imaging of Child Abuse. Baltimore, 1987, Williams & Wilkins, pp 6-20, 24-27, 221-240.

3. Howard JL, Barron BJ, Smith GG: Bone scintigraphy in the evaluation of extraskeletal injuries from child abuse. RadioGraphics 1990; 10:67-81.
4. Sato Y, Yuh WT, Smith WL. Head in jury in child abuse: evaluation with MR Imaging. Radiology 1989; 173:653.
5. Zimmerman RA, Bilavivk LT, Bruie D, et al. Interhemispheric acute subdural hematoma: a computed tomographic manifestation of child abuse by shaking. Neuroradiology 1978; 16:39-40.

49

Avascular Necrosis of the Hip

INTRODUCTION

Avascular necrosis (also called osteonecrosis or aseptic necrosis) most commonly affects the hip. Ischemic injury is probably responsible, although its exact pathophysiology is unknown. Multiple risk factors include trauma, alcoholism, sickle cell disease, steroids, and pancreatitis; no risk factors exist in many patients.[3] Untreated AVN of the hip almost always worsens; subchondral fracture, collapse of the femoral head, and secondary arthritis result. Imaging helps to detect early hip AVN, monitor its evolution, and guide therapy.

Plain films, magnetic resonance imaging (MR), and nuclear bone scanning play a role in the workup.

Costs: hip plain films, $69; hips complete MR, unenhanced, $873; hips screening coronal MR, $400; bone scan, SPECT, $651.

PLAN AND RATIONALE

The adult with suspected AVN of the hip:

Step 1: Hip Radiographs

By the time AVN is detected on hip radiographs, the disease is usually advanced. However, hip films are appropriate in the initial workup, because they may be diagnostic and also help to exclude a hip fracture.

If hip radiographs are negative or demonstrate unilateral AVN:

Step 2: Magnetic Resonance Imaging

MR is the most sensitive imaging test for detection of early hip AVN. Even if radiographs detect unilateral AVN, MR is indicated to check for an earlier stage of AVN **on the contralateral side**; 20% to 50% of AVN is bilateral.[1,2]

MR can screen asymptomatic individuals at high risk. A single series of screening coronal images is rapid and relatively inexpensive; if these are positive, additional images follow.[1] Although some authorities advocate a bone scan before MR, screening MR provides much more anatomic information, is more specific, and is priced comparably to a SPECT bone scan. MR also determines the exact location and extent of disease, which may help the orthopedic surgeon plan therapy (see **ADDITIONAL COMMENTS**). Serial MRs can monitor the efficacy of therapy.

The child with suspected idiopathic AVN (Legg-Calve-Perthes disease):

Step 1: Hip Radiographs

Legg-Calve-Perthes (LCP) disease, or idiopathic avascular necrosis of the capital femoral epiphysis, most commonly affects young males (4 to 8 years old). Plain films should be first. Findings of LCP include medial widening of the joint space, subchondral fracture, and increased density of the femoral capital epiphysis.[3]

If hip radiographs are negative but early LCP is suspected:

Step 2: Magnetic Resonance Imaging

MR should follow plain fims in the child with a high clinical suspicion of LCP. MR is highly accurate for detecting and staging the disease and for monitoring a therapeutic response. Furthermore, MR produces excellent anatomically detailed images of both hips and can define other causes of hip pain **involving both bone and soft tissue. Sedation may be required in many cases,** since scanning times are relatively long.

Despite its sensitivity, **occasionally MR will be negative in strongly suspected early LCP**. A nuclear bone scan is then appropriate.

Step 2: Nuclear Bone Scan

The bone scan is highly sensitive for early LCP,[3] but unlike MR, it does not visualize the soft tissues, and the anatomic detail of the images is poor.

Technetium-99m methylene diphosphonate (Tc-99m-MDP) is injected intravenously, and 2 hours later the skeleton is scanned by a gamma camera. Tc-99m-MDP accumulates in bone in proportion to bone metabolism and blood flow. When the study is augmented by single photon emission computed tomography (SPECT), its sensitivity is markedly increased. Unfortunately, SPECT virtually doubles the cost of the study.

Unlike adults with AVN, a minority of children with early LCP will have a normal MR yet a positive bone scan, manifested by a focal area of decreased Tc-99m-MDP accumulation in the capital femoral epiphysis.[3]

If the bone scan is also normal, the workup ends.

SUMMARY AND CONCLUSIONS

1. Hip radiographs should be first in suspected AVN.
2. If hip radiographs are negative or demonstrate unilateral AVN **in an adult or child**, MR is appropriate. A screening MR—a single series of coronal images of both hips—is rapid and relatively inexpensive. If AVN is present, the MR findings are usually specific.
3. If hip radiographs and MR are negative yet early LCP is strongly suspected **in a child**, a SPECT bone scan should be considered.
4. MR more accurately stages LCP than a bone scan, defines various other soft tissue lesions, and can monitor the evolution of LCP and its response to therapy.

ADDITIONAL COMMENTS

- Although the bone scan—particularly with SPECT—detects AVN earlier than plain films, its false negative rate approaches 18%.[4] By the time a bone scan is positive, even if radiographs are normal, AVN may be relatively advanced.
- Very early AVN may be missed even by MR; if a patient is at very high risk for AVN and MR is negative, a bone scan might be performed, because **an occasional patient with AVN may have a falsely negative MR and a positive bone scan**[5]; alternatively, the MR could be repeated after a short interval, especially if the hip remains painful.
- Therapy of AVN of the hip is controversial. Most authorities, however, agree that **early detection of AVN is the goal, before subchondral fracture develops**. MR can determine the extent of femoral head involvement and the exact location of disease, use-

ful information to the orthopedic surgeon. Core decompression is a more conservative surgical treatment for AVN than total hip replacement; while its role in treating hip AVN remains controversial, some studies have shown a much better outcome of early core decompression when less than 25% of the femoral head is affected.[6,7]

- A few recent studies suggest that MR with intravenous contrast medium (contrast enhanced) can differentiate viable from nonviable bone, increasing the specificity of MR for early AVN.[8]

- Although CT detects AVN of the hip earlier than plain films, it is less sensitive than both MR and bone scanning and has no role in routine patient workup.

REFERENCES

1. Beltran J. MR imaging of avascular necrosis: an update. In Syllabus, Categorical Course on Body Magnetic Resonance Imaging, ACR annual meeting, Sept. 1993, pp 9-11.
2. Mitchell MD, Kundel HL, Steinberg ME, Kressel HY, Alavi A, Axel L. Avascular necrosis of the hip: comparison of MR, CT, and scintigraphy. AJR 1986; 147:67-71.
3. Goldman AB, Schneider R. Clinical pitfalls in MR imaging of the hips and pelvis. In RSNA Categorical Course in Musculoskeletal Radiology 1993, pp 155-166.
4. Mitchell DG, Rao VM, Dalinka MK, et al. Femoral head avascular necrosis: correlation of MR imaging, radiograpic staging, radionuclide imaging, and clinical findings. Radiology 1987; 162:709-715.
5. Totty WG. MR imaging of the hip. In RSNA Categorical Course in Musculoskeletal Radiology 1993, pp 127-140.
6. Lafforgue P, Dahan E, Chagnaud C, et al. Early-stage avascular necrosis of the femoral head: MR imaging for prognosis in 31 cases with at least 2 years of follow-up. Radiology 1993; 187:199-204.
7. Beltran J, Knight CT, Zuelzer WA, et al. Core decompression for avascular necrosis of the femoral head: correlation between long-term results and preoperative MR staging. Radiology 1990; 175:533-536.

8. Berg BV, Malghem J, Labaisse MA, Noel H, Maldague B. Avascular necrosis of the hip: comparison of contrast-enhanced and nonenhanced MR imaging with histologic correlation [Work in progress] Radiology 1992; 182:445-450.

SUGGESTED ADDITIONAL READING

Coleman BG, Kressel HY, Dalinka MK, et al. Radiographically negative avascular necrosis: detection with MR imaging. Radiology 1988; 168:525-528.

Collier BD, Carrera GF, Johnson RP, et al. Detection of femoral head avascular necrosis in adults by SPECT. J Nucl Med 1985; 26:479-487.

Conway WF, Hayes CW, Daniel WW. Bone marrow edema pattern on MR images: transient osteoporosis or early osteonecrosis of bone? In RSNA Categorical Course in Musculoskeletal Radiology 1993, pp 141-154.

Dalinka MK. Avascular necrosis—osteonecrosis. In Resnick D, Pettersson H, eds. Skeletal Radiology. NICER Series on Diagnostic Imaging. London, England, Merit Communications, 1992, pp 515-525.

Genez BM, Wilson MR, Houk RW, et al. Early osteonecrosis of the femoral head: detection in high-risk patients with MR imaging. Radiology 1988; 168:521-524.

Markisz JA, Knowles RJR, Altchek DW. Segmental patterns of avascular necrosis of the femoral heads: early detection with MR imaging. Radiology 1987; 162:717-720.

Palmer EL, Scott JA, Strauss HW. Practical Nuclear Medicine. Philadelphia, Saunders 1992, pp 150-152.

50

Hip Disorders in Children

INTRODUCTION

The various hip disorders of children follow a fairly typical age distribution: congenital dislocation of the hip (CDH) affects neonates and young infants; Legg-Calve-Perthes' disease, 4 to 7 year olds; slipped capital femoral epiphysis, early adolescents. Septic arthritis involves a broader age group, mostly between 6 months and 12 years of age.[1] Early diagnosis is crucial for each of these disorders; delay in treatment can result in irreversible necrosis, hip deformity/destruction, and secondary degenerative arthritis. Plain films, ultrasound (US), computed tomography (CT), magnetic resonance imaging (MR), and bone scanning play a diagnostic role.

Costs: hip ultrasound, bilateral, $201; plain films of the hips, bilateral, $87; CT, limited study, $300.

SUSPECTED CONGENITAL DISLOCATION OF THE HIP

PLAN AND RATIONALE

Risk factors for CDH include breech presentation, maternal oligohydramnios, and a positive family history; girls are more commonly affected than boys by a ratio of about 8:1.[2] Imaging is indicated when clinical suspicion is raised by physical findings (on the Ortolani or Barlow maneuvers) or by the presence of risk factors.

The imaging workup depends on the patient's age at presentation.

For infants less than 1 year of age:

Step 1: Ultrasound

US is up to 100% sensitive and specific[3] for infants with suspected CDH. Its advantages over conventional radiography include no ionizing radiation, direct visualization of the soft tissues and cartilaginous structures of the hip, and the ability to image the hip dynamically and in multiple planes **as stress is applied to initiate dislocation. This last feature gives US the unique ability to dynamically image the unstable hip, which may appear normal on static plain films.** Moreover, the femoral head does not normally ossify before 4 to 7 months of age,[2] and ossification is often delayed in patients with CDH; thus **plain films cannot directly visualize the the femoral head of a young infant.** US can also assess whether the hip can be fully and concentrically reduced and can quantify the presence and degree of acetabular dysplasia, both of which are important for treatment planning. If an experienced sonographer of infants is not available, the patient should be referred elsewhere when feasible.

For infants under 4 to 7 months, a normal US ends the workup. If infant sonography is not available, plain films combined with close follow-up are a less optimal alternative.

From 6 to 12 months progressive ossification of the femoral head limits US and the value of plain films increases; in this age group, a normal **technically adequate** US ends the workup, but plain films may be required if US is technically limited. Normal plain films end the workup.

If US or plain films indicate CDH, therapy is warranted.

For infants 1 year of age or older:

Step 1: Plain Films

As progresssive femoral head ossification occurs, the accuracy and utility of US progressively diminish; by 6 to 12 months plain films assume a primary role.[4] They can determine the location of the ossified femoral heads and the degree of dislocation and acetabular dysplasia (both usually irreversible by this age). Anteroposterior (AP) and a frog-leg lateral films may be supplemented by special additional views that initiate dislocation of an unstable hip (e.g., the Von Rosen view).

MONITORING THERAPY OF CDH:

The uncomplicated, easily reducible dislocated hip is usually treated by splinting or a harness, which maintain the hips in an abducted and externally rotated position. However, significant acetabular dysplasia and irreducibility usually require surgical intervention (open reduction and pelvic osteotomy) followed by casting. Serial imaging studies during treatment are important to ensure the continued adequacy of reduction.

US is effective for patients in a splint or harness, with a baseline plain film at some point during treatment. Evaluation of infants in a cast is more difficult; although some specialized centers advocate US through a "window" cut in the cast, limited CT through the hip joints is more accessible and reproducible. Plain films can fail to detect subtle changes or posterior dislocation during therapy, and optimal evaluation is limited by the cast material.

SUMMARY AND CONCLUSIONS

1. US of the hips is appropriate for the infant less than 1 year of age with suspected CDH. If an experienced sonographer of infants is not available, the patient should be referred elsewhere or, if this is not feasible, studied with plain films and followed closely.
2. Plain films are the first study in infants 1 year of age or older and play a complementary role at 6 to 12 months of age, as the femoral heads ossify.
3. Patients treated by operative reduction and casting should be followed by limited CT **or** US through a window in the cast; plain film evaluation is limited in these patients.
4. Patients treated by closed reduction and harness or splint are followed by US, with a baseline AP radiograph of the pelvis at some point during therapy.

ADDITIONAL COMMENTS

- **Magnetic resonance imaging (MR) has no clearly established primary role in the diagnosis and treatment of CDH.** Although MR provides a wealth of anatomic information, it does not currently offer **dynamic assessment of hip stability,** is expensive, and requires sedation or anesthesia. For these reasons, MR should be reserved for those treated patients (10% to 20%) who develop suspected osteonecrosis of the femoral head.
- Arthrography is rarely, if ever, indicated in the initial evaluation of CDH. The procedure is commonly performed intraoperatively to assess the acetabular labrum and femoral head during open reduction.

SLIPPED CAPITAL FEMORAL EPIPHYSIS (SCFE)

PLAN AND RATIONALE

Most SCFE is thought to be posttraumatic, although only 50% of patients have a history of known injury.[2] About 50% of patients have hip pain **and 25% have referred knee pain**.[2] Risk factors include renal osteodystrophy with secondary hyperparathyroidism and previous radiation therapy involving the hip.

Step 1: Plain Films

Plain films are usually diagnostic and are almost always the only exam required in suspected SCFE. Anteroposterior (AP) and frog-leg lateral views of the pelvis, including both hips, are necessary. **SCFE is usually more apparent on the frog-lateral film, which is essential.** The contralateral hip is included as a basis for comparison and to detect bilateral disease (about 25%).[1]

The femoral head typically slips posteriorly and medially with respect to the femoral neck. Plain film findings include abnormal alignment of the femoral neck and head, widening of the growth plate, and occasional regional osteoporosis. Normal plain films end the workup.

SUMMARY AND CONCLUSIONS

1. Plain films, including AP and frog-leg lateral films of both hips, are the definitive imaging study for SCFE.

ADDITIONAL COMMENTS

- CT is rarely needed in the evaluation of SCFE. Preoperatively, CT can quantify the **exact** degree and direction of slippage, but estimation by plain films is almost always sufficient.

• The goal of treatment is to prevent further slippage by stabilizing the growth plate, usually by surgically placing cannulated pins across the growth plate, although other techniques are sometimes used. CT or fluoroscopy can detect penetration of the femoral head's articular cartilage by the pins. **Manipulation and attempted reduction of SCFE are contraindicated, since this significantly increases the risk of avascular necrosis.** Most cases are pinned in situ. Prompt evaluation by an orthopedic surgeon is necessary.

THE CHILD WITH AN "IRRITABLE HIP"

PLAN AND RATIONALE

The differential diagnosis of an "irritable hip" is broad, including Legg-Calve-Perthes disease (see Chapter 49), septic arthritis, osteomyelitis, transient synovitis, and less commonly juvenile rheumatoid arthritis (JRA), fracture, and neoplasm. Imaging is indicated in the workup of all children with an "irritable hip" (i.e. refusal to bear weight on a leg, limp, and pain). The goal of imaging is to differentiate septic arthritis, which is a surgical emergency, from nonsurgical problems.

Step 1. Plain Films

An anteroposterior (AP) view is always the first step. Unilateral widening of the medial joint space of the symptomatic hip strongly suggests a joint effusion, an important yet nonspecific finding that is seen in multiple conditions: septic arthritis, osteomyelitis, hemarthrosis, JRA, osteoid osteoma, and Legg-Calve-Perthes disease.

Normal plain films in the patient with a low likelihood of septic arthritis usually end the imaging workup, although close clinical observation is warranted. However, **a normal plain film in no way excludes joint fluid, infection, or other significant lesions and therefore, in the patient with a high clinical index of suspicion for septic arthritis, ultrasound is the next appropriate step.**

An abnormal plain film in the context of strong clinical suspicion of septic arthritis will lead to either emergency drainage of the hip or US to confirm the presence of joint fluid (presumeably pus) before surgery.

Step 2: Ultrasound

US detects joint fluid, which (although nonspecific) supports the diagnosis of infection in the appropriate context. **If no fluid is present, septic arthritis is excluded with a high level of certainty,**[5] and other conditions like osteomyelitis, Legg-Calve-Perthes (LCP) disease, or retroperitoneal abscess are considered (see Chapters 43, 49, and 59). If present, joint fluid can be aspirated under US guidance, and if it is purulent, open drainage follows.[5] However, US-guided aspiration requires sedation or anesthesia; therefore, some orthopedic surgeons opt for direct emergency open surgical drainage.

SUMMARY AND CONCLUSIONS

1. Plain films are always first in the evaluation of the child with an irritable hip. Normal plain films, combined with a low clinical index of suspicion for septic arthritis, usually end the imaging workup, although close observation is warranted.

2. A high clinical index of suspicion for septic arthritis requires further imaging with US, regardless of plain film findings, unless the clinical/radiographic findings indicate a need for emergency surgery.
3. A normal hip US virtually excludes the diagnosis of septic arthritis.
4. US can guide the aspiration of joint fluid, for diagnostic purposes.

REFERENCES

1. Scoles PV. Pediatric Orthopedics in Clinical Practice, 2nd ed. St Louis, 1988, Mosby.
2. Ozonoff MB. Pediatric Orthopedic Radiology, 2nd ed. Philadelphia 1992, Saunders. 1992.
3. Boal DKB, Schwentker EP. Assessment of congenital hip dislocation with real-time ultrasound: a pictorial essay. Clinical Imaging 1991; 15:77-90.
4. Mandell CA, Harcke HT, Kumer SJ. Imaging in Pediatric Orthopaedics. Baltimore, Maryland, 1990, Aspen.
5. Zawin JK, Hoffer FA, Rand FF, Teele RL. Joint effusion in children with an irritable hip: US diagnosis and aspiration. Radiology 1993; 187:459-463.

51

Deep Venous Thrombosis

INTRODUCTION

Accurate and reliable diagnosis of deep venous thrombosis (DVT) is crucial to avoid the development of pulmonary embolism (PE; see Chapter 27). As many as 5 million cases of DVT occur in the United States annually, resulting in 120,000 to 150,000 acute thromboembolic deaths.[1,2]

The clinical evaluation of DVT is notoriously unreliable; imaging studies confirm only 50% of suspected cases.[3] Many of the "classic" signs and symptoms (leg pain, swelling, redness, a palpable "cord," Homan's sign) are both insensitive and nonspecific. For example, Homan's sign (pain on forced dorsiflexion of the foot) develops in less than one-third of patients with DVT and is absent in about half.[4] Imitators of acute DVT include cellulitis, popliteal cyst, congestive heart failure, superficial thrombophlebitis, postphlebitic syndrome, and popliteal vessel aneurysm; clearly the presumptive diagnosis of DVT suffers from low specificity. The insensitivity of clinical evaluation stems from the high incidence of asymptomatic cases.

Imaging plays a dual role: confirmation of suspected DVT before anticoagulant therapy and screening of high-risk patients (i.e., those with prolonged immobilization, recent surgery, lower extremity fracture, and joint replacement surgery) who are prone to the development of asymptomatic DVT.

Despite aggressive attempts at prevention, including prophylactic subcutaneous heparin, elastic stockings, and early postoperative ambulation, DVT is common in hospitalized patients. Indeed, 37% of asymptomatic postoperative patients have deep venous thrombosis, despite prophylactic anticoagulation.[5] Failure to detect DVT can result in death from PE, and overdiagnosis of PE can cause significant complications from unnecessary anticoagulation; therefore, routine imaging of both high risk and symptomatic patients is prudent.

The imaging approach to DVT hinges on whether the clinician believes that calf DVT is clinically significant and capable of producing significant PE. Classic teaching has been that DVT below the knee is not clinically significant and does not require treatment.[7] However, some authorities question this "classic" doctrine.[8-10] Resolution of the controversy is beyond the scope of this chapter; our goal is not to debate whether calf DVT should be treated but to provide an imaging plan that will yield the information that the clinician seeks. Ultrasound (US) and venography with intravenous contrast material (contrast venography or CV) apply.

Costs: pelvic US and bilateral leg US, with Doppler, $280; pelvic US and unilateral leg US, with Doppler, $261; CV, unilateral, $210; CV, bilateral, $341.

PLAN AND RATIONALE

(A) Suspected acute thrombosis:

If the clinician does not intend to treat calf DVT:

Step 1: Ultrasound with color Doppler

US is the most effective noninvasive means of imaging the deep venous system **from the inguinal ligament to the knee**. The deep veins of the thigh are identified and compressed by the hand-held transducer at 1 to 2 cm intervals along the length of the thigh. Thromboses can be seen directly or inferred by failure of the vein walls to collapse under gentle compression. The procedure is often supplemented by various Doppler techniques that identify moving blood. US can be performed at the bedside.

The sensitivity and specificity of US for DVT in the lower extremity (excluding the calf) are 95% and 98%.[11] **However, US is not recommended for the study of suspected calf DVT, since thrombi and veins in the calf are too small for accurate US evaluation.** Although the majority of calf clots either lyse or remain isolated, about 20% extend proximally, to the knee and beyond.[12] If one does not intend to treat calf DVT, repeat US in 3 to 5 days in patients who remain symptomatic will detect those calf clots that propagate proximally.

If the detection of calf DVT will alter treatment/management of a symptomatic patient, and in symptomatic or high-risk patients where ultrasound is not technically feasible (obesity, recent lower extremity surgery, cast):

Step 1: Contrast Venography

Contrast venography (CV) has long been considered the imaging "gold standard" for lower extremity DVT. A pedal vein is cannulated and contrast material injected, **opacifying the deep veins of the calf, thigh, and pelvis**. Thrombosis is characterized by an intraluminal "filling defect"; the proximal extent of the defect is usually identified. **CV is the study of choice for evaluation of the calf veins. However, US is comparable in accuracy at and above the knee.**

CV has several disadvantages: it is invasive and often painful, and it requires intravenous contrast material. The risk of post venography thrombosis in the legs has been variously estimated at between 2% and 31%.[13] CV is significantly more expensive than US, is not a bedside examination (a significant consideration in debilitated patients), and suffers from flow-related artifacts or nonfilling of veins that may lead to an equivocal or inaccurate study.

A negative or positive CV in a symptomatic patient ends the imaging workup. Equivocal studies can often be clarified by US if the questionable area is located at or above the knee.

(B) Suspected chronic or acute-on-chronic thrombosis:

The imaging diagnosis of chronic DVT or acute-on-chronic DVT is difficult, largely because of "postphlebitic syndrome"—the anatomic/physiologic changes that occur within the venous system after clot formation.[11] After an acute thrombosis has resolved, about 50% of veins will continue to exhibit abnormalities on US, because of clot organization and recanalization.[14] Residual findings include incomplete compressibility and thickening of vein walls as well as persistent intraluminal abnormal echoes that suggest thrombus. **These residual abnormalities limit the ability of US to differentiate between acute, chronic, and acute-on-chronic DVT. Color Doppler analysis of flow is helpful, because evaluation by compressibility is limited.**

A baseline US to document residual post-DVT changes when anticoagulation is complete is recommended, so that a significant change is more readily appreciated on subsequent studies.[15] Serial US with Doppler is currently the best available technique.

SUMMARY AND CONCLUSIONS

1. Ultrasound with Doppler should be the primary imaging modality for DVT **unless detection of calf DVT will alter patient management/treatment.** If no clot is detected, the patient is considered to be free of significant DVT and treated conservatively. Repeat US should be performed in 3 to 5 days if symptoms persist, to exclude propagation of a venous thrombosis originating in the calf. US may also be a useful supplemental study when a venogram is equivocal.

2. Venography should be performed in patients with suspected DVT **if detection of calf clot is thought to be important.** A normal venogram excludes DVT. Venography is also indicated when US is technically unfeasible or when US is equivocal.

3. Chronic venous thrombosis is currently best assessed by serial US, compared to a baseline study performed when anticoagulation therapy is complete.

ADDITIONAL COMMENTS

- Magnetic resonance imaging (MR) is comparable in sensitivity and specificity to venography for detection of calf, thigh, and pelvic DVT.[16,17] Although MR may assume a more important role in the future, its high cost and longer imaging times limit its application. MR may prove to be an accurate alternative imaging modality for chronic DVT if its cost ever approaches that of US.

- Because of the proliferation of central venous catheters for hyperalimentation and chemotherapy, upper extremity DVT has increased. Upper extremity DVT is seen in nearly 30% of patients with some types of subclavian catheters, with PE occurring in 12%.[18] Although CV is the accepted diagnostic "gold standard" for upper extremity DVT, color Doppler US, which also assesses the internal jugular vein, can be effective.[19]

- Impedance plethysmography (IPG), another noninvasive test for DVT, assesses changes in electrical resistance in the leg after occlusion of the deep venous system of the leg by a blood pressure cuff. Allegedly, the study is highly sensitive and specific for proximal thrombi but insensitive for detection of calf DVT.[20] The thrombus is not directly visualized and is inferred from nonimaging data.

- Radiolabeled antifibrin and antiplatelet antibodies have been the focus of intense research. To date, all such methods suffer from practical difficulties, like a long lag time between injection and imaging or a propensity to localize acute-but-not-chronic thrombi (or vice versa).

REFERENCES

1. Evans AJ, Sostman HD, Knelson MH, et al. Detection of deep venous thrombosis: prospective comparison of MR imaging with contrast venography. AJR 1993; 161:131-139.
2. Harmon B. Deep vein thrombosis: a perspective on anatomy and venographic analysis. J Thorac Imaging 1989; 4:15-19.
3. Ferris EJ. Deep venous thrombosis and pulmonary embolism: correlative evaluation and therapeutic implications. AJR 159:1149-1155.
4. Hirsh J, Hull RD. Venous thromboembolism: natural history, diagnosis and management. In Hirsh J, Hull RD (eds): Diagnosis of Venous Thrombosis. Boca Raton, Florida, 1987, CRC Press, pp 23-28.
5. Kalebo P, Anthmyr BA, Eriksson BI, Sazhrisson BE. Phlebographic findings in venous thrombosis following total hip replacement. Acta Radiol 1990; 3:259-263.
6. Moser KM, LeMoine JR. Is embolic risk conditioned by location of deep venous thrombosis? Ann Intern Med 1981; 94:439-444.
7. Philbrick JT, Becker DM: Calf deep venous thrombosis: a wolf in sheep's clothing? Arch Intern Med 1988; 148:2131-2138.
8. Havig O. Deep vein thrombosis and pulmonary embolism: source of pulmonary emboli. Acta Clin Scand 1977; 478:42-47.

9. Lagerstedt CI, Olsson CG, Fagher BO, et al. Need for long-term anticoagulant treatment in symptomatic calfvein thrombosis. Lancet 1985; 2:515-518.

10. Lohr JM, Kerr TM, Lutter KS, et al. Lower extremity calf thrombosis: to treat or not to treat? J Vasc Surg 1991; 14:618-623.

11. Cronan JJ. Venous thromboembolic disease: the role of US. Radiology 1993; 86:619-630.

12. Kakkar VV, Flanc C, Howe CT, Clarke MB. Natural history of postoperative deep-vein thrombosis. Lancet 1969; 2:230-232.

13. Lensing AWA, Prandon P, Buller HR, et al. Lower extremity venography with iohexol: results and complications. Radiology 1990; 177:503-505.

14. Cronan JJ, Leen V. Recurrent deep venous thrombosis: limitations of US. Radiology 1989; 170:739-742.

15. Baxter GM, Duffy P, MacKechnie S. Colour doppler ultrasound of the post-phlebitic limb: sounding a cautionary note. Clin Radiol 1991; 43:301-304.

16. Erdman WA, Jayson HT, Redman HC. Deep venous thrombosis of extremities: role of MR imaging in the diagnosis. Radiology 1990: 174:425-431.

17. Evans AJ, Sostman HD, Knelson MH, et al. Detection of deep venous thrombosis: prospective comparison of MR imaging with contrast venography. AJR 1993; 161:131-139.

18. Horattas ML, Wright DJ, Fenton AH, et al. Changing concepts of deep venous thrombosis of the upper-extremity -report of a series and review of the literature. Surgery 1988; 104:561-567.

19. Knudson GJ, Wiedemeyer DA, Erickson SJ, et al. Color doppler sonographic imaging in the assessment of upper- extremity deep venous thrombosis. AJ9 1990; 154:399-403.

20. Huisman MV, Buller HR, Cate JWT, et al. Serial impedance plethysmography for suspected deep venous thrombosis in outpatients: the Amsterdam general practitioner study. N Engl J Med 1986; 314:823-828.

52

Athletic/Traumatic Knee Injury

INTRODUCTION

Participation in athletic activities has expanded greatly over the past decade, bringing with it an increase in sports injuries; up to 75% of these involve the lower extremities, and 22% to 40% involve the knee.[1-3] A delay in diagnosis may result in chronic pain, loss of function, and scarring that complicates later surgery.

Patients with acute athletic injury of the knee typically present with nonspecific signs and symptoms, and the physical exam is often limited by pain and soft tissue swelling. Therefore imaging plays a key diagnostic role; plain films and magnetic resonance imaging (MR) are often decisive. (See Chapter 45 for a separate discussion of fractures, stress fractures, and shin splints.)

Costs: plain films, AP, lateral, and axial, $71; MR, unenhanced, $894; knee arthrogram, $344 ; CT knee arthrogram, $650.

PLAN AND RATIONALE

Step 1: Plain Films

Plain films are the first step in the imaging evaluation of

an athletic knee injury. Anteroposterior (AP), lateral, and axial ("skyline") views of the knee may be supplemented by intercondylar notch ("tunnel"), oblique, or cross-table lateral views. (The cross-table lateral view is helpful in cases of suspected occult intraarticular fracture, because demonstration of a fat-fluid level, usually in the suprapatellar bursa, caused by leakage of marrow fat into the blood-filled synovial cavity, will prompt further radiologic evaluation.)

Plain films effectively detect fracture, dislocation, soft tissue swelling, and joint effusion. However, **meniscal and tendon tears, cruciate and collateral ligament tears, articular cartilage injuries, and bone contusions are not directly detected by plain films. Furthermore, plain films seldom reveal the true extent of soft tissue injury**. Plain film abnormalities like avulsion fracture, abnormal alignment, and joint effusion are often the "tip of the iceberg." Therefore plain films are a limited screening technique.

If the index of suspicion for significant knee injury is low and plain films are negative, the imaging workup usually stops. However, when internal derangement of the knee is suspected—that is, **for evaluation of the menisci, cruciate and collateral ligaments, tendons, cartilage, and occult osseous injury**—MR is appropriate regardless of plain film findings (unless the condition warrants emergency surgery).

Step 2: Magnetic Resonance Imaging

The importance of MR in the evaluation of internal derangement of the knee cannot be overemphasized. MR defines the exact location, extent, and severity of tendinous, cartilaginous, ligamen-

tous, and osseous injury. The accuracy and sensitivity of MR in this setting are so great that many observers consider MR comparable to arthroscopy.

Although diagnostic arthroscopy is the "gold standard" against which other diagnostic modalities are judged, it is expensive, invasive, and highly operator dependent and carries a risk of complications (about 8.2%) and postoperative pain.[3] **MR is emerging as a cost-effective alternative to diagnostic arthroscopy**; a negative MR—or a positive MR that indicates nonsurgical therapy—obviates the need for arthroscopy, a procedure that costs approximately $3000.[4] Moreover, an MR study that reveals a surgical lesion provides a "road map" for the surgeon or arthroscopist. (The "road map" increases the success rate of surgery, because meniscal tears and cruciate ligament injuries in certain locations may be difficult to visualize arthroscopically.)

SUMMARY AND CONCLUSIONS

1. Plain films are always first and often end the workup.
2. MR is the appropriate next step for suspected internal derangement of the knee or where clinical signs and symptoms are not explained by—or are out of the proportion to—plain film findings.
3. MR is emerging as a less invasive cost-effective alternative to diagnostic arthroscopy, a procedure that costs approximately $3000.[4]

ADDITIONAL COMMENTS

- **MR has replaced arthrography in the evaluation of virtually all knee injuries.** However, for claustrophobic patients who cannot tolerate MR or for those who cannot tolerate MR because of cardiac pacemakers, aneurysm clips, etc., knee arthrography is a reasonable alternative **for evaluation of the menisci; the anterior cruciate ligament is much less accurately evaluated**. The knee joint is entered percutaneously and contrast material is injected along with room air, followed by X-rays in multiple positions. The procedure is mildly uncomfortable. Alternatively, claustrophobic patients can be studied on newer "open bore architecture" MR units, which are less confining, though the anatomic resolution and diagnostic accuracy of these units are limited, compared to conventional MR. Despite these limitations, most authorities believe that knee images from "open bore architecture" systems are more diagnostic than arthography.

- For evaluation of articular cartilage (e.g., chondromalacia patellae) and intraarticular loose bodies, and synovial plicae, CT-arthrography may be considered as an alternative or adjunct to MR; after intraarticular injection of contrast material and air, CT of the knee is performed.

REFERENCES

1. Backs, FJG, Erich WBM, Kemper ABA, et al. Sports injuries in school-aged children. Am J Sports Med 1989; 17:234-240.
2. Baylis WJ, Rzonca EC. Common sports injuries to the knee. Clin Podiatr Med Surg 1988; 5:571-589.
3. Nocholas JA, Rosenthal PP, Gleim GW. A historical perspective of injuries in professional football. JAMA 1998; 360:939-944.
4. Ruwe, PA, Wright J, Randall, RL, et al. Can MR imaging effectively replace diagnostic arthroscopy? Radiology 1002; 183:335-339.

SUGGESTED ADDITIONAL READING

Mink JH, Reicher MA, Crues JV III, et al. MRI of the Knee, 2nd ed. New York, 1993, Raven Press.
Berquist TH. Imaging of Sports Injuries. Baltimore, Maryland, 1992, Aspen.

53

Low Back Pain

INTRODUCTION

Low back pain (LBP) is virtually ubiquitous in American adults, affecting up to 80% at some time in their lives.[1,2] In the United States, LBP ranks second only to upper respiratory infection as a cause of a visit to a physician[3] and absence from work. It is the most common Workers Compensation claim.[4] An estimated 5.2 million Americans are disabled—about 50% permanently—from LBP,[5] and about 200,000 patients in the United States annually undergo surgery for a disc abnormality.[6]

LBP has an annual incidence of 5%, a prevalence of l5% to 20%, and a recurrence rate of about 75%.[7] Enormous direct and indirect costs are incurred in the diagnosis and treatment of LBP, estimated annually at over **$50 billion**.[8] The peak prevalence of LBP is in the fifth decade, most often beginning between 20 and 50 years of age.[7] Symptoms are often nonspecific, including pain, numbness, and weakness over the lower back, hips, and legs; the symptom complex may reflect the neurologic level of the abnormality. Etiologies include intervertebral disc pathology (degeneration, herniation, bulge), spinal stenosis, osteoarthritis of the facet (apophyseal) joints, spondylolysis, as well as neoplasm, muscle or ligamentous injury, fracture, rheumatologic disease, infection, and referred pain (e.g., kidney stone).

Diagnostic imaging is only part of the organized clinical approach to patients with LBP. Up to 95% of patients with acute LBP experience significant symptomatic improvement after conservative treatment[9,10]; **only a small percentage require sophisticated imaging**. Those with chronic or recurrent symptoms, and those in whom surgery is a therapeutic option, are more likely to benefit from imaging: **whom to image and when are controversial**.

Plain films, computed tomography without intravenous contrast material (unenhanced CT), magnetic resonance imaging with and without intravenous contrast material (enhanced and unenhanced MR), CT myelography, CT discography, and the nuclear bone scan with single photon emission computed tomography (SPECT) play a role in the workup.

Costs: plain films, AP and lateral, $68; CT, unenhanced, $467; MR, unenhanced, $849; MR, unenhanced and enhanced, $1657; CT myelography, $990; CT discography $790-$1440 (depending on the number of discs studied); bone scan, SPECT, $651.

PLAN AND RATIONALE

Step 1: Conventional Plain Films

Plain films should be the first step. **The diagnostic yield of plain films is limited; abnormalities detected on plain films are not necessarily the cause of pain, and normal plain films in no way exclude a significant abnormality. Nevertheless, plain films should not be skipped**; a specific diagnosis is sometimes possible (e.g., metastasis or fracture) and correlation of other images with the initial plain films is often useful.

The plain films are inspected for malalignment, fracture, facet joint arthritis, destructive lesions, scoliosis, spondylolisthesis, and signs of degenerative disc disease. AP and lateral views are usually sufficient. Oblique views may be required for specific suspected conditions, like spondylolysis and facet disease. Lateral flexion and extension views may be helpful when assessing for dynamic instability of the lumbar spine; the degree of degenerative spondylolisthesis may increase with flexion of the lumbar spine, which may be an indication for surgical fusion.

For patients with suspected disc herniation and nerve root compression (sciatica, radiculopathy):

Step 2: Computed Tomography or Magnetic Resonance Imaging

MR has been extensively utilized and applied to imaging virtually all diseases of the spine. **Its noninvasiveness, multiplanar imaging capability, lack of ionizing radiation, ability to detect disc degeneration in its earliest stages, and exquisite anatomic detail make MR an appealing alternative to myelography and CT. MR is more accurate than myelography and as accurate as CT in evaluating lumbar disc disease and canal stenosis.**[11] However, although most radiologists would prefer to interpret MR rather than CT when evaluating a patient for suspected disc herniation with nerve root compression, **large studies have failed to demonstrate a statistically significant difference in diagnostic accuracy between these two modalities.**[11-14] **Indeed, MR, unenhanced CT, and CT-myelography are essentially equal in diagnostic accuracy for this patient population.** The sensitivity and specificity for the three modalities are in the range of

80% and 100% and 43% and 88%, respectively.[12,15] Therefore, in view of the current significant cost difference between unenhanced CT and MR and their equivalent diagnostic efficacy in this population, we recommend unenhanced CT. (CT-myelography does not compete, because it is significantly more invasive than unenhanced CT or MR and more expensive than unenhanced CT.)

If CT reveals no abnormalities and pain persists, then causes other than disc disease, nerve root compression, spinal stenosis, and spondylolysis must be pursued; for this purpose, MR is appropriate.

For patients with suspected spinal stenosis and/or degenerative disease of the facets:

Step 2: Computed Tomography

Unenhanced CT, with contiguous axial images from L2 to the sacrum, is ideal for evaluating patients with suspected spinal stenosis.

Spinal stenosis has a variety of causes; congenital stenosis is usually asymptomatic without a superimposed acquired abnormality. Acquired causes include disc bulge/herniation, degenerative disease of the facet joints, spondylolisthesis, and hypertrophy of the ligamentum flavum; a combination of these factors is usually involved.

CT effectively demonstrates the location, severity, and extent of central canal stenosis and the relative contribution of various factors. Associated neural foraminal stenosis, a common result of facet joint disease, is also depicted. MR is probably equal to CT for assessing spinal stenosis[16]; the consensus is that MR is no better. Therefore, given the higher cost of MR, we recommend CT initially for this purpose.

If CT reveals no abnormalities and pain persists, then other causes unrelated to facet disease, spinal stenosis, disc disease, and nerve root compression must be pursued. For these purposes, MR is appropriate.

Spondylolysis—for adults:

Step 2: Computed Tomography

Spondylolysis is a defect or fracture in the pars interarticularis of a vertebra, most commonly at L5. About half are associated with spondylolisthesis, a forward slipping of the vertebral body, usually mild in degree. Plain films, including oblique views, are usually adequate for detection of spondylolysis and the presence of associated spondylolisthesis.

Unenhanced CT is effective in patients with suspected spondylolysis whose plain films are negative or equivocal; **it is clearly superior to MR for this purpose.**[17]

Spondylolysis—children and adolescents:

Step 2: Nuclear Bone Scan With Single Photon Emission Computed Tomography (SPECT)

A bone scan, with SPECT of the lumbar spine, should be considered an alternative to CT in young patients. The bone-seeking radiopharmaceutical, technetium-99m-methylene diphosphonate (Tc-99m-MDP) is injected intravenously, and 1 1/2 to 2 hours later the total body is imaged, followed by additional SPECT images of the symptomatic region(s) of the spine. The study reveals increased radiopharmaceutical uptake where bone blood flow and metabolism are increased and reflect the stress-related physiologic alterations associated with symptomatic spondylolysis.

The radiation exposure is lower for a bone scan than for CT, a significant consideration in the relatively more radiation-susceptible pediatric population; however, the anatomic resolution of the bone scan is inferior. **An abnormal bone scan is more specific in the pediatric than in the adult population; a focal "hot spot" at the symptomatic lower lumbar site very likely represents spondylolysis in a child, whereas in adults a "hot spot" could represent many conditions, like degenerative or metastatic disease.**

The failed back surgery syndrome:

Step 2: Magnetic Resonance Imaging

The failed back surgery syndrome is characterized by persistent or recurrent pain and/or functional incapacitation after spine surgery. This debilitating syndrome follows about 15% of spinal operations[18] and has numerous causes, including recurrent or residual disc herniation, epidural fibrosis, arachnoiditis, mechanical instability, and bony canal stenosis. MR, enhanced **and** unenhanced, accurately differentiates scar tissue from disk material[19,20] and is more sensitive and specific than CT. MR is also highly accurate for detecting lumbar arachnoiditis, responsible for persistent symptoms in 6% to 16% of postoperative patients[18,21]

SUMMARY AND CONCLUSIONS

1. In those patients with low back pain who require an imaging workup, plain films of the lumbar spine are first. AP and lateral views are usually adequate; oblique views should be reserved for specific indications like spondylolysis, and in special cases flexion and extension views are indicated.

2. Unenhanced CT is the appropriate next step in adult patients with suspected disc herniation, spinal stenosis, arthritis of the facet joints, and spondylolsis. MR is equivalent in diagnostic accuracy for disc herniation or spinal stenosis, but because of its higher cost it is not recommended at the present time.

3. For children and adolescents, a bone scan with SPECT is a reasonable alternative when spondylolysis is suspected. However, the bone scan is not an appropriate second step for adults, or children in whom spondylolysis is not a primary consideration; in these circumstances the study is too nonspecific.

4. MR, enhanced and unenhanced, is the study of choice for evaluation of the failed back surgery syndrome.

ADDITIONAL COMMENTS

- If and when the cost of spine MR becomes comparable to that of enenhanced CT, it will likely replace CT as the preferred method of imaging patients with LBP, because MR is highly sensitive for detecting a number of additional causes of LBP, including spinal cord lesions, marrow-replacing lesions of the vertebral column, and the earliest changes of disc degeneration.

- MRI has virtually replaced CT-myelography, an invasive procedure, for diagnosis of most spinal disorders. This procedure should be reserved for those patients whose surgeon specifically requires detailed local information before surgery. (Although many spine surgeons will operate based on MR findings alone, a significant proportion request CT-myelography.)

- Lumbar discography is a controversial procedure that is rarely indicated or utilized in the evaluation of LBP. Contrast material is injected percutaneously into the nucleus pulposus of suspected symptomatic discs. If symptoms are replicated by the injection, and if leakage of contrast material from the nucleus pulposus is demonstrated on CT, the study is interpreted as positive. This provocative test is invasive and has a risk of infection and rupture of the annulus fibrosus. It is usually reserved for those symptomatic patients who either have no demonstrable disc abnormality on other imaging studies or those who have one or more disc abnormalities with uncertainty as to which, if any, is symptomatic. The major role of discography is to demonstrate pain reproduction; the test is of questionable reliability, because similar symptoms can be provoked by injection into a normal disc.

REFERENCES

1. Kelsey J, White A. Epidemiology and impact of low back pain. Spine 1980; 5:133.
2. Nachemson A. Spinal disorders. Overall impact on society and the need for orthopedic resources. Acta Orthop Scand Suppl 1991; 241:17.
3. Cypress BK. Characteristics of physician visits for back symptoms. A national perspective. Am J Public Health 1983; 73:389-395.
4. Schellinger D. The low back pain syndrome—diagnostic impact of high-resolution computed tomography. Med Clin North Am 1984; 68:1631.
5. National Center for Health Statistics Prevalence of selected impairments. United States - 1977, series 10, No. 132. Hyattsville, Maryland, 1981, DHHS Publication (PHS) 81-1562.
6. Onik G, Maroon J, Helms C, et al. Automated percutaneous diskectomy—initial patient experience. Radiology 1987; 162:129-132.
7. Dey RA, Tsui-Wu YJ. Descriptive epidemiology of low-back pain and its related medical care in the United States. Spine 1987; 12:264-268.
8. Frymoyer JW, Cats-Baril WL. An overview of the incidences and costs of low back pain. Orthop Clin North Am 1991; 22:263-282.
9. Spitzer W, LeBlanc F, Dupuis M. Scientific approach to the assessment and management of activity-related spinal disorders. A monograph for clinicians. Report of the Quebec Task Force on Spinal Disorders. Spine 1987; 12:S1.

10. Enmann DR. Special report: on low back pain. American Society of Neuroradiology 1994; 15:109-113.
11. Modic MT, Masory KT, Boumphrey F, et al. Lumbar herniated disc disease and canal stenosis: prospective evaluation by surface coil MR, CT, and myelography. AJR 1986; 147:757-765.
12. Thornbury JR, Fryback DG, Tursk PA, et al. Disk-caused nerve compression in patients with acute low-back pain: diagnosis with MR, CT myelography, and plain CT. Radiology 1993; 186:731-738.
13. Deyo RA. Diagnostic imaging procedures for the lumbar spine. Ann Intern Med 1989; III:865-867.
14. Jackson RP, Cain JE Jr, Jacobs RR, et al. The neuroradiographic diagnosis of lumbar herniated nucleus pulposus. A comparison of CT, myelography, CT-myelography and magnetic resonance imaging. Spine 1989; 14:1362-1367.
15. Petz DM, Haddad RG. Radiologic investigation of low back pain. Can Med Assoc J 1989; 140:289-295.
16. Schnebel B, Kingston S, Watkins R, et al. Comparison of MRI to contrast CT in the diagnosis of spinal stenosis. Spine 1989; 14:332-337.
17. Grenier N, Kressel HY, Schiebler ML, et al. Isthmic spondylosis of the lumbar spine: MR imaging at 1.5 Tesla. Radiology 1989; 170:489-494.
18. Burton C, Kirkaldy-Willis W, Yong-Hing K. Causes of failure of surgery of the lumbar spine. Clin Orthop 1981; 157:191.
19. Ross J, Masary KT, Schrader M, et al. MR imaging of the postoperative spine: assessment with gadopentetate dimeglumine. AJR 1990; 155:867-872.
20. Hveftle M, Modic M, Ross J, et al. Lumbar spine: postoperative MR imaging with GD-DTPA. Radiology 1988; 167:817-824.
21. Ross J, Masaryk T, Modic M. MR imaging of lumbar arachnoiditis. AJR 1987; 149:1025.

54

Elective Workup of Myocardial Ischemia/ Coronary Artery Disease

INTRODUCTION

Coronary artery disease (CAD) has been the focus of intense and growing interest over the past 20 years. A better understanding of risk factors, new diagnostic modalities, and powerful interventions have radically changed our understanding of this condition in only one generation. Noninvasive diagnostic imaging plays a key role in selecting patients for coronary angiography and medical/surgical intervention and for assessing the effectiveness of medical, surgical, or angioplastic therapy.

Traditionally, new patients are first screened by an exercise ECG unless the **resting ECG reveals abnormalities** (like left bundle branch block or ST-T wave changes) **that preclude a valid exercise ECG.** There is a growing consensus among cardiologists that patients with **good exercise capacity** and a **normal exercise ECG** have an excellent cardiovascular prognosis—less than 1% mortality per year over a 5-year follow-up. **Thus such patients are unlikely to benefit from any additional noninvasive testing.**[1]

Among patients whose exercise ECG is equivocal or abnormal, follow-up imaging is likely to be most revealing and cost effective when **the pretest likelihood of CAD is intermediate or high.** Such patients with a **strongly abnormal exercise ECG** often proceed directly to angiography, whereas those whose exercise ECG is **equivocal or borderline** usually proceed to noninvasive imaging for clarification.

A currently unresolved issue is whether the exercise ECG should remain the initial exam, before noninvasive imaging, in those patients with an intermediate or high pretest likelihood of CAD. Since such patients with an abnormal or equivocal exercise ECG may progress to imaging, it can be argued that the exercise ECG should be bypassed in favor of noninvasive imaging as the first exam. A counter argument holds that even in intermediate- or high-risk patients many exercise ECGs will be normal, with good exercise capacity, obviating the need for further, more expensive tests. The current tendency among many cardiologists is to proceed directly to noninvasive imaging. Resolution of this argument, which focuses on the value of the exercise ECG, is beyond the scope of this book.

Imaging techniques that evaluate the coronary arteries are categorized as "noninvasive" or "invasive." The **non-invasive techniques** include **nuclear myocardial perfusion imaging** (SPECT thallium or SPECT Tc-99m-sestimibi) and **stress echocardiography**; the current "gold standard" is coronary angiography, which is much more invasive and expensive. **Noninvasive imaging** can confirm or exclude myocardial ischemia with sufficient confidence to select patients for the definitive coronary angiogram.

Costs: nuclear myocardial perfusion imaging, stress and rest, $646; stress echocardiogram, $389; coronary angiogram, $2172.

PLAN AND RATIONALE

Recent comparisons between state-of-the-art nuclear myocardial perfusion imaging and stress echocardiography suggest that their sensitivities and specificities are roughly equal in patients who present no special technical difficulties.[2] Therefore, a rational choice depends on their relative cost and availability. Almost invariably stress echocardiography is the less expensive of the two, although it may be limited technically by advanced COPD. **Thus in the initial imaging evaluation for CAD, where this technical limitation is absent:**

Where state-of-the-art digital echocardiography is available:

Step 1: Stress Echocardiography

The stress echocardiogram is based on the fact that myocardial ischemia—the unbalancing of myocardial oxygen supply and demand—is manifested almost immediately by decreased contractility (hypokinesis) and that this hypokinesis persists for at least 1 minute. Therefore, sonographic images of the heart will reveal localized or generalized motion abnormalities if generated within 1 minute of sufficient exercise.

The patient is exercised on a treadmill, under the supervision of a cardiologist, according to a graded exercise routine. When exercise capacity or 85% to 90% of maximal heart rate is achieved, the patient is removed from the treadmill and imaged while supine; the images require only superficial contact between a hand-held transducer and the skin of the anterior chest wall. Preexercise baseline and postexercise images in multiple planes are compared, and the left ventricular ejection fraction is estimated. In addition, valvular function, pericardial thickness, and myocardial thickness are easily assessed.

For patients who are unable to exercise—because of obesity, orthopedic problems, pulmonary disease, peripheral vascular disease, etc.—pharmacologic stress is available; infusion of vasodilators (dipyridamole or adenosine) or sympathomimetic agents (dobutamine) can unbalance myocardial oxygen supply and demand, producing ischemia manifested by hypokinesis.[3] Dobutamine is particularly cost effective, since it is much less expensive than the other pharmacologic stressors.

Where state-of-the-art digital echocardiography is unavailable:

Step 1: Nuclear Myocardial Perfusion Imaging

Nuclear myocardial perfusion imaging is based on the fact that various radiopharmaceuticals are rapidly extracted from the circulation by the myocardium, according to myocardial perfusion. Underperfused areas are seen by a nuclear camera as regions of reduced radiopharmaceutical uptake. Perfused regions represent viable myocardium, whereas underperfused areas may represent scar and/or "hibernating" myocardium. ("Hibernating myocardium" refers to ischemic muscle that does not extract radiopharmaceutical from the blood or contract normally; such tissue, however, is viable and can resume normal contractility and metabolism if revascularized.)

Although thallium-201 (Tl-201) was for a generation the radiopharmaceutical of choice, it has largely been supplanted by technetium-99m (Tc-99m) sestimibi. Moreover, "planar" images have been replaced by far more sophisticated single photon emission computed tomography (SPECT).

Both Tl-201 and Tc-99m-sestimibi studies require two intravenous injections, and both are combined with treadmill stress, according to a graded exercise protocol. The exam is more time consuming than stress echocardiography since the rest and the stress images each require 30 to 40 minutes. These time requirements, added to the high cost of the radiopharmaceutical itself, raise the total cost of the procedure.

Nuclear myocardial perfusion imaging visualizes the myocardium itself; **perfusion is correlated directly with radiopharmaceutical uptake, rather than inferred from secondary hypokinesis.** Nonetheless, the sensitivity and specificity of SPECT myocardial perfusion studies are probably about the same as those of stress echocardiography[2]; thus both exams are an effective follow-up to the stress ECG.

Important disadvantages of nuclear myocardial perfusion imaging, as opposed to stress echocardiography, are that the ejection fraction is not presently calculated nor is information provided regarding the cardiac valves or pericardium. When patients are unable to exercise, the same pharmacchologic agents used in stress echocardiography are effective stressors for nuclear myocardial perfusion imaging.

Neither stress echocardiography nor myocardial perfusion imaging addresses the detailed anatomy of the vascular compromise that causes myocardial ischemia. Thus when intervention is planned, coronary angiography is necessary.

Step 2: Coronary Angiography

Because of its high specificity, coronary angiography is the imaging "gold standard" for coronary artery disease, but its expense and morbidity preclude indiscriminate use.

For coronary arteriography, a specially designed catheter

is inserted via a percutaneous femoral artery puncture (Judkins technique) or a brachial arteriotomy (Sones technique) and passed retrograde into the proximal aorta. Contrast material is injected into each coronary artery during rapid radiographic filming.

The coronary circulation is well visualized by the angiogram, showing atheromatous change, stenoses, and collaterals. During the same procedure, contrast material injection into the left ventricle produces images of the chamber during the cardiac cycle. These films are useful for evaluating valvular lesions, ventricular wall motion, intraventricular thrombi, and ejection fraction. Regions of reduced (hypokinetic), absent (akinetic), and paradoxical (dyskinetic) wall motion are identified. While the catheter is in place, pressure readings across the cardiac valves are recorded.

Cardiac catheterization and coronary angiography are invasive procedures with uncommon, but potentially serious, complications. These include cardiac perforation, major arrhythmias, hemorrhage, hypotension, vascular thrombosis or dissection, cerebral embolism, myocardial infarction, and death. Moreover, the usual cautions regarding radiographic contrast material apply.

SUMMARY AND CONCLUSIONS

1. Coronary angiography is the "gold standard" for the evaluation of coronary artery disease because of its exquisite demonstration of coronary arterial anatomy. However, it is expensive and invasive. Therefore, non-invasive imaging should precede the angiogram, to select patients for this procedure, except in emergency situations, such as some acute myocardial infarctions, in which an occlusion must be demonstrated immediately to facilitate interventional therapy (e.g., percutaneous transluminal coronary angioplasty).

2. The stress echocardiogram and nuclear myocardial perfusion study are roughly equivalent in sensitivity and specificity for coronary artery disease, except in cases where echocardiography is technically limited, particularly in COPD. Echocardiography visualizes myocardial hypokinesis as a function of perfusion, whereas nuclear perfusion imaging visualizes radiopharmaceutical uptake as a direct correlate of perfusion. Both studies can effectively select patients for coronary angiography.

3. **Because of its lower cost, we suggest the stress echocardiogram as the procedure of choice for an initial evaluation when digital state-of-the-art equipment is available. However, in the presence of advanced COPD, nuclear perfusion imaging is usually preferable.**

4. Advantages of the stress echocardiogram include its ability to evaluate valvular function, myocardial thickness, the pericardium, and the ejection fraction.

5. Both exams are feasible in patients who are unable to exercise; the heart can be stressed by pharmacologic means.

6. Both studies are also useful in the evaluation of medical and/or surgical therapy.

ADDITIONAL COMMENTS

- Obesity limits both echocardiography and myocardial perfusion imaging. If the excess body fat is chiefly distributed over the abdomen, buttocks, and legs, the limitations are minimal, but chest-wall fat presents major technical problems. Most imagers believe that moderate chest wall fat is less of an inhibitor to nuclear studies. Truly massive obesity is incompatible with either test.

- The "noninvasive" evaluation of myocardial ischemia by either stress echocardiography or nuclear myocardial perfusion imaging involves exercise, which has risks. It has been estimated that one fatality and two nonfatal complications occur per 10,000 tests.

- Computed tomography (CT) may soon contribute in a major way to the evaluation of myocardial ischemia, as ultrafast "cine" CT capability becomes more readily available. Ultrafast CT scanners produce high-resolution "slice" images in **milliseconds** and have visualized the proximal coronary arteries after **a peripheral intravenous injection of contrast material**.

- Some authorities have advocated cardiac fluoroscopy to identify coronary artery calcifications. They note a strong correlation of coronary artery disease and calcifications in patients less than 50 years old but a weaker correlation in the elderly, in whom coronary calcifications are common. Coronary artery calcification is even better deteced by CT. Systematic use of this observation for diagnosing coronary artery disease is not widespread but may increase as ultrafast ("cine") CT scanners proliferate.

- Magnetic resonance (MR) has great potential in the evaluation of tissue ischemia, but as yet the technique is not clinically applicable.

REFERENCES

1. Chaitman BR. Exercise ECG testing. Myocardial Perfusion Imaging, Part I. The American Journal of Cardiology Continuing Education Series. Cahners Healthcare Communications, 1993.
2. Zoghbi WA. Echocardiography In Iskandrian AS, ed. Myocardial Perfusion Imaging, Part I. The American Journal of Cardiology Continuing Education Series. Cahners Healthcare Communications, 1993.
3. Verami SM, Mahmarian JJ. Nonexercise stress testing, In Iskandrian AS, ed. Myocardial Perfusion Imaging, Part I. The American Journal of Cardiology Continuing Education Series. Cahners Healthcare Communications, 1993.

55

Cardiac Ejection Fraction

INTRODUCTION

An important measure of cardiac performance is the ejection fraction (EF), that portion of the ventricular volume ejected in systole. Numerically, this fraction is the end–diastolic volume, minus the end-systolic volume, divided by the end–diastolic volume.

The EF is **calculated** by nuclear ventriculography and cardiac angiography but **estimated** by echocardiography. Nuclear ventriculography and echocardiography are non-invasive, whereas angiography requires peripheral vascular puncture, retrograde passage of a catheter into the heart, and injection of contrast material.

Costs: nuclear ventriculogram, $358; echocardiogram, $316.

PLAN AND RATIONALE

When a precise, numerical EF is required and valvular function, pericardial disease, and myocardial thickness are not at issue:

Step 1: Nuclear Ventriculogram

In certain patients, particularly those undergoing

chemotherapy, **a quantitative determination of ejection fraction** is required to monitor cardiotoxic drug effects. The nuclear ventriculogram is well suited to this purpose.

Some of the patient's red blood cells are labeled with technetium-99m (Tc-99m), and the chest is imaged by a nuclear camera, which records radioactivity in the heart during different phases of the ECG. The computer constructs a series of individual images, each representing a slightly different phase of the cardiac cycle. The cycle—from systole through diastole—is displayed as a "movie," called a "multi-gated acquisition" (MUGA) study, and the ejection fraction is calculated.

By appropriate positioning, all ventricular segments except part of the left ventricular posterior wall may be imaged for an accurate assessment of regional contraction. Hypokinesis, akinesis, and dyskinesis are easily detected, and chamber size can be estimated.

A "stress" nuclear ventriculogram compares the EF before and during exercise as an estimate of cardiac reserve. In young adults who have undergone chemotherapy as children, serial monitoring by "stress" nuclear ventriculography can detect those persons whose heart has suffered significant permanent cardiotoxicity, despite good cardiac function at rest. This determination is important because **heavy exercise has caused sudden death in some of these young adults.**

Nuclear ventriculography does not define the cardiac valves, the pericardium, or the myocardium itself, since the blood pool, rather than the myocardium or endocardium, is visualized.

When an approximate estimate of ejection fraction is satisfactory and information regarding valvular function, pericardial disease, and myocardial thickness may be useful:

Step 1: Echocardiography

Ultrasound of the heart (echocardiography) is a sophisticated method of cardiac imaging, useful for evaluating the motion of the cardiac valves and ventricular walls, pericardial thickness, and myocardial thickness. In fact, in most cases it is the most cost-effective method of evaluating myocardial contractility as an indication of myocardial ischemia in response to exercise (see Chapter 54, Elective Workup of Myocardial Ischemia/Coronary Artery Disease).

In the great majority of institutions, at the time of this writing, **the ventricular EF is estimated—rather than calculated—by echocardiography.** From a practical standpoint, this estimate **usually** fulfills the clinician's requirements, but a nuclear ventriculogram remains the procedure of choice when strict quantitation is required. The echocardiogram is preferable when a good estimate of EF is satisfactory, and information involving the valves, pericardium, and myocardial thickness may be valuable.

A new generation of echocardiographic equipment quantitates the EF, generating numerical values that are competitive with the nuclear study.

SUMMARY AND CONCLUSIONS

1. Radionuclide ventriculography and echocardiography are noninvasive methods of determining the ventricular EF.
2. When a **precise quantitation** of EF is required, as in the **monitoring of chemotherapy patients for cardiotoxicity**, the nuclear ventriculogram is preferable.
3. When a **good estimate of the EF is satisfactory and information regarding the cardiac valves, pericardium, and myocardial thickness** may be useful, echocardiography is effective.

4. A new generation of echocardiographic equipment quantitates the EF.

ADDITIONAL COMMENTS

- Severe COPD and obesity may technically impede echocardiography, but COPD does not affect nuclear ventriculography, and obesity is a minor impediment unless massive. Therefore, **the EF in such patients is better determined by the nuclear technique.**
- The cardiac angiogram requires catheterization of the aorta and injection of radiographic contrast material into the left ventricle. During the cardiac cycle, rapid-sequence radiographs are obtained. The ejection fraction is calculated from the change in size of the contrast material–filled ventricle, directly measured from the films, during systole and diastole. This invasive procedure correlates well with the nuclear ventriculogram.
- Gated magnetic resonance imaging (MR) has produced images of the heart that reveal regional wall motion, anatomic and valvular lesions, pericardial disease, and myocardial infarctions. Furthermore, the EF can be calculated. Thus MR combines the best features of nuclear imaging and echocardiography, but its higher cost and limited availability have delayed MR's expansion into the clinical arena.
- CT may soon contribute to the clinical determination of EF as ultrafast (cine) CT scanners proliferate. Ultrafast scanners visualize the contrast material-filled cardiac chambers with excellent anatomic resolution during systole and diastole. Highly accurate EFs are calculated and wall motion defined.

SUGGESTED ADDITIONAL READING

Mettler FA, Guiberteau MJ. Essentials of Nuclear Medicine Imaging, ed 3. Philadelphia, 1991, Saunders, pp.123-131.

Palmer EL, Scott JA, Strauss WH. Practical Nuclear Medicine. Philadelphia, 1992, Saunders, pp 71-75, 103-119.

56

Pericardial Effusion

INTRODUCTION

Pericardial effusion can be defined by chest radiography, sonography, computed tomography (CT), and magnetic resonance imaging (MR). The expense and sensitivity of these techniques vary enormously. In practical terms, chest films and sonography dominate the workup.

Costs: plain chest films, PA and lateral, $59; chest MR, unenhanced, $789; chest CT, unenhanced, $429; echocardiogram, $316.

PLAN AND RATIONALE

Steps 1 and 2: Echocardiography and Chest Radiographs

A normal chest film does not exclude pericardial effusion, and sizable effusions often produce a large "cardiac silhouette" that could represent cardiomegaly, effusion, or both. Thus chest films are insensitive and rarely specific for this condition, and an additional study is indicated **following any serious clinical or radiographic suspicion.** (An initial chest film remains mandatory, however, to exclude intrathoracic conditions whose symptoms mimic those of pericardial effusion and to define or characterize associated lesions.)

Echocardiography (sonography of the heart) is highly sensitive and specific for pericardial fluid; images of the pericardium and heart are generated by scanning over the anterior chest wall, and the quantity of fluid can be accurately estimated. **Thus a negative echocardiogram ends the imaging workup unless there is strong clinical suspicion of a small loculated effusion** (small loculated effusions may escape detection because of limited sonographic access to certain portions of the pericardium).

Echocardiography can be a portable, bedside examination and can guide the drainage of effusion for diagnosis and/or therapy. However, dressings and wounds from recent surgery may interfere with placement of the sonographic transducer on the skin surface; **in such unusual cases, or when small loculated effusions are suspected, CT or MR may help.**

Step 3: Magnetic Resonance Imaging or Computed Tomography

MR with electrocardiographic "gating" gathers imaging data during selected phases of the cardiac cycle, reducing the motion blur of the beating heart; it generates highly detailed images of the heart and pericardium. Pericardial effusions are invariably clearly defined, but the exam is costly compared to sonography. MR is especially useful for detecting loculated effusions and for differentiating hemorrhagic from nonhemorrhagic effusions.

CT can reveal pericardial thickening but often cannot differentiate pericardial thickening caused by tumor or inflammation from uncomplicated effusion.

SUMMARY AND CONCLUSIONS

1. An initial chest film is appropriate when pericardial effusion is suspected, to exclude thoracic conditions that could mimic an effusion and to define or characterize associated lesions. The chest film cannot rule out small effusions, and sizable effusions usually produce a large "cardiac silhouette" that is nonspecific.

2. Echocardiography is appropriate if there is any clinical or radiographic suspicion of pericardial effusion. It is accurate, noninvasive, inexpensive, quick, and portable. The procedure can localize and quantitate pericardial fluid and may guide percutaneous drainage for diagnosis and/or therapy.

3. CT or "gated" MR, if available, should follow when sonography is negative, equivocal, or technically limited and strong clinical suspicion of pericardial effusion remains.

SUGGESTED ADDITIONAL READING

Braunwald E. Pericardial disease. In Wilson JD, et al. Harrison's principles of internal medicine, 12th ed. New York, 1991, McGraw-Hill, pp 981-987.

Higgins CB. Essentials of Cardiac Radiology and Imaging. Philadelphia, 1992, Lippincott, pp 35, 267, 419-422.

Isner JM, Carter BL, Bankoff MS, Kinstam MA, Salem DN. Computed tomography in the diagnosis of pericardial heart disease. Ann Intern Med 1982; 7:473-479.

Lane EJ, Carsky EW. Epicardial fat: lateral plain film analysis in normals and in pericardial effusion. Radiology 1968; 91:1-5.

Mulvagh SL, et al. Usefulness of nuclear magnetic resonance imaging for evaluation of pericardial effusions, and comparison with two-dimensional echocardiography. Am J Cardiol 1989; 64:1002-1009.

Olson, MC, Posniak HV, McDonald V, Wisniewski R, Moncada R. Computed tomography and magnetic resonance imaging of the pericardium. RadioGraphics 1989; 9:633-639.

Sechtem U, Tscholakoff D, Higgins CB. MRI of the abnormal pericardium. AJR 1986; 147:245-252.

Part VII
GENERAL

57

Metastatic Cancer with an Unknown Primary

INTRODUCTION

Metastatic cancer with an unknown primary is the eighth most common presentation of malignancy[1]; **knowledge of the primary site is useful only when it can affect clinical management.** Presenting metastatic site(s) may be the lymph nodes, liver, pleura, bones, or central nervous system. Because of this variability, virtually any imaging study potentially applies; therefore, the search must be focused by clinical factors.

The most direct approach is biopsy and histologic study of a metastatic lesion. The following discussion assumes that the primary site remains unknown after a history and physical exam, laboratory studies including serum tumor markers like CEA, complete blood count, urinalysis, and stool exam for occult blood, a chest film, and biopsy of a metastatic site.[2]

A chest film is universally recommended because it is inexpensive, noninvasive, and straightforward. For many years it was commonly believed that a normal chest film effectively excludes the lungs as the source of a primary neoplasm that has already metastasized; this belief has been disproved by computed tomography (CT), which not infrequently detects primary mediastinal or hilar cancers that have already metastasized, despite a normal chest film. One might, therefore, conclude that CT is an appropriate part of the workup, but we do not recommend CT because the identification of a lung primary tumor will not significantly alter patient management.

Survival of patients with metastatic cancer of unknown origin is short, averaging 3 to 7 months. Even at autopsy a primary is found less than 50% of the time. The most common primary sites are the pancreas and lung, two organs whose metastases are incurable. **The cost-effective imaging workup is best confined to finding those primary cancers that can present as metastatic disease for which relatively effective therapy is available.** These are (1) squamous cell lesions of the oropharynx and nasopharynx, which present as high- or middle-cervical adenopathy, and (2) neoplasms of the prostate, neural crest, germ cells, breast, thyroid, and ovary, which may present is a variety of ways, symptomatically unrelated to the primary site.

Costs: neck CT, enhanced, $495; neck MR, enhanced, $989; abdominal and pelvic CT, enhanced, $840; mammogram, $119.

PLAN AND RATIONALE

Metastatic high or middle cervical adenopathy of squamous cell origin:

Step 1: Computed Tomography or Magnetic Resonance Imaging

CT can demonstrate submucosal lesions of the oral cavity and nasopharynx that may be missed by direct inspection and endoscopy, and the study will also reveal the extent of lymphadenopathy.[3]

MR may also have a role in detecting occult primary head and neck cancer, but because the exam is more costly than CT, it is reserved for those cases in which CT is equivocal or technically inadequate; to date there are no definitive controlled studies comparing these two modalities for this specific problem.[4]

If CT or MR are normal, the imaging workup ends.

Metastatic undifferentiated carcinoma or adenocarcinoma of unknown primary site:

Step 1: Abdominal and Pelvic Computed Tomography

Abdominal and pelvic CT will define the primary site in about one-third of cases. The most common lesion is a pancreatic mass. If CT of the abdomen and pelvis is negative, further study of this region (e.g., by sonography) is very unlikely to demonstrate a treatable lesion.[4] However, if there are subsequent specific symptoms that require imaging as a guide to palliation (e.g., bowel obstruction) studies of the GI tract are appropriate.[4]

SUMMARY AND CONCLUSIONS

1. An initial chest film is appropriate in every patient undergoing workup for suspected metastatic disease without a known primary, before biopsy of the suspected metastatic site.

2. When biopsy of enlarged middle or high cervical nodes shows metastatic cancer of squamous cell origin and endoscopic exam of the mouth and nasopharynx fails to find a primary site, CT or MR may be helpful.

3. When no primary site of origin of metastatic or undifferentiated adenocarcinoma is evident clinically, abdominal and pelvic CT is the next step.

ADDITIONAL COMMENTS

- Quality of life and cost efficacy both demand a rapid imaging workup that will find those lesions amenable to effective treatment. It has been unfortunately true that many patients with metastatic disease from an unknown primary site spend many days and dollars in a futile search for a primary tumor that, even if found, would prove untreatable.

- Imaging of the patient with nonspecific constitutional signs or symptoms that may be caused by an otherwise occult primary cancer is unproductive if specific areas of interest cannot be identified clinically.

- Although metastatic breast carcinoma is a common disease amenable to treatment, presentation as metastatic disease **with an occult primary site** is decidedly rare. In such cases mammograms are virtually always fruitless. **However, if there is palpable axillary lymphadenopathy, mammography may be helpful in detecting a clinically occult ipsilateral breast carcinoma.**[2,5] Biopsy of any mammographic abnormality defined should precede an axillary biopsy.

- Negative mammography does not completely exclude an occult primary breast cancer, but unfortunately additional radiologic exams are usually not helpful.[2]

- Bone scans are abnormal in nearly half of patients who present with metastatic cancer of unknown origin. While bone scans are potentially useful for staging or locating a favorable site for biopsy or palliative radiotherapy, they do not detect occult **primary** bone malignancies; these will have presented clinically by the time of a scan.

- In the absence of suggestive clinical findings like occult GI bleeding or hematuria, the yield from contrast studies of the bowel and urinary tract is so low that they cannot be recommended.
- Patients presenting with **low cervical or supraclavicular lymph nodes** are most likely to have lung or gastrointestinal cancer, not occult primary head and neck cancer.
- Thyroid imaging is reserved for those patients with a palpable thyroid nodule or elevated thyroglobulin (see Chapter 66, Thyroid Mass/Thyroid Enlargement).
- Any mass detected in any specific organ—for example, a pancreatic mass detected by abdominal CT—can be a primary or a metastasis. Thus the search for a primary site ultimately depends on biopsy of lesions defined by imaging.

REFERENCES

1. Diggs CH. Cancer of unknown primary site: deciding how far to carry evaluation. Postgrad Med 1989; 86:186-191.
2. Greenberg BR, Lawrence HJ. Metastatic cancer with unknown primary. Med Clin North Am 1988; 72:1055-1065.
3. Dillon WP, Harnsberger HR. The impact of radiologic imaging on staging of cancer of the head and neck. Semin Oncol 1991; 18:64-79.
4. Bitran JD, Ultmann JE. Malignancies of undetermined primary origin. Dis Month 1992; 38:217-260.
5. Leibman AJ, Kossoff MB. Mammography in women with axillary lymphadenopathy and normal breasts on physical examination: value of detecting occult breast carcinoma. AJR 1992; 159:493-495.

SUGGESTED ADDITIONAL READING

Didolkar MS, Fanous N, Elias EG, Moore RH. Metastatic carcinomas from occult primary tumors. A study of 254 patients. Ann Surg 1977; 186:625-630.

Kagan AR, Steckel RJ. Diagnostic imaging in clinical cancer management: metastases from unknown primary tumors. Invest Radiol 1988; 23:545-547.

Maichel AG. Cancer of unknown primary: a retrospective study based on 109 patients. Am J Clin Oncol 1993; 16:26-29.

McMillan JH, Levine E, Stephens RH. Computed tomography in the evaluation of metastatic adenocarcinoma from an unknown primary site: a retrospective study. Radiology 1982; 143:143-146.

Osteen RT, Kopf G, Wilson RE. In pursuit of the unknown primary. Am J Surg 1978; 135:494-498.

Steckel RJ, Kagan AR. Metastatic tumors of unknown origin. Cancer 1991; 67:1242-1244.

58

Abdominal and Pelvic Masses in Children

INTRODUCTION

Abdominal masses in children are often incidentally discovered by a parent or during a routine physical exam. Imaging can confirm the presence of a mass, localize it to a major abdominal space or organ, define its extent, and suggest a probable cause.

Plain films, ultrasound (US or sonography), contrast material studies of the gut, computed tomography (CT), magnetic resonance imaging (MR), intravenous pyelography (IVP), voiding cystourethrogram (VCUG), nuclear renal scan, nuclear hepatobiliary scan (HIDA), nuclear labeled leukocyte (WBC) scan, and nuclear pertechnetate scan may all play a role.

Costs: abdominal plain film, $57; upper GI series, $160; barium enema, $147; IVP, $168; VCUG, $121; abdominal MR, unenhanced, $823; abdominal MR, enhanced, 943; pelvic MR, unenhanced, $811; pelvic MR, enhanced, $931; abdominal US, $201; pelvic US, $184; abdominal and pelvic CT, enhanced, $840; chest CT, enhanced, $498; renal scan, $257; nuclear WBC scan, $505; HIDA scan, $225; nuclear Meckel's diverticulum scan, $177; liver biopsy, US guided, $511; liver biopsy, CT guided, $802.

PLAN AND RATIONALE

Step 1: Plain Abdominal Film

An abdominal radiograph can reveal the general location of a mass, fat or calcifications within the mass (like teeth in a teratoma), and evidence of gastrointestinal tract obstruction. It also examines the bones of the spine and pelvis, sometimes revealing associated anomalies or unsuspected metastases.

When the plain abdominal film suggests a GI tract–related mass:

Step 2: Upper GI Series or Enema with Contrast Material

Masses associated with the GI tract, especially those involving obstruction (e.g., intussusception or volvulus) are best defined by studies of the upper GI tract or colon with contrast material. **The suspected level of obstruction determines the appropriate exam.**

Emergency bowel studies are indicated if there is obstruction without evidence of bowel perforation. Often, no further presurgical imaging is needed.

When the plain abdominal film shows a mass that appears unrelated to the GI tract:

Step 2: Sonography, Followed by Computed Tomography or Magnetic Resonance Imaging in Selected Patients

Sonography is the radiologic test of choice for evaluating abdominal and pelvic masses in children.

Sonographic detail is superior to that of CT **in small patients:** most infants and children have little body fat to interfere with sonography, tissue planes are ideally demonstrated, and images are generated in multiple planes. Unlike CT, sonography requires no oral or intravenous contrast material, usually requires no sedation, and delivers no ionizing radiation.

Initially, sonography confirms the presence of an abnormal mass. It then localizes and characterizes the mass in terms of its organ oranatomic compartment of origin and its nature (cystic, solid, or complex—i.e., cystic and solid). Also, with color Doppler, sonography can evaluate the vascularity of a mass. **The sonogram is therefore invaluable when the exact origin and character of the mass are unknown; however, we stress that sonography can be bypassed in favor of CT if the plain films and clinical data clearly indicate that the mass is malignant.**

If the abdominal film and sonogram is normal, the imaging workup ends.

If the sonogram is equivocal, then CT or MR is required for confirmation. (In children, an equivocal sonogram with a palpable abdominal mass is quite uncommon.) In fact, in many cases a mass is sufficiently localized and characterized by sonography so that biopsy and/or surgery can follow directly.

Further imaging follows according to the clinical, radiographic, and sonographic localization of the mass. Certain general features of MR and CT bear mentioning before their place in the workup of specific masses is addressed. CT remains central to the workup; unlike sonography, CT is not hampered by gas or bone, and CT visualizes **the retroperitoneum** better than sonography, especially in older children. CT demonstrates calcifications and necrosis better than MR. Moreover, CT with intravenous contrast material (contrast enhanced) can estimate tumor vascularity. Nonetheless, the role of MR in the workup of pediatric abdominal and pelvic masses is expanding, and in some instances MR has replaced CT, because it images in multiple planes, without ionizing radiation. This multiplanar capability is particularly useful when **the exact origin** of a mass—for example, renal versus adrenal—is in dispute. MR also reveals direct extension of a mass into the subarachnoid space and metastatic replacement of bone marrow.

CT and MR are often complementary, and both usually require sedation in infants and young or uncooperative children for a high-quality study.

Hepatobiliary mass suggested by sonogram:

*(A) If the mass is **primarily solid:***

Step 1: Magnetic Resonance Imaging and/or Computed Tomography

Most solid pediatric hepatic masses are hepatoblastomas, particularly in older children, although hepatocellular carcinomas can occur in young children. About two-thirds of solid hepatic masses in children are malignant.[1] CT can define the intrahepatic and extrahepatic extent of tumor, adenopathy, and invasion of major blood vessels. However, MR more accurately determines the resectability of primary liver tumors in children and may be preferable to CT.[2] The choice of CT and/or MR should be made in consultation with the surgeon, pediatric oncologist, and radiologist.

CT (or US) guidance may be used to biopsy liver masses in children (see Chapter 61, Percutaneous Invasive Guided Biopsy). Currently, MR is not amenable to biopsy guidance.

Additional imaging studies prior to surgery may be indicated. For example, a bone scan should be performed in children with hepatocellular carcinoma.[3]

(B) If the mass is **cystic:**

A cystic mass in the portal region is probably a choledochal cyst. Usually identified by the first decade of life, only 30% of children present with the classic triad of intermittent jaundice, pain, and an abdominal mass.[2] For clarification, a nuclear hepatobiliary scan is effective.

Step 1: Nuclear Hepatobiliary Scan

After peripheral intravenous injection, technetium-99m hepatobiliary iminodiacetic acid (Tc-99m-HIDA) is extracted from the blood by the liver and excreted into the bile ducts. HIDA will usually fill a choledochal cyst, confirming the diagnosis. (See Chapter 1, Acute Cholecystitis, for a more complete discussion of HIDA.)

Renal mass suggested by sonogram:

Hydronephrosis, usually demonstrated convincingly by sonography, is the most common cause of an abdominal mass in the neonate. Other renal masses found in children include multicystic dysplastic kidney, malignant tumors like Wilms', and rarer conditions like nephroblastomatosis.

(A) If the mass is **hydronephrosis:**

(See Chapter 18, Obstructive Uropathy and Chapter 22, Urinary Tract Infections/Pyelonephritis in Infants and Children.) If the renal mass is hydronephrosis, vesicoureteral reflux is often the cause. (Reflux may be suggested during initial sonography, if the collecting system dilates when the child voids.) However, a negative sonogram does not exclude vesicoureteral reflux; a VCUG is essential.

Step 1: Voiding Cystourethrogram

The bladder is catheterized and contrast material is introduced under fluoroscopy; the presence or absence of retrograde flow of contrast material into the ureters (reflux) is assessed, and the urethra is examined during voiding for abnormalities (e.g., posterior urethral valves, found in males).

If reflux is identified, the hydronephrosis is explained, but if no reflux is identified, then the dilated renal collecting system may be due to obstruction at either the ureteropelvic junction or, less commonly, the ureterovesical junction. An IVP differentiates between these two sites.

Step 2: Intravenous Pyelogram

After intravenous injection, contrast material is filtered by the kidneys and excreted, opacifying the urinary tract. The site of obstruction causing hydronephrosis is defined. Sometimes only questionable obstruction is apparent. In such cases, or to follow the results of reparative surgery, a nuclear diuretic renal scan can be extremely useful.

Step 3: Nuclear Diuretic Renal Scan

After intravenous injection, technetium-99m diethylen-etriamene pentaacetic acid (Tc-99m-DTPA) is concentrated and excreted by the kidneys. Nuclear images reveal the kidneys and collecting systems; although the anatomic resolution is inferior to that of the IVP, **renal uptake, excretion, and drainage can be quantified.**

By quantifying the "wash-out" of radiopharmaceutical from the collecting systems after a Lasix-induced fluid load, **patulous but not obstructed pelvocalyceal systems are differentiated from those that are truly obstructed.**

The absolute and fractional glomerular filtration rate (GFR) of each kidney is accurately calculated. This measurement is a crucial determinant of renal function and is used to follow pediatric patients who have had reparative surgery for vesicoureteral reflux and/or urinary tract obstruction.

*(B) If the **renal** mass is **solid:***

Wilms' tumor is the most common solid abdominal tumor in children.[1] Although some surgeons will operate on the basis of the sonogram alone, additional imaging is occasionally needed. **Any solid renal mass should be considered malignant until proven otherwise.**

Step 1: Computed Tomography

CT with intravenous contrast material defines the extent of the lesion, adenopathy, and renal vein or inferior vena cava tumor thrombus. The contralateral kidney (5% of Wilms' tumors are bilateral) and liver (a common site of metastases) are also examined. If the malignant nature of the lesion is obvious from imaging or is confirmed by biopsy, then workup of the chest follows.

Step 2: Chest Computed Tomography

Chest CT is appropriate to find pulmonary metastases, which are found in 10% of children presenting with Wilms' tumor.

(C) **Multicystic dysplastic kidney** *suggested by sonogram:*

Multicystic dysplastic kidney is a congential lesion associated with extreme disorganization of renal tissues that do not function. In most instances the diagnosis is obvious on the initial sonogram, but uncommonly the appearance can be confused with—or overlap—extreme hydronephrosis secondary to congenital obstruction at the ureteropelvic junction.

Step 1: Nuclear Renal Scan

The nuclear renal scan can usually differentiate multicystic dysplastic kidney from obstructive lesions, because the former never function at all,[4,5] whereas almost all obstructive lesions function to some extent. The scan also evaluates the GFR of the contralateral kidney, an important consideration when only one functioning kidney is present.

(D) **Probable renal mass** *suggested by sonogram*

Step 1: Magnetic Resonance Imaging

When the renal origin of a mass is questionable, the multiplanar imaging capability of MR is invaluable, because MR can separate adjacent but contiguous organs (e.g., the kidney and adrenal) Like CT, MR can reveal liver metastases, and unlike CT it can easily detect intraspinal extension of tumor.[1,6] Moreover, MR can show invasion of bone marrow, a sensitive indicator of bone metastases.

Retroperitoneal (nonrenal) mass suggested by sonogram:

The most common childhood retroperitoneal nonrenal mass is neuroblastoma. Although they can lie anywhere along the sympathetic chain, most abdominal neuroblastomas are located in the adrenal. Other less common tumors such as lyphoma and teratoma also arise in the retroperitoneum.

The initial sonogram usually defines the extrarenal location of the tumor and in many cases demonstrates its extent, adenopathy, or hepatic metastases, but CT and/or MR are more accurate in this regard.[6]

(A) When the origin of the tumor is clearly **retroperitoneal:**

Step 1: Computed Tomography

CT clearly delineates the extent of tumor, adenopathy, and metastases including those to the liver. The response to therapy can be followed. Depending on the type of tumor, additional imaging tests may be needed. For example, in neuroblastoma a bone scan is mandatory, because the bone marrow is a favored site of tumor metastases.

(B) When the origin of the tumor **may be** *retroperitoneal or adrenal (nonrenal):*

Step 1: Magnetic Resonance Imaging (see above, [D] Probable Renal Mass Suggested by Sonogram)

Pelvic mass suggested by sonogram:

(A) If the pelvic mass is **cystic:**

A pelvic mass in an older child is often an ovarian cyst; in an infant, hydrometrocolpos.[1] The inital sonogram usually defines the nature of the lesion and confirms that other organs are normal. Additional imaging is usually unnecessary.

(B) If the pelvic mass is primarily **solid or complex:**

A complex mass (both cystic and solid) may represent an ovarian tumor. Solid pelvic masses are most commonly neuroblastomas or teratomas. (Both neuroblastomas and teratomas may have characteristic calcifications on the initial plain film; in fact, the plain film appearance of some teratomas is pathognomonic.)

CT is the next exam; MR is complementary in some cases.[7]

Step 1: Computed Tomography or Magnetic Resonance Imaging

Because a solid pelvic mass is often malignant, CT is appropriate to visualize the relationship of the tumor to adjacent pelvic structures and survey the remainder of the abdomen for adenopathy, tumor implants, and liver metastases. MR is an alternative favored by some, because it delivers no ionizing radiation. However, most centers continue to prefer CT, reserving MR for those cases in which specific problems must be solved before biopsy; usually, these involve the separation of the lesion from adjacent organs, a task well suited to the multiplanar imaging capability of MR.

Gastrointestinal-related mass suggested by sonogram:

Although some GI-related abdominal masses will be diagnosed by a combination of plain films and contrast material studies, others, like mesenteric and duplication cysts, may be defined by the sonogram. Abdominal and pelvic abscesses and lymphoma can be of GI origin.

(A) When a GI-related mass could be a **Meckel's diverticulum:**

Step 1: Nuclear Tc–99m Pertechnetate Scan

Tc-99m pertechnetate injected intravenously concentrates in gastric mucosa, including the ectopic gastric mucosa often present in symptomatic Meckel's diverticula. (See Chapter 10, Chronic Gastrointestinal Bleeding in the Adult, for a complete discussion of Meckel's diverticula and the Tc-99m-pertechnetate scan.)

*(B) When a GI-related mass could be **lymphoma:***

Step 1: Computed Tomography

CT is the test of choice for defining suspected or known abdominal/pelvic lymphoma. CT defines tumor extent, nodal, hepatic, pelvic, and retroperitoneal involvement. After a positive biopsy, the chest should be studied for metastases.

*(C) When a GI-related mass could be an **abscess:***

Step 1: Computed Tomography

CT surveys the entire abdomen and pelvis for abnormal collections that in the appropriate setting may represent an abscess. CT can also guide needle aspiration and catheter drainage of abdominal and pelvic abscesses.

Step 2: In-111-Labeled Leukocyte Scan

If CT fails to demonstrate an abscess and clinical suspicion persists, a labeled leukocyte study frequently succeeds. Leukocytes are harvested from the patient's blood and labeled with In-111- or Tc-99m-HMPAO (see Chapter 59, Occult Bacterial Infection, for a discussion of these radiopharmaceuticals). Reinjected into the patient, the labeled cells localize in collections of pus where their presence is detected by the nuclear camera.

SUMMARY AND CONCLUSIONS

1. The plain abdominal film often indicates the general location of a palpated mass, reveals calcifications, and evaluates the GI tract for obstruction. A normal plain film does not exclude a mass.

2. In the absence of GI obstruction, sonography is next, to confirm the presence of a mass, localize it, and characterize it.

3. Based on sonographic findings, additional imaging may or may not be needed. CT is usually the next step, but the radiologist should be consulted, because in some specific circumstances MR is better.

4. Imaging should be tailored according to the organ system(s) involved and clinical factors, because in the abdomen and pelvis a very wide range of additional options is available, including nuclear renal scans, Tc-99m–pertechnetate scans, contrast material studies of the GI tract, radiolabeled leukocyte scans, the VCUG, and the IVP.

ADDITIONAL COMMENTS

- Most cystic abdominal/pelvic masses in children are benign, whereas most solid abdominal/pelvic masses in children are malignant.
- **In selected instances, CT and/or MR may be indicated as the next step after plain films, as opposed to sonography, particularly when the clinical suspicion of a malignant solid neoplasm is high.**

- Fifty-seven percent of abdominal "masses" in children are enlarged organs without a pathologic mass (organomegaly).[1]
- Hepatic hemangioma or hemangioendothelioma may be suspected from the clinical presentation and initial sonogram. Additional studies, including contrast-enhanced CT and a technetium-99m-labeled red cell nuclear scan are helpful for confirmation.
- Almost three-fourths of abdominal masses in neonates are either multicystic dysplastic kidneys or hydronephrotic kidneys.[1]
- Abdominal masses are now not infrequently discovered by prenatal sonograms. After delivery, the workup proceeds with plain films, followed by sonography.[1]
- Adrenal hemorrhage in the neonate has a characteristic appearance on sonography. Occasionally, a repeat sonogram is necessary to differentiate this lesion from neonatal adrenal neuroblastoma.
- The occasional nonobstructing intraperitoneal mass or abdominal wall lesion, such as urachal cyst or mesenteric cyst, can often be identified and characterized on the sonogram; surgery is usually needed for removal and for confirmation.
- Angiography now has a very limited role in the routine evaluation of abdominal and pelvic masses in children.

REFERENCES

1. Mahaffey SM, Ryckman FC, Martin LW. Clinical aspects of abdominal masses in children. Semin Roentgenol 1988; 23:161-174.
2. Boechat MI, Kangarloo H, Gilsanz V. Hepatic masses in children. Semin Roentgenol 1988; 23:185-193.
3. Stomper PC. Cancer Imaging Manual. Philadelphia, 1993, Lippincott.
4. Teele RL, Share JC. The abdominal mass in the neonate. Semin Roentgenol 1988; 23:175-184.

5. Donaldson JS, Shkolnik A. Pediatric renal masses. Semin Rogentgenol 1988; 23:194-204.
6. Daneman A. Adrenal neoplasms in children. Semin Roentgenol 1988; 23:205-215.
8. Surratt JT, Siegel MJ. Imaging of pediatric ovarian masses. RadioGraphics 1991; 11:533-548.

SUGGESTED ADDITIONAL READING

Hayden CK Jr, Swischuk LE. Pediatric Ultrasonography. Baltimore, 1987, Williams & Wilkins.
Kirks DR, ed. Practical Pediatric Imaging: Diagnosic Radiology of Infants and Children, ed 2. Boston, 1991, Little, Brown, Chapters 7, 8.
Sty JR, Wells RG. Other abdominal and pelvic masses in children. Semin Roentgenol 1988; 23:216-231.

59

Occult Bacterial Infection

INTRODUCTION

When clinical or laboratory findings suggest occult bacterial infection, the chest, abdomen, or pelvis is usually the source. Chest radiography is the first imaging procedure. Two additional studies, abdominal/pelvic computed tomography (CT) and autologous radiolabeled leukocyte (WBC) scanning, may be valuable.

Costs: chest films, PA and lateral, $59; abdominal and pelvic CT, enhanced, $840; nuclear WBC scanning, $505.

PLAN AND RATIONALE

Step 1: Chest Radiograph

Inflammatory disease in the chest does not necessarily produce localizing signs. Lack of physical findings or complaints related to the thorax does not exclude pneumonia and other parenchymal, pleural, or mediastinal disease. Chest radiographs (PA and lateral) are mandatory.

If chest films fail to find a source of infection, CT of the abdomen is appropriate.

Step 2: Computed Tomography of the Abdomen/Pelvis

The abdomen is by far the most common source of occult infection, if thoracic disease has been excluded radiographically.

The abdomen is surveyed from the diaphragm to the pelvic floor. Adequate opacification of the bowel by oral contrast material is essential. Moreover, intravenous contrast material, concentrated and excreted by the kidneys, opacifies the urinary tract, helping to differentiate the kidneys, ureters, and bladder from pelvic or retroperitoneal inflammatory masses.

If an abnormal fluid collection that may represent pus is defined, the interventional radiologist may successfully drain it, without the need for laparotomy (see Chapter 61, Percutaneous Invasive Guided Biopsy), but if CT is normal or equivocal, a nuclear autologous leukocyte scan is appropriate.

Step 3: Nuclear Radiolabeled Autologous Leukocyte Scan

A nuclear radiolabeled autologous leukocyte (WBC) scan may detect intraabdominal pus collections missed by CT. Moreover, the WBC study can often clarify an equivocal CT by differentiating fluid-filled bowel from an abscess. Also, **the nuclear exam is a total body survey** that reveals unsuspected lesions in the head, neck, and extremities, as well as in the abdomen.

Leukocytes are harvested from 30 ml of the patient's blood and labeled with indium-111-oxine (In-111-oxine) or technetium-99m-hydroxymethylpropyleneamine oxime (Tc-99m-HMPAO); the cells are injected intravenously, and their migration to infected sites is monitored by a nuclear scan. Eighteen to 24 hours must elapse between injection of In-111-oxine-labeled WBCs and scanning, but scanning can begin only 2 hours after injection of Tc-99m-HMPAO-labeled WBCs.

In general, Tc-99m-HMPAO WBC scans excel for detecting lesions in the head and extremities, whereas In-111-oxine WBCs are favored for surveying the abdomen, lungs, and thorax, because some Tc-99m-HMPAO WBCs are normally seen in the lungs, gut, and bladder, confounding scan interpretation. Nonetheless, some nuclear physicians favor Tc-HMPAO WBCs for evaluating the abdomen, because of the much briefer interval between injection and scanning. **When a radiolabeled WBC scan is contemplated, the choice of isotope should be discussed with the nuclear physician, so that options can be considered in light of the urgency of the case and probable infection source.**

SUMMARY AND CONCLUSIONS

1. Even without thoracic symptoms, chest films are crucial in the search for occult infection.
2. Most occult infections outside of the thorax are in the abdomen and pelvis; therefore, abdominal/pelvic CT is appropriate after chest radiographs.
3. An abnormal fluid collection defined by CT, consistent with an abscess, can often be successfully drained by the interventional radiologist.
4. If CT is normal or equivocal, a total body radiolabeled WBC scan can be definitive. The proper radioisotope should be determined in consultation with the nuclear physician.

ADDITIONAL COMMENTS

- Many nuclear imagers believe that a radiolabeled WBC scan is appropriate after the initial chest film, **before abdominal CT,** on the grounds that **extraabdominal lesions are also imaged by total body scans.** Against this argument is the superior anatomic resolution of CT and the fact that a positive abdominal WBC scan is usually followed by CT, to provide better anatomic definition before drainage. Thus the choice of a WBC study versus abdominal CT is controversial; often the two are complementary.

- Upright chest films in the radiology department are almost always superior to portable films, despite the time and inconvenience for the patient and nursing staff that they entail.

- Although CT is favored over ultrasound for a general abdominal survey, in some patients, like pregnant women and young children, where radiation exposure should be severely limited, ultrasound is a reasonable alternative.

- Agranulocytic patients occasionally require a WBC scan. Heterologous (donor) leukocytes have been successfully used. Present leukocyte harvesting and labeling methods, however, inadvertently include some erythrocytes. **Therefore, donors and recipients must be ABO- and Rh-matched**. Moreover, if the patient has previously received white cell transfusions, more specific matching may be required. Such situations are best discussed between the hematologist and nuclear physician. The utmost precautions, of course, must apply, in view of the possibility of transfering bloodborne infections from donor to recipient.

- When there is a **probable source of abdominal infection**, like appendicitis, Tc-99m–HMPAO WBCs excel; the confounding effect of faint normal gut activity is overcome by scanning very early, **1 hour after WBC injection,** before normal gut activity appears. This strategy is unsuitable for a general abdominal survey, because it somewhat degrades overall scan quality, but is effective when a particular focus, like the right lower quadrant, is suspect. Moreover, early imaging is crucial in the emergency setting of possible appendicitis.

- Unless the appendix is ruptured, CT is often normal or equivocal in acute appendicitis. In most cases a decision regarding surgery is made without any imaging beyond the initial abdominal plain films; CT or a WBC study is appropriate when additional support for surgery is required.

- Gallium-67 citrate is a viable pharmaceutical for oncologic imaging and the study of some infections (see Chapter 43, Osteomyelitis), but it is unsatisfactory for a total body survey in occult bacterial infection.

SUGGESTED ADDITIONAL READING

Allan RA, Sladen GE, Bassingham S, Lazarus C, Clarke SEM, Fogelman I, Clarke L. Comparison of simultaneous 99m-TcHMPAO and 111-In oxine labelled white cell scans in the assessment of inflammatory bowel disease. Eur J Nucl Med 1993; 20:195-200.

Palmer EL, Scott JA, Strauss WH. Practical Nuclear Medicine. Saunders, Philadelphia, 1992, pp 350-354.

60

Recurrent Ovarian and Colorectal Carcinoma

INTRODUCTION

Colorectal carcinoma is the third most common noncutaneous malignancy in the United States, with a yearly mortality of 58,000. Ovarian cancer is the primary cause of gynecologic cancer death and the most frequent cause of cancer death in women, with a yearly mortality of 13,000. The detection of recurrence is vital to effective surgery and chemotherapy for palliation and, in some cases, for attempted cure.

Traditionally, the search for recurrent ovarian or colorectal cancer has been dominated by computed tomography (CT), along with other imaging studies—like intravenous pyelography, barium studies, and sonography—tailored to organ-specific symptoms. Recently, a radiolabeled monoclonal antibody that reacts with a tumor cell surface antigen expressed by most colorectal and ovarian carcinomas has been FDA approved for clinical use; this antibody, "Oncoscint" (Satumomab Pendetide), may alter the traditional approach.

Costs: abdominal and pelvic CT, enhanced, $840; nuclear Oncoscint scan, $1,735.

PLAN AND RATIONALE

Step 1: Computed Tomography

In the patient without specific organ-related symptoms or abnormal laboratory studies, CT remains the primary imaging exam for detection of recurrent ovarian or colorectal carcinoma. CT is also appropriate when serum tumor markers are rising in the asymptomatic patient.

The imaging workup usually ends if abdominal/pelvic CT is normal or demonstrates new soft tissue masses, lymphadenopathy, or liver lesions. However, even after CT difficult management problems sometimes arise that Oncoscint may resolve.

Step 2: Oncoscint Nuclear Scan

Nabi and Doerr[1] cite the following indications for Oncoscint:

1. Rising serum tumor markers in the presence of an otherwise negative workup, **including CT**.
2. Determining whether an apparently isolated and resectable extrahepatic abdominal or pelvic recurrence is truly solitary.
3. Differentiating recurrent neoplasm from postsurgical or postradiation changes.
4. Confirming equivocal findings of neoplasm on CT or other imaging studies (barium enema, etc.).
5. Determining the extent and location of neoplasm in the presence of rising serum tumor markers, as an alternative to "second look" surgery.

The antibody is labeled with indium-111 (In-111) and injected intravenously over several minutes; the patient is closely monitored for allergic reactions. Less than 4% of patients experience side effects, and these are usually mild and transient. The sole contraindication to Oncoscint injection is known allergy to mice or to mouse biologic products. The whole body is scanned at 72 hours and sometimes also at 96 or 120 hours.

About 40% of patients injected with Oncoscint develop human antimouse antibody (HAMA). Because circulating HAMA can degrade subsequent studies (by reacting with injected antibody before it reaches the tumor target), and because the reaction between HAMA and Oncoscint could theoretically be serious, **Oncoscint is now FDA approved as a single use agent only.** Note also that HAMA may interfere with the accuracy of CEA and CA-125 testing.

Published studies suggest that Oncoscint is **inferior to CT for detecting intrahepatic metastases yet superior to CT in detecting extrahepatic abdominal and pelvic tumor recurrences. However, false negatives do occur, and therefore a negative Oncoscint study should not alter patient management. False positive Oncoscint studies are distinctly uncommon;** in one study 97% of positive scans were confirmed at surgery and only seven biopsy-confirmed false positive lesions were found in 192 patients.[2] Despite these encouraging published results, we caution that **Oncoscint is expensive and that a number of nuclear physicians have encountered more false negative scans in their experience than in the literature.** Therefore, the study should be considered only according to the above indications; moreover, we consider guidelines 1, 2, and 4 to be stronger than 3 or 5.

SUMMARY AND CONCLUSIONS

1. In the asymptomatic patient with either normal laboratory values or rising serum tumor markers, CT is the appropriate initial imaging study.

2. After CT, complex management problems can sometimes be resolved by a radiolabeled monoclonal antibody product, marketed as Oncoscint.
3. **Oncoscint should never be used as a screen;
   moreover, a negative Oncoscint study is of no
   clinical significance and should not alter patient
   management.**
4. **Oncoscint is approved for a single use only**,
   because 40% of patients develop HAMA, which can
   theoretically interfere with a second study and/or cause
   a clinically significant allergic reaction. However, FDA
   approval for a second use is probable, after the patient's
   serum is checked for the presence of HAMA.
5. A previous history of allergy to mouse protein is an
   absolute contraindication to Oncoscint administration.

ADDITIONAL COMMENTS

- Oncoscint is the first FDA-approved tumor-seeking
  radiolabeled monoclonal antibody, but many others have
  been developed, and some are well into clinical trials.
  The field of imaging with radiolabeled monoclonal antibodies, known as "immunoscintigraphy" or "radioim-
  munoimaging," is sure to expand rapidly in the next
  decade. Related products, including tumor-avid and
  other receptor-avid peptides, are pending approval.

SUGGESTED ADDITIONAL READING

Collier BD, Nabi HA, Doerr RJ, et al. Immunoscintigraphy performed with In-111-labeled CYT-103 in the management of colorectal cancer: comparison with CT. Radiology 1992; 185:179-186.
Doerr RJ, Nabi HA, Krag D, et al. Radiolabeled antibody imaging in
the management of colorectal cancer: results of a multicenter clinical study. Ann Surg 1991; 214:118-124.
Galandiuk S, Wieand HS, Moertel CG, et al. Patterns of recurrence
after curative resection of carcinoma of the colon and rectum. Surg
Gynecol Obstet 1992; 174:27-32.

Nabi HA, Doerr RJ. Radiolabeled monoclonal antibody imaging (immunoscintigraphy) of colorectal caners: current status and future perspectives. Am J Surg 1992; 163:448-456.

Surwit, EA, Childers, JM, Krag DN, et al. Clinical assesmenrt of In-111-CYT-103 immunoscintigraphy in ovarian cancer. Gynecol Oncol 1993; 48:285-292.

61

Percutaneous Invasive Guided Biopsy

INTRODUCTION

Radiologically guided needle biopsy has become a standard method of obtaining tissue from virtually any organ; in reliability and accuracy it is competitive with surgical biopsy, is often safer, and is invariably less expensive.

Guidance methods include fluoroscopy, ultrasound (US), and computed tomography (CT).

Costs: Costs vary according to the site biopsied and the guidance method; see individual chapters.

PLAN AND RATIONALE

Indications

Percutaneous needle biopsy can determine (1) the histology of a mass, (2) whether residual tumor tissue after therapy is viable, (3) whether there is tumor recurrence, and (4) if masses are metastatic (for tumor staging). Culture material from possibly infected sites can be obtained. **The technique is ideal for patients who refuse surgery or are poor surgical risks.**

Guided biopsy is usually an outpatient procedure and

requires no major patient preparation. Contraindications include an uncorrected bleeding diathesis or inability of the patient to cooperate. Each potential percutaneous needle biopsy should be discussed with the radiologist.

Imaging Guidance Methods

Imaging localizes the needle. Various techniques apply, depending on the site and size of the lesion. If they can be localized in two planes, chest lesions can be biopsied **fluoroscopically** with a high degree of accuracy and low complication rate.

Outside of the chest, **ultrasound is the method of choice,** if the lesion and its access route can be adequately visualized, because US **continuously visualizes the needle and the target.** US applies best to relatively large, superficial or cystic lesions; however, some imagers report high diagnostic accuracy for even solid, small, deep abdominal lesions. The technique is unsuitable if the lesion is obscured by overlying bowel gas or bone. Endoluminal US with a transvaginal or transrectal probe can guide biopsy in the female pelvis or the prostate.

Computed tomography is appropriate for lesions that are small or deep, lie close to vital organs, and are inaccessible to US or fluoroscopy. However, CT does not continuously image the biopsy needle; serial scans are necessary as the needle advances. Newer, faster (spiral) CT scanners have decreased the time requirement for serial scans; nonetheless, CT remains the most time consuming, cumbersome, and expensive of the biopsy methods.

Risks/Complications

Mortality from guided biopsy is extremely rare. In the chest, pneumothorax occurs not infrequently but seldom requires a chest tube. In the abdomen, the risk of hemorrhage and infection is very low.

Most lesions can be biopsied with a 22-gauge needle that traverses bowel or solid organs with minimal risk of bleeding or infection. Larger bore cutting needles that obtain a tissue core are appropriate, if the lesion is believed to be not highly vascular and is easily accessible. Tumor implantation along the needle tract is theoretically possible but exceedingly rare.

SUMMARY AND CONCLUSIONS

1. Percutaneous needle biopsy under radiologic guidance is an accurate, safe, established method for obtaining tissue or culture material from nearly any organ.
2. The technique uses fluoroscopy, ultrasound, or CT.
3. Material obtained is usually suitable for cytology and culture and frequently for histology.
4. Communication between the referring physician, radiologist, and pathologist is necessary for optimal patient selection and good results. In some circumstances, open surgical biopsy may be preferred.

ADDITIONAL COMMENTS

- When the vascularity of a lesion is in question, CT with a bolus injection of intravenous contrast material before biopsy can demonstrate a lesion's vascularity and avoid a potentially dangerous biopsy that might bleed excessively. In the liver, where hemangiomas are common, a lesion suspicious for hemangioma should be studied with a nuclear RBC scan (see Chapter 5, Hepatic Metastases).
- Magnetic resonance (MR) guidance biopsy is not feasible at the present time but may be possible in the future.

SUGGESTED ADDITIONAL READING

Charboneau JW, Reading CC, Welch TJ. CT and sonographically guided needle biopsy: current techniques and new innovations. AJR 1990; 154:1.

Matalon TAS, Silver B. US guidance of interventional procedures. Radiology 1990; 174:43-47.

Mueller PR, van Sonnenberg E. Interventional radiology in the chest and abdomen. N Engl J Med 1990; 322:1364-1374.

Murphy TP, Dorfman GS, Becker J. Use of pre-procedural tests by `interventional radiologists. Radiology 1993; 186:213-220.

Reading CC, Charboneau JW, Felmlee JP, James EM. Sonographically guided percutaneous biopsy of small masses. AJR 1988; 151:189-192.

62

Sinusitis

INTRODUCTION

"Sinusitis" is infection, usually bacterial, of one or more of the paranasal sinuses.[1] There are more than 31 million cases yearly in the United States.[2]

Acute bacterial sinusitis follows a viral upper respiratory infection and presents with fever, rhinorrhea, facial pain, halitosis, and purulent nasal secretions. Similar, but less acute, symptoms occur in recurrent or chronic disease.[3]

Uncomplicated acute sinusitis is usually apparent clinically, and imaging studies are unnecessary.[1,4] However, plain films may be helpful in equivocal cases, and computed tomography (CT) now plays a vital role in the evaluation of patients with chronic sinusitis who are under consideration for endoscopic sinus surgery (ESS). Also, in selected patients with complications of sinusitis, magnetic resonance imaging (MR) may be helpful.

Costs: sinus series, complete, $81; sinus series, limited (3 views or less), $50; sinus CT, unenhanced, $405; sinus CT, enhanced, $593; sinus CT, unenhanced and enhanced, $676; MR, unenhanced, $869.

PLAN AND RATIONALE

For adults or adolescents with questionable acute sinusitis:

Step 1: Standard Sinus Series

A standard four-view sinus series is simple and relatively inexpensive. Unfortunately, the accuracy of this study is limited. An air-fluid level is the only completely reliable radiographic sign of acute sinusitis. Moreover, the ethmoid sinuses, which are most commonly affected, are inadequately evaluated.[5] **Thus a negative sinus series does not completely exclude sinusitis.**

If the study is positive, the disease is treated with antibiotics, and follow-up imaging is rarely required. If the study is negative or equivocal, symptoms persist for weeks to months, and empirical antibiotic therapy is ineffective, then chronic sinusitis may have developed, and CT is usually definitive (see *For adults or adolescents with chronic sinusitis, when endoscopic sinus surgery is considered*, **Step 1: Computed Tomography,** below, or *For children with chronic sinusitis*, **Step 1: Computed Tomography**, below).

For young children with questionable acute sinusitis:

Step 1: Limited Sinus Series

Sinusitis is particularly common in small children. The signs and symptoms of acute sinusitis in these patients are different than in adults and older children; fever may be absent and otitis media is frequently present. A two-view study (a Waters view—a frontal view with the X-ray beam angled upward—and a lateral view) is inexpense, limits radiation, and is helpful for confirmation.[6] Even in children as young as 1 year of age, an air-fluid level in the maxillary sinus is a reliable indicator of acute sinusitis.[6,7]

Usually no further imaging is necessary. However, if the study is negative or equivocal, symptoms persist for weeks to months and empirical antibiotic therapy is ineffective, then chronic sinusitis may have developed, and CT is usually definitive (see *For children with chronic sinusitis,* **Step 1: CT,** below).

For adults or children with complicated acute sinusitis:

Step 1: Computed Tomography with Intravenous Contrast Material

The complications of acute sinusitis may be serious and even life-threatening. Infection may spread to the orbit and the intracranial cavity, causing meningitis, abscess, subdural empyema, and thrombophlebitis.

If complications of acute sinusitis are present or suspected, emergency CT with intravenous contrast material (contrast enhanced) is appropriate to examine the sinuses, orbits, and adjacent brain.

In most cases of complicated sinusitis, CT is sufficient, but when aggressive fungal infection, meningitis, and vascular thrombosis are suspected, MR is more effective.

Step 2: Magnetic Resonance Imaging with Contrast Material

The multiplanar imaging capability of MR reveals any extension of sinus infection into the orbit and adjacent brain, especially in cases of aggressive fungal infection.[2] MR is superior to CT for the evaluation of meningeal infection and vascular thrombosis. However, MR should not precede CT, because CT better displays the complex bony anatomy of the paranasal sinuses, orbits, and skull base; the infection originates in—and propagates from—bony cavities.

For adults or adolescents with chronic sinusitis, when endoscopic sinus surgery is considered:

Step 1: Computed Tomography

"Chronic sinusitis" is sinusitis persisting beyond 3 months or recurrent episodes of acute sinusitis. CT is helpful in chronic sinus disease, particularly as a precursor to endoscopic sinus surgery (ESS). ESS represents a major advance for individuals who fail conservative therapy. Patients are selected for ESS on the basis of both nasal endoscopy and CT.

For this purpose CT images are most revealing in the coronal plane, and thus the study is usually ordered as a "coronal CT." However, details of the exam should be left to the radiologist in consultation with the ENT surgeon. To optimize CT, patients should complete a course of antibiotics, decongestants, and antihistamines; if allergic disease is suspected, topical steroids are appropriate. Immediately before imaging a nasal decongestant is administered and the nose emptied by blowing.[8] **These maneuvers eliminate reversible findings**.

CT reveals the detailed bony anatomy of the paranasal sinuses, defining obstructions or anatomic variations that impede drainage and predispose to intractable infection.

For children with chronic sinusitis:

Step 1: Computed Tomography

Children with chronic sinusitis often have cough, rhinorrhea, and otitis media.[9] Asthma, cystic fibrosis, and immunodeficiency are predisposing factors. The disease is usually managed conservatively, without imaging, but if the diagnosis is equivocal and symptoms are severe and/or debilitating, CT may reveal obstructions or anatomic variations that impede drainage and predispose to intractable infection. As in adults or adolescents, CT is most often revealing in the coronal plane, but details of the study are best left to the radiologist in consultation with the ENT surgeon. ESS can be curative if conservative therapy repeatedly fails.

SUMMARY AND CONCLUSIONS

1. Acute uncomplicated sinusitis in adults and older children is usually apparent clinically, and imaging studies are usually not indicated. In equivocal cases, a standard sinus series is helpful, although the accuracy of sinus radiographs is somewhat limited.
2. Imaging is also seldom necessary in children with suspected acute sinusitis, although a limited sinus series may be helpful, particularly since the diagnosis of sinusitis in children may be more difficult than in adults and older children.
3. Adults or children with suspected or definite complications of acute sinusitis should have emergency CT with intravenous material and, for some further complications, MR. CT and MR are complementary in this setting.
4. The cause of chronic sinusitis, which can be significant or even debilitating, can often be elucidated by CT. The study should be tailored to the individual patient, after consultation between the ENT surgeon and the radiologist.

ADDITIONAL COMMENTS

- A single Waters view of the sinuses is an inadequate study. If imaging of uncomplicated acute sinus disease in adults is indicated, a complete sinus series is appropriate.

- Some institutions favor limited screening CT for chronic sinusitis. Although the cost and radiation dose of a limited CT are much lower than for a standard CT, **local but very significant disease can be missed by this technique**.[2] Thus most imagers consider limited CT an unacceptable compromise.

- The sphenoid sinus and its drainage route are optimally evaluated by **axial rather than coronal** images. Sinus anatomy is sufficiently complex that the optimal CT approach should be determined by consultation between the ENT surgeon and the radiologist.

- CT is helpful in further assessing patients who have not clinically responded to ESS.

- CT is also very valuable to image suspected or clinically evident complications of ESS, such as orbital injury or cerebrospinal fluid leak.

- MR, especially with intravenous contrast material, can often differentiate between inflammatory sinus disease and tumor. Otherwise, MR has a very limited role in the study of uncomplicated sinus disease.

REFERENCES

1. Williams JW Jr, Simel DL. Does this patient have sinusitis? Diagnosing acute sinusitis by history and physical examination. JAMA 1993; 270:1242-1246.
2. Yousem DM. Imaging of sinonasal inflammatory disease. Radiology 1993; 188:303-314.
3. Druce HM. Diagnosis of sinusitis in adults: history, physical examination, nasal cytology, echo, and rhinoscope. J Allergy Clin Immunol 1992; 90:436-441.
4. Fireman P. Diagnosis of sinusitis in children: emphasis on the history and physical examination. J Allergy Clin Immunol 1992; 90:433-436.
5. Mafee MF. Imaging for sinusitis (letter). JAMA 1993; 270:2687.
6. Swischuk LE, Hayden CK Jr, Dillard RA. Sinusitis in children. RadioGraphics 1982; 2:241-244.
7. Barnes PD, Wilkinson RH. Radiographic diagnosis of sinusitis in children. Pediatr Infect Dis J 1991; 10:628-629.

8. Babbel RW, Harnsberger HR. A contemporary look at the imaging issues of sinusitis: sinonasal anatomy, physiology, and computed tomography techniques. Semin US CT MR 1991; 12:526-540.
9. Lazar RH, Younis RT, Parvey LS. Comparison of plain radiographs, coronal CT, and intraoperative findings in children with chronic sinusitis. Otolaryngol Head Neck Surg 1992; 107:29-34.

SUGGESTED ADDITIONAL READING

Diament MJ. The diagnosis of sinusitis in infants and children: x-ray, computed tomography, and magnetic resonance imaging. J Allergy Clin Immunol 1992; 90:442-444.

Mafee MF. Imaging methods for sinusitis. JAMA 1993; 269:2608.

Mafee MF, Chow JM, Meyers R. Functional endoscopic sinus surgery: anatomy, CT screening, indications, and complications. AJR 1993; 160:735-744.

McCaffrey TV. Functional endoscopic sinus surgery: an overview. Mayo Clin Proc 1993; 68:571-577.

Som PM. The paranasal sinuses: nonneoplastic disorders. In Som PM, Bergeron RT, eds. Head and Neck Imaging, ed 2. St Louis, 1992, Mosby, pp 114-166.

Zinreich SJ. Imaging of chronic sinusitis in adults: x-ray, computed tomography, and magnetic resonance imaging. J Allergy Clin Immunol 1992; 90:445-451.

Zinreich SJ, Kennedy DW, Rosenbaum AE, Gayler BW, Kumar AJ, Stammberger H. Paranasal sinuses: CT imaging requirements for endoscopic surgery. Radiology 1987; 163:769-775.

Part VIII
ENDOCRINE

63

Adrenal Masses/Adrenal Endocrine Syndromes

INTRODUCTION

Adrenal masses or extraadrenal tissue with adrenal function (like extraadrenal pheochromocytoma) may present with a variety of clinical syndromes. Each syndrome requires a different imaging sequence.

In endocrine conditions associated with **benign** hyperfunctioning adrenal tissue—notably Cushing's syndrome, primary aldosteronism, and pheochromocytoma—imaging can localize and define the responsible lesion. Also, imaging can identify **malignant** hyperfunctioning adrenal tissue and **both benign and malignant** nonhyperfunctioning tissue.

Adrenal imaging falls into two categories: (1) anatomic and (2) anatomic/functional. Computed tomography (CT), ultrasound (US or sonography), magnetic resonance imaging (MR), adrenal venous sampling, I-131-metaiodobenzyl guanidine (MIBG), and I-131-iodocholesterol all play a role.

Costs: abdominal CT, unenhanced, $362; abdominal US, $201; abdominal MR, unenhanced, $823; MIBG, $362; adrenal venous sampling, $3028; iodocholesterol, $386.

ANATOMIC

Computed Tomography

CT nearly always identifies normal adrenals and accurately defines adrenal masses as small as 0.5 cm. Although a few lesions—adrenal cysts and myelolipomas—have typical CT characteristics, the great majority are not fully characterized by CT alone. Clinical and laboratory data are necessary for a specific diagnosis.

Ultrasound

Although US does not routinely identify the adrenals, on occasion it defines the adrenal origin of an abdominal mass better than CT, because the transverse sections of CT may fail to reveal the separation between a large adrenal mass and the upper pole of a kidney; unlike CT, sonography can image in multiple (not only transverse) planes. Nonetheless, ultrasound is **not** an appropriate **screen** for adrenal masses in the adult; in children, however, sonography is more useful, because of the relative paucity of fat in the child's abdomen and retroperitoneum.

Magnetic Resonance Imaging

MR is an adjunctive study for adrenal masses but has a role in helping to differentiate between pheochromocytoma, metastases, and adenomas.

FUNCTIONAL/ANATOMIC

Adrenal Venous Sampling

This study involves placement of a catheter, introduced

via percutaneous transfemoral venipuncture, into the right and left adrenal veins. Injection of contrast material visualizes the veins, and blood samples are drawn from each, and from the inferior vena cava, for analysis of hormone levels. The exam is effective for lateralizing functioning lesions, but the procedure can be technically difficult and is invasive.

Nuclear Medicine Studies

(A) For the adrenal medulla: I-131-metaiodobenzylguanidine (MIBG)

The pheochromocytoma-seeking compound MIBG is highly effective for localizing intra- and extraadrenal pheochromocytomas. The radiopharmaceutical is injected intravenously, and the thorax, abdomen, and pelvis are imaged at 1, 2, and 3 days. The technique is safe and non-invasive. However, MIBG is available only in large medical centers and provides severely limited **anatomic** information compared to CT or MR; in other words, it can locate pheochromocytomas but provides no information on the status of adjacent tissue, blood supply, vascular invasion, etc.

(B) For the adrenal cortex: I-131 iodocholesterol or "NP-59"

Adrenal cortical scintigraphy involves intravenous injection of I-131- iodocholesterol. This radiolabeled precursor of cortisol accumulates in corticosteroid-producing tissue, demonstrated 5 to 6 days later on the nuclear scan. The uptake is especially intense when corticosteroid synthesis is elevated. I-131-iodochocholesterol has a limited role in localizing **functioning or hyperfunctioning adrenal tumors** and in differentiating these from nonfunctioning metastases and nonfunctioning primary adrenal carcinomas.

Adrenal cortical imaging has declined sharply in recent years because of CT's sensitivity for detecting the adrenal enlargement characteristic of adenomas, metastases, and primary carcinomas. In fact, this pharmaceutical is now unavailable in even major university nuclear medicine departments.

PLAN AND RATIONALE

The imaging of adrenal masses depends on the hormonal pattern observed clinically and biochemically.

Cushing's Syndrome

Cushing's syndrome may develop from adrenal cortical hyperplasia (70%) or adrenal neoplasm—adenoma (20%) or carcinoma (10%). All of these usually enlarge the adrenals. The imaging goal is to localize a functioning neoplasm, if present, for curative surgery. **Cortisol-producing tumors are usually large, and almost all will be detected by CT.** CT of the adrenals is rarely falsely positive. **Similarly, a negative CT usually excludes a cortisol-producing mass.** The accuracy of CT in diagnosing an adrenal cortisol-producing tumor approaches 100%. **Therefore, if CT is normal, the workup for a functioning adrenal cortisol-producing mass usually ends.** However, in the **rare** circumstance of a negative or borderline CT but very strong clinical/laboratory evidence of a functioning cortisol-producing neoplasm, adrenal vein sampling or nuclear scanning with I-131-iodocholesterol is appropriate. I-131-iodocholesterol will accumulate in the hyperfunctioning tissue with a high degree of sensitivity and specificity, and it is preferable to venous sampling, because the study is completely noninvasive, **but its relative unavailability may leave adrenal**

venous sampling as the sole imaging option. A normal or borderline CT, followed by a normal I-131-iodocholesterol study or normal venous sampling, ends the workup.

Primary Aldosteronism

Adenomas cause 80% of primary aldosteronism; most of these are less than 2 cm in diameter. **High-resolution CT, with very thin transverse sections, will detect most adenomas.** After nodular adrenal enlargement is detected by CT, some investigators recommend surgery without further imaging, because false positive CTs are uncommon; others prefer a confirmatory exam (I-131-iodocholesterol scanning or adrenal venous sampling) before surgery.

Despite its efficacy in cortisol-producing tumors, **a negative CT does not exclude aldosteronoma** and, in the presence of compelling clinical evidence, should always be followed by an additional study, either I-131-iodocholesterol or adrenal venous sampling. I-131-iodocholesterol is available in only a few large medical centers. If I-131-iodocholesterol is available, dexamethasone suppression should be used to prove that a nodule is autonomous; dexamethasone is administered prior to the scan, supressing ACTH secretion and reducing I-131-iodocholesterol uptake on the **normal** side, but the abnormal—**autonomous**—side will hyperaccumulate I-131-iodocholesterol regardless of low ACTH levels. The study is about 90% sensitive and 90% specific for aldosteronoma. A negative nuclear exam is followed by adrenal venous sampling only when clinical evidence is very strong. Adrenal venous sampling, when positive, is more specific than a nuclear study for this tumor, **and since the nuclear scan is often unavailable, adrenal venous sampling is usually the next step after a negative CT.**

Pheochromocytoma

About 90% of pheochromocytomas are located in the adrenals (10% bilateral), but 10% are extraadrenal, involving paraaortic or paracaval sympathetic nervous tissue. Unusual locations include the chest (1%) and urinary bladder (1%). Malignant pheochromocytomas can metastasize widely.

CT of the abdomen is the initial study for suspected pheochromocytoma, because most intraadrenal pheochromocytomas are large and easily detected. However, If CT is normal and clinical evidence of pheochromocytoma is compelling, MIBG is appropriate.

Shapiro has emphasized the importance of careful screening before patients are subjected to imaging: **"Neither MIBG scintigraphy nor any other imaging procedure should be an initial screening test for pheochromocytoma,** and patients selected for study should be those in whom there is a reasonable suspicion of pheochromocytoma based on the presence of: (a) labile, severe, or uncontrolled hypertension and/or spells manifested by headache, palpitations, sweating, or abdominal pain; (b) elevated basal plasma norepinephrine and/or persistent elevated urinary excretion rates for catecholamines; (c) historical, clinical, or laboratory evidence for syndromes in which pheochromocytomas occur with increased frequency (multiple endocrine neoplasia [MEN] 2a or 2b, neurofibromatosis and von Hippel-Lindau disease) but who manifest only minor symptoms and/or intermittent or borderline laboratory abnormalities for pheochromocytoma."[1]

Traditionally, CT has been the primary imaging study for pheochromocytoma. **Although CT is effective in the study of sporadic intraadrenal lesions, with sensitivity and specificity exceeding 90%, MIBG is certainly superior in detecting extraadrenal, recurrent,**

and malignant lesions. Even if an adrenal lesion has been demonstrated by CT, MIBG may be useful in disclosing unsuspected metastatic or multicentric disease. Thus in the great majority of cases a rational approach indicates **initial abdominal CT, followed by MIBG if CT is normal, borderline, or does not fully explain the endocrine syndrome.** Moreover, the search for **extraadrenal, malignant, or recurrent pheochromocytoma** is best undertaken by MIBG.

The role of MR is currently not defined; although the study can often differentiate pheochromocytomas from adenomas and metastases, it is best reserved for those very unusual puzzling cases in which CT and MIBG are not definitive.

Incidental Adrenal Mass

A problem arising from the frequent application of CT is the incidental, nonfunctioning adrenal mass. Autopsy series have revealed grossly visible nonfunctioning adenomas in 2% to 9% of adults (the higher numbers probably include macronodular hyperplasia as well as nonfunctioning adenomas). A study of 2,200 patients who had abdominal CT showed that 0.6% had incidental nonhyperfunctioning adrenal masses; 50% of these masses were less than 3 cm in diameter. The likelihood that an incidental mass is an adrenal carcinoma is relatively remote. **Therefore, in the absence of adrenal hyperfunction or known malignancy, small incidentally discovered adrenal masses should be followed by CT in 2 to 3 months. This follow-up will almost always exclude the rare primary carcinoma, which usually grows very rapidly**. If the mass is greater than 5 cm, it should be surgically removed. If the mass is 3 to 5 cm, it is indeterminate, and various management schemes are advocated.

An incidentally discovered adrenal mass, in the context

of a known primary neoplasm elsewhere, may represent a metastasis. **(Carcinomas of the lung and breast metastasize frequently to the adrenals.) If CT is not specific, MR may be helpful,** although, unfortunately, there is overlap between the appearance of benign and malignant lesions on MR also. Percutaneous adrenal biopsy under CT guidance is the most accurate method of differentiating nonhyperfunctioning adenomas from metastases.

SUMMARY AND CONCLUSIONS

1. The appropriate imaging modality for a suspected adrenal lesion depends on the patient's endocrine status.
2. In Cushing's syndrome, CT alone almost always defines or excludes adenomas. Adrenal venous sampling and I-131–iodocholesterol adrenal cortical scanning (if available) will clarify relatively rare selected cases.
3. CT will detect most aldosteronomas; a confirmatory study may be needed, because the lesion is usually very small. A negative CT does not exclude aldosteronoma. If necessary, adrenal venous sampling or I-131–iodocholesterol adrenal cortical nuclear scanning, with dexamethasone supression, is appropriate after CT.
4. For pheochromocytoma, CT is usually be the first imaging test. MIBG is as accurate as CT and is more accurate than CT in detecting metastatic or extraadrenal lesions. Thus MIBG, if available, may be the first test, with CT as a follow-up for further anatomic information. In unusual selected cases, MR is helpful after both CT and MIBG.
5. The incidental mass, in the patient with no known neoplasm, is followed when small and removed when large.
6. In the context of a known malignancy elsewhere, an adrenal mass is suspicious for a metastasis.

REFERENCES

1. Shapiro B, Copp JE, Sisson JC, Eyre PL, Wallis J, Beierwaltes WH. Iodine-131 metaiodobenzylguanidine for the locating of suspected pheochromocytoma: experience in 400 cases. J Nucl Med 1985; 26:576-585.

SUGGESTED ADDITIONAL READING

Dunnick NR. Adrenal imaging: current status. AJR 1990; 154:927-936.

Dunnick NR, Doppman JL, Gill JR Jr, Strott CA, Keiser HR, Brennan MF. Localization of functional adrenal tumors by computed tomography and venous sampling. Radiology 1982; 142:429-433.

Ferris EJ, Seibert JJ. Adrenal gland. In Ferris EJ, Seibert JJ, eds. Multiple lmaging Procedures, vol 4, Urinary tract and adrenal glands. New York, 1980, Grune & Stratton, pp 473-520.

Francis IR, Glazer GM, Shapiro B, et al. Complementary roles of CT scanning and 131-I-MIBG scintigraphy in the diagnosis of pheochromocytoma. AJR 1983; 141:719-725.

Francis IR, Gross MD, Shapiro B, Korobkin M, Quint LE. Integrated imaging of adrenal disease. Radiology 1992; 184:1-13.

Newhouse JH. MRI of the adrenal gland. Urol Radiol 1990; 12:1-6.

Rossi P, Young IS, Panke WF. Techniques, usefulness and hazards of arteriography of pheochromocytoma: review of 99 cases. JAMA 1968; 205:54733.

Shapiro B, Sisson JC, Kalf V, et al. The location of middle mediastinal pheochromocytomas. J Thorac Cardiovasc Surg 1984; 87:814-820.

Thrall JH, Freitas JE, Beierwaltes WH. Adrenal scintigraphy. Semin Nucl Med 1978; 8:23-41.

64

Thyroid Nodule/Thyroid Enlargement

INTRODUCTION

The workup of thyroid nodules and diffuse thyroid enlargement differs. In nodular disease the diagnostic thrust is to differentiate benign from malignant nodules, whereas in diffuse enlargement imaging helps to narrow a wide range of benign diagnostic options.

Traditionally, imaging was used to establish whether nodular lesions in the thyroid region were actually part of the thyroid gland and, if so, what they probably represented. However, in recent years fine-needle aspiration biopsy (FNAB) has largely supplanted imaging. A thorough discussion of FNAB is beyond the scope of this book; nonetheless, ample evidence supports the view that in the patient who is not hyperthyroid **nodules that are clearly in the thyroid gland should undergo initial FNAB rather than imaging.** Those that are malignant go directly to surgery, while those that are benign are followed clinically; reaspiration of benign lesions is necessary only if the lesion grows. "Suspicious" cytology is associated with malignancy about 20% of the time and also mandates surgery. Thus the role of imaging is to clarify those cases in which the cytologic specimen is nondiagnostic, to work up a thyroid mass when expert cytopathology is unavailable, or to establish whether a nodule is actually in the thyroid.

Even in the event of a nondiagnostic specimen, rebiopsy is often more cost effective than imaging. Ultrasound (US or sonography) can play a role in a few selected circumstances.

Patients with clinical or chemical hyperthyroidism, however, should have thyroid function tests, sometimes followed by a radioiodine uptake and often a thyroid scan, even if their thyroid is nodular.

Costs: thyroid scan, $124; thyroid biopsy, US-guided, $380; thyroid biopsy, unguided, $171.

PLAN AND RATIONALE

NODULAR THYROID DISEASE

If a nodule or nodules are clearly in the thyroid on palpation and the patient is not hyperthyroid:

Step 1: Fine Needle Aspiration Biopsy, Unguided

FNAB usually requires no imaging guidance. It is safe, minimally invasive, and productive, yielding diagnostic material about 85% of the time. The cytopathologic interpretation, in good hands, is 95% accurate. Therefore, malignant and "suspicious" lesions are directed to surgery, whereas benign lesions are followed. Indeterminate or nondiagnostic specimens can be referred for rebiopsy, usually under ultrasound guidance.

Step 2: Ultrasound-Guided FNAB

The majority of nodules that are rebiopsied under ultrasound guidance yield diagnostic material. However, a small minority remain indeterminate, and for these cases radionuclide scanning can be helpful.

If fine-needle aspiration biopsy of a thyroid nodule is inconclusive, if the procedure and/or expert cytopathology is unavailable, or if the patient is hyperthyroid:

Step 1: Nuclear Thyroid Scan

An intravenous injection of technetium-99m pertechnetate ($TcO4^-$) is followed by images of the neck. Frequently, the neck is reimaged after the nuclear physician has placed a marker on any palpable lesion.

If the palpable lesion is in the thyroid, the workup diverges according to the nuclear findings. By and large, **truly functional ("hot") nodules can safely be considered benign and do not require surgery, whereas nonfunctional or poorly functional ("cold" or "cool" nodules) may be cysts or neoplasms and require surgery.**

(A) Solitary cold or cool nodule:

A solitary hypofunctioning nodule is ominous, especially if it is hard. Depending on the size of the lesion and the patient population, the likelihood of malignant neoplasm is between 15% and 40%. Benign cold nodules are either cysts, nonfunctioning adenomas, or partly cystic and partly solid benign lesions like degenerating adenomas; because the true cysts are not malignant and because sonography is capable of defining cysts, a sonogram is sometimes suggested after the nuclear scan to differentiate benign cysts from possibly malignant solid lesions. **However, sonography cannot establish benignancy with a high degree of confidence, and a histologic or cytologic diagnosis is mandatory. Therefore we do not recommend sonography as a next step.**

(B) Multiple cold and/or cool nodules:

Multiple well-defined hypofunctioning nodules in an otherwise normal gland may also represent malignant neoplasm and should be pursued histologically, especially if they are hard on palpation. Most of these lesions will be benign adenomas or cysts superimposed on a finely multinodular adenomatous goiter, too subtle to detect by palpation or nuclear scanning.

(C) Irregular cold or cool area:

A hard, irregular cold area or a hard, cold area distorting the gland is ominous and could indicate either malignant neoplasm, scar (secondary to previous inflammation, hemorrhage, or trauma), or atypical adenoma. Histologic diagnosis is required.

(D) Solitary hyperfunctioning nodule:

A solitary hot nodule is usually a hyperfunctioning benign adenoma, especially if it suppresses the remainder of the gland, by producing enough T4 to reduce thyroid stimulating hormone (TSH) production by feedback inhibition. Although the chance of malignancy in a single hyperfunctioning nodule is very, very low, a few cases have been reported. Nonetheless, most endocrinologists prefer to follow such cases clinically and, if indicated, treat with radioiodine to ablate the nodule and repeat the thyroid scan only if the lesion enlarges.

(E) Multiple hot nodules:

Multiple, very clearly defined hyperfunctioning nodules and faint or absent visualization of the remainder of the thyroid gland indicate Plummer's disease. In this condition several separate areas of the thyroid develop autonomy, producing sufficient thyroid hormone to suppress the remainder of the gland by reducing TSH by feedback inhibition. The hyperfunctioning lesions may or may not produce enough hormone to cause clinical hyperthyroidism. Autonomy of these nodules may be proved by reimaging after a course of T3 (T3 suppression test). Statistically, the chance of malignancy in one of several hyperfunctioning (hot) nodules is virtually nil, so further imaging is unnecessary, except to follow their regression after radioiodine therapy. Histologic diagnosis is not appropriate.

(F) Enlarged inhomogeneous gland:

An enlarged, inhomogeneous gland with multiple patchy, poorly defined areas of increased and decreased function is frequently termed a "multinodular goiter." "Multinodular goiter" literally means "an enlarged gland with many nodules," and, strictly speaking, it is a descriptive rather than a diagnostic term. In common medical usage, however, "multinodular goiter" has become synonymous with "multinodular colloid adenomatous goiter," a pathologic entity in which the thyroid gland is partly replaced by cysts, poorly functioning normal tissue resembling adenomas, fibrosis-compressed normal tissue, and possibly calcification or hemorrhage. The condition is frequently familial and typical on palpation (rubbery and nodular), with a characteristic imaging appearance: an enlarged, inhomogenous gland with areas of hypofunction interspersed between areas of normal function. The poorly functioning (cold) areas in multinodular colloid adenomatous goiter have traditionally been considered to have a very, very low incidence of malignancy, but recent evidence suggests that as many as 4% may be malignant. **Therefore, histologic diagnosis of a cold lesion that is hard, growing, or dominant is prudent, even in a multinodular gland.**

A condition that may mimic multinodular colloid adenomatous goiter on imaging is chronic (Hashimoto's) thyroiditis, which merits no further imaging.

If a nodule in the thyroid region may or may not be intrathyroidal:

Step 1: Sonogram

Sonography clearly defines the thyroid gland and establishes whether a palpable nodule is intra- or extrathyroidal. Not infrequently, the sonogram proves that a palpable "nodule" is, in fact, a prominent lobe of the normal thyroid gland, ending the workup.

Sonography can establish whether a nodule is solid, cystic, or "complex" (mixed solid and cystic), but **even lesions that are primarily cystic can be malignant; therefore, no sonographic appearance can establish benignancy with a high degree of confidence.**

If the nodule is extrathyroidal, it is worked up like any other soft tissue mass. If a true intrathyroidal nodule is located, FNAB is appropriate.

DIFFUSELY ENLARGED THYROID

Step 1: Nuclear Thyroid Scan

An intravenous injection of technetium-99m pertechnetate ($TcO4^-$) is followed by images of the neck. The typical patterns observed when the gland is enlarged include the following.

(A) Enlarged homogeneous hot gland:

A diffusely enlarged homogeneous gland with **increased** TcO4$^-$ accumulation strongly suggests Graves' disease. Elevated serum hormone levels, low TSH levels, and a high radioiodine uptake are confirmatory. Graves' disease requires neither further imaging nor histology.

Rarely, this scan pattern may result from a metabolic defect in thyroid hormone synthesis after iodide is trapped (e.g., an organification or coupling defect). In these cases, serum thyroid hormone levels will be low and the patient will be euthyroid or hypothyroid; TSH is accordingly high, with subsequent enlargement of the gland (compensatory goiter) and intense TcO4$^-$ trapping. The radioiodine uptake may be low or high, depending on the site of the metabolic defect: if iodine is properly organified, the uptake will be high, but if organification is defective, the uptake will be normal to low, because the trapped radioiodine will soon leave the thyroid.

Synthesis defects may be idiopathic or may accompany Hashimoto's thyroiditis or recovering subacute thyroiditis. Further imaging usually is not required.

(B) Enlarged homogeneous gland with normal TcO4^2 uptake:

A diffusely enlarged, homogeneous gland with **normal** TcO4$^-$ accumulation could represent early, developing Graves' disease ("euthyroid Graves' disease"), in which the gland is in a borderline state between normal function and autonomous hyperfunction and may later progress to flagrant hyperthyroidism. Radioiodine uptake will usually be "upper normal." Correlation with serum thyroid hormone levels is useful to confirm developing hyperthyroidism, but a test of thyroid autonomy, the TRH (thyrotropin-releasing hormone) level, is virtually diagnostic.

A diffusely large, homogenous gland could also represent a stage of Hashimoto's disease, recovering subacute thyroiditis, a normal variant, or simply a very finely multinodular colloid goiter, in which the nodules are so small as to be unpalpable and beyond the resolution threshold of the nuclear camera. None of these conditions warrants histologic diagnosis.

(C) Large faint gland:

A large, tender gland with poor $TcO4^-$ uptake, barely visualized on the scan, is characteristic of subacute thyroiditis. Usually the serum thyroid hormone levels are high, while radioiodine uptake is low (or virtually absent). Further imaging or histology is unnecessary.

SUMMARY AND CONCLUSIONS

1. **In the patient who is not hyperthyroid, FNAB should precede all imaging.** The cytopathologic results of FNAB can direct patients to surgery or non-surgical follow-up.
2. When FNAB yields nondiagnostic material, ultrasound-guided FNAB is usually successful.
3. Ultrasound can precede FNAB **when it is important to determine whether a lesion is actually in the thyroid.**
4. Where FNAB and expert cytopathology are unavailable and when repeat guided FNAB is nondiagnostic, radionuclide scanning of a nodule can be helpful.
5. In the hyperthyroid patient with one or more nodules, a thyroid scan after basic thyroid function tests is usually more valuable than FNAB, because the thyroid often contains one or more "hot" nodules that will not require biopsy and because the scan patttern is a helpful guide to proper therapy.

6. Radionuclide scanning is the procedure of choice for workup of a diffusely enlarged thyroid.

ADDITIONAL COMMENTS

- The population with childhood head and neck radiation is at a higher risk for thyroid malignancy than the general population. These radiation-induced malignancies sometimes present as multiple cold nodules. **Therefore, multiple cold nodules in a previously radiated patient virtually always require a tissue diagnosis.**
- In the nuclear medicine community the proper follow-up of a solitary "hot" nodule is somewhat controversial. A few nuclear imagers have pointed out that hyperfunctioning benign adenomas are relatively well differentiated and will trap TcO4$^-$ **and organify radioiodine,** whereas the very, very rare malignant hyperfunctioning nodule will **trap pertechnetate but fail to organify radioiodine**, permitting a second scan with radioiodine to differentiate between them. Thus some imaging authorities recommended a follow-up radioiodine scan for **each solitary hot nodule**; this plan represents minority opinion, and since secondary factors—like firmness of the lesion on palpation, history of the lesion, **and growth rate**—influence the decision, each solitary hot nodule should be discussed individually between the clinician and the imager.
- Occasionally, two thyroid diseases can coexist (e.g., Graves' disease superimposed upon a preexistent colloid adenomatous goiter.) In these cases FNAB can exclude malignancy, but a thyroid scan may also be necessary to arrive at an endocrinologic diagnosis.

SUGGESTED ADDITIONAL READING

Belfiore A, La Rosa GL, La Porta GA, Giuffrida D, Milazzo G, Luppo L, et al. Cancer risk in patients with cold thyroid nodules: relevance of iodine intake, sex, age, and multinodularity. Am J Med 1992; 93:363-369.

Charkes ND. Nodular goiter. Semin Nucl Med 1971; 1:316-333.

Gharib HG. Fine needle aspiration biopsy of thyroid nodules. Mayo Clin Proc 1994; 69:44-49.

Hamburger JI. Application of the radioiodine uptake to the clinical evaluation of thyroid disease. Semin Nucl Med 1971; 1:287-300.

Jones EM, Charboneau SW. High-frequency (10 MHz) thyroid ultrasonography. Semin US CT MR 1985; 6:294-309.

Khan O, Ell PJ, Maclennan KA, Kurtz AB, Williams ES. Thyroid carcinoma in an autonomously hyperfunctioning thyroid nodule. Postgrad Med J 1981; 57:172-175.

Pinsky S, Ryo UY. Thyroid imaging: a current status report. In Freeman LM, Weissmann HS, eds. Nuclear Medicine Annual. New York, 1981, Raven Press, pp 157-194.

Simeone JF, Daniels GH, Mueller PR, Maloof F, van Sonnenberg E, Hall DA, O'Connel RS, Ferrucci JT Jr, Wittenberg J. High-resolution real-time sonography of the thyroid. Radiology 1982; 145:431-436.

Turner JW, Spencer RP. Thyroid carcinoma presenting as a pertechnetate "hot" nodule but without I-131 uptake: case report. J Nucl Med 1976; 17:223.

65

Parathyroid Adenoma

INTRODUCTION

Traditionally, parathyroid adenomas are characterized by clinical and laboratory findings. Although magnetic resonance imaging (MR), computed tomography (CT), and ultrasound (US) can define adenomas with a sensitivity of 60% to 75%, neck exploration without previous imaging is favored by most surgeons on the grounds that surgery is required regardless of imaging results, and exploration is over 90% successful. However, adenomas can be multiple or ectopic and occasionally the postsurgical patient presents with recurrent symptoms; reexploration can be technically difficult and unsuccessful. A recently developed nuclear method, using technetium-99m-sestimibi (MIBI) effectively localizes parathyroid adenomas and promises to expedite reexploration.

Costs: MIBI with SPECT, $632.

PLAN AND RATIONALE

MIBI, originally developed for myocardial perfusion imaging, concentrates in certain well-perfused noncardiac tissues, including some neoplasms, and can define small parathyroid adenomas missed by more complex nuclear methods and by CT.[1,2]

The thyroid gland itself is well defined by MIBI, but the dynamics of MIBI "washout" differ for thyroid and parathyroid tissue; early (almost immediate) nuclear images of the thoracic inlet reveal uptake **in the thyroid gland and parathyroid adenomas, whereas images 1 hour later reveal only the parathyroid adenomas.**

If MIBI is positive, most surgeons will operate without further imaging.

SUMMARY AND CONCLUSIONS

1. A MIBI scan is the procedure of choice for detecting recurrent parathyroid adenomas before second surgery.
2. Many surgeons will operate on the basis of a MIBI scan alone, in the proper clinical context.

ADDITIONAL COMMENTS

- MIBI has replaced the older, more complex, less sensitive nuclear methods, which used a combination of thallium-201 and technetium-99m pertechnetate.
- MIBI has also successfully defined parathyroid carcinomas and hyperplasia, in addition to adenomas.[2,3]

REFERENCES

1. Taillefer R, Boucher Y, Potvin C, Lambert R. Detection and localization of parathyroid adenomas in patients with hyperparathyroidism using a single radionuclide imaging procedure with technetium-99m-sestimibi (double-phase study). J Nucl Med 1992; 33 (10):1801-1807.
2. OsmanagaogluK, Schelstraete K, Lippens M, Obrie E., De Feyter I. Visualization of a parathyroid adenoma with Tc-99m MIBI in a case with iodine saturation and impaired thallium uptake. Clin Nucl Med 1993; 18 (3):214-216.
3. Parathyroid imaging—current status and future prospects (editorial comment) J Nucl Med. 1992; 33 (10):1807-1809.

66

Breast Imaging

Julie L. Barudin, M.D., Susan G. Orel, M.D.,
Rosalind H. Troupin, M.D.

INTRODUCTION

Breast cancer is the most common cancer of American women,[1] and 183,000 new cases are expected in 1994. It is the leading cause of cancer death in women under age 54, and the second most common in women aged 55 to 74. Risk factors include age, early menarche, late menopause, nulliparity, family or personal history of breast cancer, and previous biopsy-proven atypical hyperplasia or lobular neoplasia. The etiology of breast cancer has remained elusive, its incidence is rising, and our only hope of prevention to date is early detection by screening—including monthly breast self-examination, yearly examination by a health care practitioner, and mammography, the only imaging modality proven to decrease mortality from breast cancer.[2-4]

Mammography's two distinct functions, **screening** and **diagnosis**, should be clearly differentiated. **Screening mammography is the imaging of asymptomatic women** to detect early, clinically occult breast cancer. **Diagnostic mammography is the workup of a patient with clinical symptoms or signs** (like localized pain, lumps, or nipple discharge) **or further evaluation after an abnormal screening exam.** Diagnostic mammography is perhaps better termed "diagnostic breast imaging" because it may include supplemental mammographic views as well as other modalities (ultrasound [US], magnetic resonance imaging [MR], or galactography).

Costs: screening mammogram, bilateral, $100; breast US, $150; breast cyst aspiration, $250; preoperative breast needle localization, $300; galactography, $150; breast MR, $1000; breast core biopsy, stereotactic, $1000; breast open excisional biopsy, $3000.

PLAN AND RATIONALE

Screening mammography

Step 1: Physician Recommendation

The most important first step for clinicians is to recognize their critical role in recommending mammography.[5,6] Most American women are not screened according to appropriate guidelines, primarily because their physicians fail to urge them to undergo the procedure. In this context, clinicians should refer only to facilities performing high-volume, high-quality mammography (in the United States, previously accredited by the American College of Radiology, now monitored and regulated by the FDA).

Step 2: Screening Guidelines

Seventy-five percent of breast cancers occur in women without known risk factors; therefore, screening mammography is recommended for **all** women, following age guidelines, which are periodically debated and revised.

Currently, the American College of Radiology, American Cancer Society, and American College of Obstetricians and Gynecologists recommends **for all women**:

Age 35:	**Baseline mammography**
Age 40–50:	**Mammography every 1 to 2 years**
Age 50 and above:	**Yearly mammography**

For a woman with a first-degree relative who developed premenopausal breast carcinoma, most authorities recommend that screening be initiated 5 to 10 years before the age at which her relative was afflicted.

Step 3: Patient Education

Some women resist screening mammography because they are not experiencing any breast symptoms; they need to understand that the goal of screening is to detect early, clinically occult cancer, at a curable stage, before mastectomy is necessary. Others resist because they fear allegedly painful compression during the procedure; they should be reassured that most women experience a tolerable discomfort—not pain—during the few moments of necessary breast compression and that this discomfort may be minimized by undergoing mammography immediately after a menstrual cycle. Finally, some women avoid screening mammography because they fear that radiation might actually **induce** breast cancer. **Mammography is, in fact, safe. All analyses of the risk of radiation-induced breast cancer are based on populations that received *extremely high doses***—atomic bomb survivors,[7] patients radiated for benign breast disease,[8] and sanitarium patients who repeatedly underwent fluoroscopy.[9] These doses are many orders of magnitude higher than those of modern mammography (100 to 2000 rad.[10], compared to 0.2 rad or less, respectively). **The risk of mammography is negligible compared to its benefits.**[10] Nonetheless, the extremely small theoretical risk is likely to be higher for young breast tissue; this consideration, coupled with the low incidence of breast cancer in young women and mammography's diagnostic limitations in young, dense, glandular breasts, justifies screening mammography along age-based guidelines.

Step 4: Anticipation of "Call Backs" in Screening

Where rapid-flow, reduced-cost screening mammography is practiced, images are usually interpreted after the patient has left the facility, and a few patients (less than 10%) will be contacted to return for additional views. This call back **does not necessarily mean that there is a highly suspicious lesion**; rather, it often proves that a finding is *not* worrisome. **Therefore, to avoid unnecessary anxiety, every patient should be alerted to the possibility that she may be asked to return for additional views.**

Step 5: Providing "Outside" Films

Internal breast anatomy varies enormously, so comparison to a prior baseline is invaluable. The clinician should therefore emphasize to the patient that **old** mammograms are extremely important for comparison and that if she has had previous mammograms elsewhere, she should attempt to make them available to the radiologist, preferably when she undergoes her mammogram.

Step 6: Follow-up

The **screening** mammogram will result in a recommendation for:

a. Continued routine screening or
b. Call back

The clinician's role is to ensure that the screening study is performed, to be aware of the radiologist's interpretation and recommendations, and to act on these recommendations.

Diagnostic mammography

(A) Patient with equivocal or suspicious screening exam:

Step 1: Patient Education/Involvement

After screening mammography, a few patients will be asked to return for additional images, which may include spot compression, magnification, and rotated tailored views to establish whether a lesion is really present, and, if so, to clarify its location and characteristics. Sometimes, instead of additional mammographic views, the radiologist will ultrasound (US) the abnormality to determine whether it is a cyst. In most practices the radiologist contacts the patient to arrange for this call-back visit.

Step 2: Follow-up

The call-back visit for supplemental imaging will result in a recommendation for:

a. Return to routine screening
b. Biopsy (see **Interventional Procedures,** below)
c. Short interval follow-up (usually 6 months)

As in screening mammography, the clinician's role is to see that the study is performed, to be aware of the radiologist's final interpretation and recommendations, and to act on these recommendations.

(B) Patient with a palpable abnormality:

Step 1: Physical Exam

The clinical setting and characteristics of the palpable lesion are extremely important in selecting the next step. **The patient's age is particularly critical**.

Step 2: Evaluation: Tailored by Age Group

1. ***Under age 30:*** Both aspiration (usually by the clinician) or US (by the radiologist) can establish that the palpable lesion is a simple cyst; if so, the workup is complete and the patient can return to routine screening. **It is extremely important to note that US is not an effective screening technique;** US should be used only as a **directed** exam, to evaluate a palpable or mammographically defined abnormality. When requesting breast US for a palpable lesion, one must be sure to indicate its precise location so that US will be appropriately directed.

If a simple cyst is **not** confirmed, then a unilateral, single-view mammogram is appropriate to seek calcifications suspicious for malignancy. (However, even this single view is not recommended if the patient less than 20 years old.[11]) If the single view reveals suspicious calcifications, bilateral mammography should be completed to exclude a lesion in the contralateral breast, and the patient progresses to biopsy (see ***Interventional Procedures,*** below).

2. ***Age 30 to 35:*** If there is no strong family history of breast cancer, the protocol for women age 30 and under applies.

If a first-degree relative has had breast cancer, then the protocol for women age 35 and older applies.

3. *Age 35 and older:* A bilateral mammogram is performed first. If the mammogram is negative or nonspecific, attention is directed toward establishing whether the palpable lesion is a cyst. Both aspiration (usually by the clinician) or US (by the radiologist) can establish that the lesion is a simple cyst; if so, the workup is complete and the patient can return to routine screening. **It is extremely important to note that US is not an effective screening technique. US should be used only as a directed exam, to evaluate** a palpable or mammographically defined abnormality. When requesting breast US for a palpable lesion, one must be sure to indicate its precise location so that US will be appropriately directed.

If the palpable lesion is not a cyst or if other noncystic lesions are defined, the patient progresses to biopsy (see *Interventional Procedures,* below).

Step 3: Be Aware of False Negatives in Mammography

The false negative rate of mammography is approximately 10% to 15%, depending on patient age. Most of these "misses" occur because a noncalcified cancer is obscured by dense fibroglandular tissue. The mammographic report generally alerts the clinician to the breast tissue density in each case. **Any clinically suspicious mass should be biopsied despite negative or nonspecific results from breast imaging.**

(C) Patient with unilateral nipple discharge:

Most patients with nipple discharge have benign disease. However, discharge from one nipple only, especially from one duct orifice only, can herald a malignancy. The discharge is especially worrisome if it is bloody or watery.

Step 1: Unilateral Mammogram

Mammography is a good starting point, and it can be unilateral if the patient has been screened regularly. If the study reveals a suspicious mass, biopsy is appropriate (see *Interventional Procedures*, below); if not, a galactogram can be helpful.

Step 2: Galactogram

Galactography, or ductography, involves cannulating the discharging duct with a blunt needle and injecting a very small amount of contrast material. A filling defect within the duct or an abrupt cut-off of the ductal drainage system can indicate a malignancy; the galactogram is an excellent presurgical "road map."

(D) Patient with breast pain:

Step 1: If Localized Pain, Consider Mammography or Ultrasound

Although breast pain is an extremely unlikely presentation for cancer, a limited mammogram or directed US may define a reason for **localized pain**, such as a distended cyst. (Usually, breast pain is the result of diffuse fibrocystic changes and hormonal influences.)
   If breast pain is diffuse, US is not helpful.

(E) Patient with mastitis and suspected abscess:

Step 1: Consider Ultrasound

Mastitis/suspected abscess is the one situation in which US of the entire breast is appropriate. If the breast is painful, swollen, red, and tense, there may be an abscess in addition to diffuse mastitis, and US may detect it and guide drainage.

Step 2: Mammography, if the Patient Does Not Respond to Treatment

Mammography is difficult and even cruel for the patient with **true** mastitis, because the compression needed for high-quality imaging is extremely painful to inflamed breasts. If probable mastitis does not respond to antibiotic treatment, however, mammography must be performed to rule out underlying tumor causing a pseudoinflammatory clinical presentation. **Moreover, inflammatory cancer and mastitis may be mammographically identical.**

(F) Patients with augmentation implants:

Women with implants are at risk for two totally separate entities: cancer and prosthesis rupture. These women are at the same risk for breast cancer as the remainder of the population, but imaging accuracy is unfortunately compromised by the prosthesis.

Step 1: Mammography with Extra Views

Women with breast augmentation must be monitored for suspicious lesions according to the same guidelines as women without implants. However, their exam requires special implant displacement views in addition to routine projections. The patient should be aware that her mammogram involves more filming, will take longer, and should not be at a screening facility or mobile unit. If a suspicious lesion is discovered, the standard procedures for a patient without implants are followed.

If prosthesis rupture is suspected, mammography may reveal silicone droplets and granulomas secondary to extracapsular extravasation. However, a tailored additional workup may be necessary, including other imaging modalities.

Step 2: Ultrasound and/or Magnetic Resonance Imaging

In consultation with the radiologist, a tailored imaging workup can be developed for the individual patient. US and MR are capable of demonstrating more subtle intracapsular ruptures than mammography. No imaging modality can currently demonstrate the traces of microscopic or molecular silicone that are under investigation as a cause of hyperimmune collagen-vascular disease.

(G) Patient who is pregnant or lactating:

Step 1: For a Palpable Lump, Ultrasound

A palpable mass during late pregnancy or lactation is often a galactocele. US is the most appropriate imaging procedure because it can define a cystic lesion, ending the workup. A solid lesion requires biopsy.

Mammography is avoided in these patients because of possible fetal radiation exposure and because mammograms of dense lactating breasts are nondiagnostic (because of edema, hyperemia, and glandular hypertrophy).

Step 2: Return to Routine Screening

In the asymptomatic patient, routine screening should be delayed for 4 to 6 months after lactation ceases, to permit subsidence of the physiologic density.

(H) Male patients:

Step 1: Mammogram

Although breast cancer is uncommon in males, it does represent 1% of all breast cancers. In a man with a palpable breast mass, bilateral mammography is appropriate. Gynecomastia is sometimes highly distinctive mammographically; in other instances it cannot be distinguished from cancer and a biopsy is necessary (see ***Interventional Procedures***, below).

Interventional Procedures

Mammography, although quite sensitive, is not highly specific; three-fourths of mammographically directed surgical biopsies performed in the United States are for benign disease. (This ratio is approximately the same for clinically triggered surgical biopsies.) Therefore, if 183,000 cases of breast cancer are newly diagnosed each year, **approximately 732,000 biopsies are performed**. The total cost of a surgical biopsy, including pathology, the procedure, ambulatory unit care, operating room charges, and presurgical testing, approximates $3000. Therefore, approximately $1.65 **billion** are spent each year on biopsies of benign tissue! Breast biopsies also entail a large psychologic cost, paid by the patient in the form of anxiety. Only about one-third of the cost of a breast screening program is due to mammography itself; the remainder is due to the biopsies generated.[12]

Surgical excisional biopsy of a nonpalpable mammographic abnormality must be preceded by needle localization. On the day of surgery, the patient begins in the radiology suite, where a needle, mammographically guided, is inserted into the lesion. Once the location of the needle is confirmed by mammography, a thin hook wire is threaded through the needle, and the needle is withdrawn. (The hook at the wire's end anchors it in the breast.) The surgeon is guided by this wire to the abnormality, with the help of the final films from the localization procedure. After excisional biopsy the specimen must be radiographed to ensure that the mammographic abnormality was excised.

Within the past decade, percutaneous needle biopsy of nonpalpable breast lesions has been pursued in an effort to decrease the economic and psychological costs of excisional biopsy. Percutaneous needle biopsy must be differentiated from needle localization. **Needle biopsy involves sampling the tissue through a needle, whereas needle localization refers to placing a needle (and ultimately a wire) to direct surgical excision.**

Typically, a percutaneous needle biopsy costs approximately one-third of an open excisional biopsy and is minimally invasive. Appropriate indications for these techniques are still under development and comprehensive investigation. For lesions with an extremely high probability of benignity in a woman whose compliance is anticipated, close mammographic follow-up (6, 12, and 24 months) is recommended. Lesions with a high probability of malignancy, in the patient who requests breast conservation, raise issues of margin assessment and microinvasion, better assessed by excisional biopsy. A large middle range of lesions, **likely** to be benign but warranting pathologic study, should be well suited to needle biopsy.

Percutaneous needle biopsy for nonpalpable breast

lesions can take the form of fine needle aspiration (FNA) or 14-gauge "core biopsy"; the latter provides tissue for **histology** rather than **cytology** and has a lower failure rate caused by insufficient sampling. Guidance can be mammographic or, if the lesion is visible on US, sonographic. For mammographic guidance, a technique called **stereotaxis** is used, employing a computer to triangulate the precise three-dimensional position of the lesion.

SUMMARY AND CONCLUSIONS

1. Screening mammography is the imaging of asymptomatic patients to look for clinically occult cancer and should be performed for all women, according to age guidelines. It is the only imaging modality proven to reduce mortality from breast cancer. The false negative rate of mammography (approximately 10% to 15%) must always be remembered, and **a negative mammogram should never preclude biopsy of a clinically suspicious lesion.**

2. The majority of women in the United States are not being screened according to the recommended guidelines. Urging by clinicians is the single most effective way to increase compliance.

3. **Patient education/involvement is crucial.** The patient should understand the favorable prognosis of early breast cancer, the importance of old baseline films, and the safety of mammography. She needs to know that a call back often excludes, rather than proves, the need for biopsy.

4. Diagnostic mammography, better termed diagnostic breast imaging, is the workup of a symptomatic patient or the patient with an abnormal screening exam. The correct approach for each individual patient should be tailored conjointly by the clinician and the radiologist.

5. Percutaneous needle biopsy of nonpalpable lesions, guided by stereotactic mammography or US, is often an alternative to excisional biopsy, offering decreased cost and morbidity of tissue diagnosis.

REFERENCES

1. Boring CB, Squires TS, Tong T, Montgomery S. Cancer statistics, 1994. CA Cancer J 1994; 44:7-26.
2. Verbeek ALM, Holland R, Sturmans F, Hendriks JHCL, Mravunac M, Day NE. Reduction of breast cancer mortality through mass screening with modern mammography. Lancet 1984; 1222-1224.
3. Andersson I, Aspegren K, Janzon L, et al. Mammographic screening and mortality from breast cancer: the Malms mammographic screening trial. Br Med J 1988; 297:943-948.
4. Tabar L, Gad A, Holmberg LH, et al. Reduction in mortality from breast cancer after mass screening with mammography. Lancet 1985; 829-832.
5. Sienko DG, Hahn RA, Mills EM, et al. Mammography use and outcomes in a community: the Greater Lansing area mammography study. Cancer 1993; 71:1801-1809.
6. Fajardo LL, Saint-Germain M, Meakem TJ III, Rose C, Hillman BJ. Factors influencing women to undergo screening mammography. Radiology 1992; 184:59-63.
7. Tokunga M, Norman JE, Asano M, et al. Malignant breast tumors among atomic bomb survivors, Hiroshima and Nagasaki, 1950-1974. J Natl Cancer Inst 1979; 62:1347-1359
8. Mettler FA, Hempelmann LG, Dutton AM, et al. Breast neoplasms in women treated with X-rays for acute postpartum mastitis: a pilot study. J Natl Cancer Inst 1969; 43:803-811.
9. Boice JD, Monson RB. Breast cancer following repeated fluoroscopic examinations of the chest. J Natl Cancer Inst 1977; 58:823-832.
10. Feig SA, Ehrlich SM. Estimation of radiation risk from screening mammography: recent trends and comparison with expected benefits. Radiology 1990; 174:638-647.
11. Feig SA. Breast masses: mammographic and sonographic evaluation. Radiol Clin North Am 1992; 30:67-92.
12. Cyrlak D. Induced costs of low-cost screening mammography. Radiology 1988; 168:661-663.

Part X
MISCELLANEOUS

67

Impotence

INTRODUCTION

Impotence is the inability of a man to achieve or maintain an erection that is adequate for sexual intercourse. It affects an estimated 10 to 20 million males in the United States.[1] Although the incidence of impotence greatly increases over age 50, it is not a normal consequence of aging.

The mechanism of erection is complex and only partially understood, but a new understanding of impotence and new therapies have substantially improved the management of the disorder. Numerous factors—vascular, neurologic, endocrine, systemic, and psychologic—may be responsible, in addition to surgery, trauma, or medications.

Costs: not listed; imaging is not recommended except in exceptional cases.

PLAN AND RATIONALE

The emphasis in treating impotence has shifted to conservative management. Hormonal replacement, papaverine injections into the corpora cavernosa, vacuum constriction devices, and penile implants are usually tried **before any routine radiologic imaging**.[1-3]

Additional imaging—Doppler ultrasound of the cavernosal arteries, cavernosometry/cavernosography, and angiography of the iliac vessels and the internal pudendal arteries—is not cost effective and usually does not influence patient management; therefore, it is not routinely recommended.[1,3,4] These studies are limited by few "normal" standards and do not necessarily determine which patients will benefit from vascular surgery. They should be performed only at centers with special interest and expertise in the impotence workup on patients who are serious candidates for vascular surgery. **Because the results of both arterial and venous surgery in most older men have been poor, ultrasound of the penis, cavernosometry/cavernosography (see Additional Comments), and selective arteriography of the internal pudendal artery should be reserved for relatively young men with a history of pelvic trauma, who may have a focal arterial stricture or who are believed to have a congenital anomaly like an arteriovenous malformation. These represent a small minority of patients with impotence.**[1,4-8]

SUMMARY AND CONCLUSIONS

1. Routine radiologic imaging of impotent men is **not** recommended because the diagnosis of arterial and/or venous insufficiency **usually does not** change patient management.
2. The best candidates for vascular surgery are young men with a history of pelvic trauma or who are believed to have a congenital vascular anomaly. Doppler ultrasound exam of the cavernosal arteries of the penis, cavernosometry/cavernosography, and arteriography may be appropriate.

ADDITIONAL COMMENTS

- For cavernosometry/cavernosography, saline is infused into the corpora cavernosa, after the intracavernosal injection of papaverine; pressure is recorded as the flow of saline into the penis is increased and when the flow is stopped, after an erection is achieved. Contrast material is then infused into the corpora cavernosa to check for abnormal leakage into the venous system during erection.
- Doppler studies assess both the penile arterial and venous systems. Blood flow in both cavernosal arteries is measured before and after intracavernosal injection of paperverine.

REFERENCES

1. NIH Consensus Development Panel on Impotence. NIH consensus conference: impotence. JAMA 1993; 270:83-90.
2. Morley JE, Kaiser FE. Impotence: the internist's approach to diagnosis and treatment. Adv Intern Med 1993; 38:151-168.
3. Jeffcoate WJ. The investigation of impotence. Br J Urol 1991; 68:449-453.
4. Steers WD. Impotence evaluation. J Urol 1993; 149:1248.
5. Krane RJ, Goldstein I, de Tejada IS. Impotence. N Engl J Med 1989; 321:1648-1659.
6. Morgantaler A. Current diagnosis and management of impotence. Com Ther 1991; 17:25-30.
7. Thomas RH. The imaging of impotence. West J Med 1992; 156:299-300.
8. Delcour C, Wespes E, Vandenbosch G, Schulman CC, Stryven J. Impotence: evaluation with caversonography. Radiology 1986; 161:803-806.

SUGGESTED ADDITIONAL READING

Benson CB, Vickers MA Jr, Aruny J. Evaluation of impotence. Semin US CT MR 1991; 12:176-190.
Fitzgerald SW, Erickson SJ, Foley WD, Lipchik EO, Lawson TL. Color doppler sonography in the evaluation of erectile dysfunction. RadioGraphics 1992; 12:3-7.

Hattery RR, King BF Jr, Lewis RW, James EM, McKusic MA. Vasculogenic impotence: duplex and color doppler imaging. Radiol Clin North Am 1991; 29:629-645.

Krysssiewicz S, Mellinger BC. The role of imaging in the diagnostic evaluation of impotence. AJR 1989; 153:1133-1139.

Lue TF. Erectile dysfunction: problems and challenges. J Urol 1993; 149:1256-1257.

Rosen MP, Schwartz AN, Levine FJ, Greenfield AJ. Radiologic assessment of impotence: angiography, sonography, cavernosography, and scintigraphy. AJR 1991; 157:923-931.

Wespes E, Schulman C. Venous impotence: pathophysiology, diagnosis, and treatment. J Urol 1993; 149:1238-1245.

Glossary

Angiography: blood vessel imaging.

Angioplasty: dilation of a narrowed blood vessel; the interventional radiologist dilates the vessel by the percutaneous transluminal approach, manipulating a special catheter introduced percutaneously. The introduction site is usually in the groin and may be distant from the vascular lesion.

Antegrade pyelogram: study of the urinary tract by injection of contrast material into the renal collecting system by transcutaneous puncture or through a nephrostomy tube.

Arteriovenous malformation (AVM): a vascular lesion, probably congenital, composed of abnormal arteries and veins. These lesions can produce symptoms and signs characteristic of other space occupying masses, but they also affect organ function by virtue of their abnormal blood flow.

AVM: abbreviation for arteriovenous malformation.

AVN: abbreviation for avascular necrosis.

Barium enema: a radiographic study in which barium, in suspension, is introduced per rectum under direct fluoroscopic visualization to define lesions of the colon. In most cases air is introduced after the barium, to produce an "air-contrast" or "double-contrast" study. Air-contrast studies are superior for demonstrating small lesions like polyps.

BE: abbreviation for barium enema.

CAT scan: abbreviation for computed axial tomography scan; synonym for computed tomography; CT is preferred to this obsolete term.

Cholecystokinin (CCK): a short-acting agent previously delivered intravenously to empty the gallbladder before a nuclear hepatobiliary iminodiacetic acid (HIDA) study, because an empty gallbladder fills more easily with HIDA. Most nuclear medicine departments have abandoned CCK in favor of morphine, injected intravenously after the common bile duct is visualized; morphine potentiates gallbladder filling by raising back pressure in the extrahepatic ducts.

Cold: a nuclear medicine term for nonradioactive.

Computed axial tomography: synonym for computed tomography.

Computed tomography (CT): the imaging technique that produces transaxial images of body "slices" by directing an X-ray beam through the body at many angles; the attenuation of the beam by body structures is indicated by the intensity of the beam striking special radiation detectors, which produce electrical impulses proportional to beam intensity. Computer storage and manipulation of the electrical impulses reconstruct an image that is more sensitive to small radiographic density changes than standard X-rays, is amenable to recall and optimization at any time, and is displayed in the transaxial projection as "slices" or "cuts." Newer units, called "spiral" or "helical" CT, acquire data much more rapidly and in such a way that image reconstruction and display in multiple planes, including a three-dimensional display, is feasible.

Contrast material: any chemical introduced into a space for the purpose of changing the radiopacity or "signal characteristics" of that space for imaging. The term most often applies to iodinated organic compounds delivered intravenously and excreted by the kidneys via glomerular filtration, but strictly speaking many other products, including barium and gadolinium-based compounds, are contrast materials.

Contrast resolution: the ability to discern small differences in radiographic density; computed tomography is superior in contrast resolution to conventional radiography.

CT: abbreviation for computed tomography.

CT arterial portography (CTAP): computed tomography performed during the injection of contrast material directly into the superior mesenteric artery. An angiographer places the catheter. This method increases the sensitivity of CT for detection of liver metastases and primary liver tumors.

CTAP: abbreviation for CT arterial portography.

DEXA: abbreviation for dual X-ray absorptiometry

Diethylenetriaminepenta-acetic acid (DTPA): a metal chelating agent excreted by glomerular filtration; technetium-99m-DTPA is a common radiopharmaceutical for renal scanning.

Digitized: converted to a numerical form for computer storage or arithmetic manipulation.

Diisopropyl iminodiacetic acid (DISIDA): a chemical variant of hepatobiliary iminodiacetic acid (HIDA), the nuclear pharmaceutical used for hepatobiliary imaging.

DISIDA: abbreviation for diisopropyl iminodiacetic acid.

DPA: abbreviation for dual photon absorptiometry.

DTPA: abbreviation for diethylenetriaminepenta-acetic acid.

Dual photon absorptiometry (DPA): a technique of estimating bone mass of the lumbar spine or hip, based on the absorption of gamma rays aimed at the anatomic area in question. Although no isotope is injected into the patient, the study is usually performed in nuclear medicine departments.

Dual X-ray absorptiometry (DEXA): a technique of estimating bone mass of certain regions, typically the lumbar spine or hip, based on the absorption of X-rays aimed at the anatomic area in question. Although no isotope is injected into the patient, the study is usually performed in nuclear medicine departments.

Dye: a radiographic term loosely applied to contrast material.

Echo planar: a new generation of ultrafast magnetic resonance software able to generate images in milliseconds, eliminating motion blur caused by respiration, peristalsis, and cardiac pulsations.

Echocardiography: sonography of the heart, usually applied to the diagnosis of pericardial effusion, valvular disease, ventricular wall motion, or estimation of the ejection fraction.

Ejection fraction: that portion of the ventricular volume ejected in systole. Mathematically, the ejection fraction is the end–diastolic volume minus the end-systolic volume divided by the end-diastolic volume.

Endorectal sonogram: sonography performed with a transducer in the rectum. This method produces superior images of the prostate and is especially useful to guide transrectal prostatic biopsy.

Endoscopic retrograde cholangiopancreatography (ERCP): an endoscopic technique involving passage of the endoscope through the mouth, esophagus, and stomach into the duodenum and then cannulation of the ampulla of Vater; contrast material injected in a retrograde fashion fills the pancreatic and bile ducts. Radiographs provide excellent ductal visualization.

Endoscopic ultrasound (EUS): ultrasound performed with a transducer in the tip of a catheter introduced into the gut—for example, the distal esophagus or duodenum.

Enhanced: with intravenous contrast material, usually referring to computed tomography or magnetic resonance imaging.

Enhanced CT: computed tomography performed during

or after intravenous contrast material infusion. The opacification of vascular spaces, renal concentration and excretion of contrast material, and the diffusion of contrast material across injured capillaries into the interstitium reveal lesions that are sometimes invisible to unenhanced CT.

Enteroclysis: a special small bowel examination, in which barium, air, water, and sometimes methylcellulose are carefully introduced into the proximal jejunum via naso-duodenal tube.

ERCP: abbreviation for endoscopic retrograde cholangiopancreatography.

EUS: abbreviation for endoscopic ultrasound.

Fast spin echo: a newer generation of magnetic resonance software that substantially decreases scan time; fast spin echo equipment decreases scanning time and is convenient but is not fast enough to eliminate motion blur (see echo planar).

Gallium-67: an intermediate half-life radionuclide that accumulates in inflammatory foci and some neoplasms, notably lymphoma, after peripheral intravenous injection; uptake in both neoplastic and inflammatory lesions reduces the specificity of gallium scans, and gastrointestinal excretion sometimes obscures abdominal lesions. Gallium-67 scans for infection have been largely replaced by labeled autologous leukocyte studies.

Gamma camera: the standard nuclear instrument for producing images of the in vivo radiobiodistribution of previously administered pharmaceuticals; these images constitute "scans."

Gamma scintigraphy: synonymous with nuclear scanning.

Gantry: the physical opening or "portal" through which a patient passes for a CT study.

Gastrograffin: a water-soluble radiographic contrast material usually used for gastrointestinal opacification.

Gated: images synchronized with motion of the heart (cardiac gating) or the lungs (pulmonary gating), so that the images are free from motion blur.

GFR: abbreviation for glomerular filtration rate.

GHA: abbreviation for glucoheptonate.

Glucoheptonate (GHA): a five-carbon organic molecule similar to glucose; bonded to technetium-99m, this compound is concentrated and excreted by the kidneys. Because parenchymal renal visualization is better with glucoheptonate than diethylenetriamine penta–acetic acid (DTPA), the compound is preferred for visualization of the renal cortex.

Guided biopsy: percutaneous needle biopsy performed under direct visualization with fluoroscopy, ultrasound, or computed tomography. With sonographic or fluoroscopic guidance, the needle, normal structures, and the lesion are visualized during the biopsy, greatly diminishing uncertainty in needle placement and reducing risk. Tissue for cytology or histology can be obtained at less expense than by surgery.

Hepatobiliary iminodiacetic acid (HIDA): the original technetium-99m-labeled nuclear pharmaceutical for hepatobiliary imaging; after intravenous injection, the compound is cleared by the liver and excreted into the biliary tree, with visualization of the common duct, gallbladder, and duodenum. Many chemical relatives, including diisopropyl iminodiacetic acid and paraisopropyl iminodiacetic acid, are now in clinical use, but in most nuclear medicine departments "HIDA" is the generic term for all of these.

Hexamethylpropylene amine oxime (HMPAO): the best current brain scanning agent. This lipid-soluble compound is also an excellent white cell label that competes with In-111-oxine-WBC studies for osteomyelitis of the extremities.

HIDA: abbreviation for hepatobiliary iminodiacetic acid, also a general term loosely applied to any of its current analogs for nuclear gallbladder/biliary tract imaging.

HMPAO: abbreviation for hexamethylpropylene amine oxime, a white cell label when chelated to Tc-99m.

Hot: a nuclear medicine term for radioactive.

I-123: abbreviation for iodine-123.

I-125: abbreviation for iodine-125.

I-131: abbreviation for iodine-131.

Indium-111 (In-111): an intermediate half-life isotope; when chelated by oxine, indium-111 is an effective leukocyte label.

Indium-111-oxine: the radiopharmaceutical used for labeling polymorphonuclear neutrophilic leukocytes for in vivo abscess localization.

Intravenous pyelogram (IVP): a urinary tract study; radiographs of the kidneys, ureters, and bladder are obtained after intravenous injection of iodinated contrast material that is cleared from the circulation by glomerular filtration. Synonym for IVU (intravenous urogram).

Iodine-131 total-body metastatic thyroid carcinoma search: a method for detecting functioning metastatic thyroid cancer. The exam requires careful preparation and is most effective when endogenous thyroid-stimulating hormone levels are high, in order to stimulate radioiodine uptake by metastases.

Isodense: having the same density as surrounding tissue; in computed tomography an isodense lesion cannot be differentiated from surrounding tissue without special techniques such as enhancement with intravenous contrast material.

Isotope imaging: synonym for nuclear imaging.

Isotopes: atomic species having the same atomic number (number of protons) but different atomic weights (atomic mass numbers—i.e., protons plus neutrons).

IVU: abbreviation for intravenous urogram, synonym for IVP.

KUB: abbreviation for kidneys, ureters, bladder; the term KUB refers to a plain films of the abdomen, because a plain film is the initial study for many conditions that affect the urinary tract.

Labeled leukocytes: the best current agent for localization of occult bacterial infection by nuclear methods. Both In-111-oxine and Tc99m-HMPAO are useful as radiolabels.

Liver–spleen scan: a nuclear method of imaging the liver and spleen. Radiolabeled microcolloid particles are injected intravenously and taken up by the hepatic and splenic reticuloendothelial system.

Low osmolar contrast material: a new formulation of iodinated contrast material that is associated with far fewer untoward effects than conventional contrast materials. Many—but not all—of these agents are also "nonionic." The cost of low osmolar agents is much more than the cost of conventional agents.

MAA: abbreviation for macroaggregated albumin.

Macroaggregated albumin (MAA): very small albumin particles; when labeled with technetium-99m, macroaggregated albumin particles (Tc-99m-MAA) are an excellent and inexpensive lung scanning agent, because they trap in the pulmonary capillary bed, distributing according to pulmonary arterial blood flow.

Magnetic resonance angiography (MRA): a sophisticated method of MR imaging that produces good visualization of blood vessels without the need for contrast material or catheterization. MRA is expected to replace some conventional angiographic procedures.

Magnetic resonance imaging (MR or MRI): noninvasive technique that images body structures without ionizing radiation of any type, through analysis of signals emitted by body tissue, after the anatomic area under study is placed in magnetic field and perturbed by pulses of radiofrequency energy.

MDP: abbreviation for methylene diphosphonate.

Metaiodobenzylguanidine (MIBG): a radiopharmaceutical that localizes in certain neoplasms of neural crest origin, specifically pheochromocytoma and neuroblastoma.

Methylene diphosphonate (MDP): a small organic phosphate molecule; technetium-99m MDP is the most widely used and probably most effective skeletal scanning agent.

MIBG: abbreviation for metaiodobenzylguanidine.

MR (I): abbreviation for magnetic resonance (imaging).

MRA: abbreviation for magnetic resonance angiography.

MUGA: abbreviation for multigated acquisition study.

Multigated acquisition study (MUGA): a nuclear ventriculogram created by collecting imaging data from defined portions of the cardiac cycle, by computer synchronization of the gamma camera and the electrocardiogram, so that images of the cardiac cycle can be constructed and displayed as a multiframe "movie."

Nonionic contrast material: a newer formulation of iodinated contrast material that is associated with far fewer untoward effects than conventional contrast material; the lower incidence of side effects is probably due to their low osmolarity rather than their nonionicity. The cost of nonionic and low osmolar agents is much more than the cost of conventional contrast materials.

Nuclear magnetic resonance (NMR): obsolete synonym for magnetic resonance imaging (MRI).

Nuclear medicine: the analysis of organ structure and function by imaging the radiobiodistribution of administered radiopharmaceuticals, the determination of radionuclide levels in various body fluids, and the determination of blood levels of many chemical substances by radioimmunoassay.

Nuclear medicine imaging: that part of the broader field of nuclear medicine that consists only of imaging.

Nuclide: the current preferred term for isotope; strictly speaking, a nuclide is an atomic species, whereas a radioactive atomic species is a radionuclide.

OCG: abbreviation for oral cholecystogram.

Oncoscint: the commercial name for a radiolabeled antibody imaging agent that reacts with a cell surface antigen of ovarian and colorectal carcinoma.

Oral cholecystogram (OCG): the classic radiographic study for visualizing the gallbladder and defining gallbladder stones; orally administered contrast material is absorbed into the circulation and excreted by the liver, filling the gallbladder via the cystic duct. For visualization, the gallbladder wall must absorb water but not contrast material, thereby concentrating the contrast material. Gallbladder stones stand out as radiolucencies against the contrast medium. The oral cholecystogram has been almost entirely replaced by gallbladder sonography.

Percutaneous angioplasty: synonym for percutaneous transluminal angioplasty.

Percutaneous transhepatic cholangiogram (PTC): a radiographic method of imaging the bile ducts; the liver is punctured through the abdominal wall and contrast material is injected into a peripheral duct through a thin needle.

Percutaneous transluminal angioplasty (PTA): dilation of a narrowed, diseased blood vessel, usually by a balloon catheter. The special catheter is introduced via percutaneous puncture, usually in the groin, and threaded through appropriate vessels to the lesion.

Pericholecystic edema: fluid around the gallbladder demonstrated by ultrasound; this sign may indicate acute cholecystitis but may be mimicked by noninflammatory fluid originating elsewhere (e.g., ascites).

Pertechnetate: the term for technetium-99m in one of its common oxidation states, $TcO4^-$; $TcO4^-$ is usually the chemical state of technetium-99m obtained from an in-house generator, and although this chemical configuration is purposefully altered for the preparation of various technetium-labeled radiopharmaceuticals, pertechnetate itself is excellent for imaging the thyroid gland and Meckel's diverticula.

PET: abbreviation for positron emission tomography.

Positron emission tomography (PET): a nuclear technique for imaging certain cyclotron-produced radionuclides (positron emitters); this method can study the critically important elements of living tissue (e.g., oxygen and nitrogen) that have no radioactive isotopes suitable for conventional nuclear imaging. The technique requires an on-site cyclotron for isotope production (the isotopes are generally too short-lived for shipping) and a special positron camera.

PTC: abbreviation for percutaneous transhepatic cholangiogram.

QCT: abbreviation for quantitative CT.

Quantitative CT (QCT): a method of measuring bone mass of the spine with CT. The method competes with DEXA.

Radiographic density: the ability of any substance to attenuate an X-ray beam.

Radionuclide: a radioactive nuclide—i.e., a radioactive atomic species.

Radionuclide imaging: synonym for nuclear medicine imaging.

Real-time sonography: a method of continuously and instantaneously displaying sonographically visualized internal anatomy as the transducer moves across the body's skin surface. The method is analogous to viewing a subject through the viewfinder of a camera as the camera moves, as opposed to later examining single still photographs obtained one at a time. Virtually all sonography is now real time.

Red blood cell scan: a term that describes various nuclear procedures, all based on imaging the patient's radiolabeled blood pool. Imaging the cardiac blood pool produces a ventriculogram, imaging the abdominal blood pool can reveal a GI bleed, imaging the liver with SPECT can detect hemangiomas, etc.

Retrograde pyelogram: study of the urinary tract by retrograde injection of contrast material into the distal ureter via a catheter placed by a urologist after cystoscopy.

SBO: abbreviation for small bowel obstruction.

Signal characteristics: a term that indicates how a particular tissue or fluid appears on an MR image.

Single photon emission computed tomography (SPECT): an outgrowth of nuclear medicine requiring a special gamma camera that produces images of the in vivo radiobiodistribution of previously injected pharmaceuticals as "slices" of the organ under study. The slices can be in the frontal, transaxial, or sagittal projection. Conventional radionuclides (not positron emitters) are used.

Sono: short for sonogram; synonym for ultrasound.

Sonogram (sono): synonym for ultrasound.

Spatial resolution: the ability to discern fine anatomic detail by imaging.

SPECT: abbreviation for single photon emission computed tomography.

Spiral CT: a new gerneration of ultrafast CT scanners that acquire data fast enough to eliminate motion blur, even from respiration, peristalsis, and cardiac pulsations. Spiral scanners acquire "volume data," so that images can be reconstructed in multiple planes and even in three dimensions. When coupled with a peripheral intra-venous injection of contrast material, spiral CT can visu-alize many vascular structures and promises to replace some conventional angiographic procedures.

Sulfur colloid: the pharmaceutical used for nuclear liver-spleen scanning when labeled with technetium-99m.

Surface coil: an augmentation of standard MR that pro-duces superior images of a specific anatomic site—like the knee—by applying a small metal coil over the imaged area. The coil functions as both a transmitter and a receiver of RF signals.

T1-weighted image: a magnetic resonance image in which fat is light and cerebrospinal fluid is dark.

T2-weighted image: a magnetic resonance image in which cerebrospinal fluid is light.

Tc-99m: abbreviation for technetium-99m.

Tc-99m-MAA: abbreviation for technetium-99m macroaggregated albumin, the lung-scanning agent.

Tc-99m-MDP: abbreviation for technetium-99m-meth-ylene diphosphonate, the most common bone-scanning agent.

Technegas: a nuclear product for assessing lung ventilation, using submicronsize technetium-99m-labeled carbon particles.

Technetium-99m (Tc-99m): the most clinically useful radionuclide in nuclear imaging, with a short half-life (6 hours) and a gamma ray energy (140 KeV) almost ideal for gamma camera imaging. Technetium-99m is avail-able around the clock in all nuclear medicine depart-ments, because it is produced in-house from molybde-num-99/–technetium-99m generators. The chemistry of this radionuclide allows it to be combined with mol-ecules that are organ specific, for example, MDP (bone-seeking), HIDA (hepatobiliary), and DTPA (renal).

Tomography: a method for imaging slices of tissue in a given plane. Originally, the term "tomography" referred simply to the radiographic technique, but current technology has created radiographic computed tomography (CT), single photon emission computed tomography (SPECT), and positron emission tomography (PET). Moreover, magnetic resonance (MR) images are tomographic.

Transaxial: the plane obtained by slicing the body perpendicular to its long (head-to-foot) axis; this plane examines the body the way one would examine a loaf of bread by slicing it.

Transrectal ultrasound: ultrasound of the prostate and seminal vesicles with a sound beam originating from an intrarectal transducer. Accurate, relatively noninvasive prostate biopsies can be performed with a special attachment to the intrarectal probe.

Transvaginal ultrasound (TVU): ultrasound of the female pelvis with a sound beam originating from an intravaginal transducer. The technique produces better images of the pelvis and adnexa than conventional ultrasound.

TVU: abbreviation for transvaginal ultrasound.

Ultrasonography: the technique of ultrasound.

Ultrasound: the method of obtaining diagnostic medical images of internal anatomy by bombarding the area of interest with an ultrasound beam and reconstructing the returning sound (echoes) into an image.

Unenhanced: without benefit of contrast material, referring to computed tomography and magnetic resonance imaging.

Unenhanced CT: computed tomography performed without benefit of intravenous contrast material.

VCUG: abbreviation for voiding cystourethrogram.

Ventilation scan: images of the lungs performed during ventilation with a radioactive gas, to obtain information on alveolar ventilation and air trapping. In some centers, radioactive aerosol particles have been very successfully used instead of radioactive gas (xenon-133). A newer method, using submicron size carbon particles, known as Technegas, will probably replace all other gas or aerosal procedures.

Ventriculogram: an imaging study of the ventricles designed to determine their ejection fractions and define their wall motion. Nuclear, sonographic, and angiographic methods can produce ventriculograms.

Vesicoureteral reflux (VUR): retrograde filling of the ureters by urine from the bladder.

Voiding cystourethrogram (VCUG): a radiographic study of the bladder and urethra that defines the anatomy of the lower urinary tract and establishes the presence or absence of vesicoureteral reflux. A complete VCUG requires filling of the bladder with contrast material instilled through a transurethral catheter and fluoroscopic observation of voiding.

VUR: abbreviation for vesicoureteral reflux.

Index